2015

The Year Book of ORTHOPEDICS®

Editor-in-Chief

Bernard F. Morrey, MD

Professor of Orthopedics, Mayo Graduate School of Medicine; Professor of Orthopedics, University of Texas, Health Science Center, San Antonio, Texas

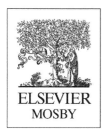

ELSEVIER
MOSBY

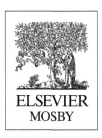

ELSEVIER
MOSBY

Vice President, Global Medical Reference: Mary E. Gatsch
Senior Clinics Editor: Jennifer Flynn-Briggs
Developmental Editor: Barbara Cohen-Kligerman
Production Supervisor, Electronic Year Books: Donna M. Skelton
Electronic Article Manager: Mike Sheets
Illustrations and Permissions Coordinator: Dawn Vohsen

2015 EDITION

Composition by TNQ Books and Journals Pvt Ltd, India
Printing/binding by Sheridan Books, Inc.

Editorial Office:
Elsevier, Inc.
Suite 1800
1600 John F. Kennedy Blvd
Philadelphia, PA 19103-2899

International Standard Serial Number: 0276-1092
International Standard Book Number: 978-0-323-35549-0

Editorial Board

Paul M. Huddleston III, MD
Assistant Professor of Orthopedic Surgery and Neurosurgery; Chair, Division of Spine Surgery, Mayo Clinic College of Medicine, Rochester, Minnesota

Peter S. Rose, MD
Associate Professor of Orthopedic Surgery, Mayo Clinic College of Medicine, Rochester, Minnesota

Stephen A. Sems, MD
Consultant, Department of Orthopedic Surgery; Chair, Division of Orthopedic Trauma Surgery; Assistant Professor of Orthopedic Surgery, Mayo Clinic, Rochester, Minnesota

Stephen D. Trigg, MD
Assistant Professor of Orthopedics, Mayo Graduate School of Medicine, Rochester, Minnesota; Consultant in Orthopedic Hand Surgery, Mayo Hospital, Jacksonville, Florida

Table of Contents

Journals Represented

Journals represented in this YEAR BOOK are listed below.

Acta Orthopaedica
American Journal of Sports Medicine
Anaesthesia
Anesthesiology
Annals of the Rheumatic Diseases
Arthroscopy
Bone and Joint Journal
British Journal of Radiology
British Journal of Sports Medicine
Canadian Journal of Surgery
Canadian Medical Association Journal
Clinical Journal of Pain
Clinical Journal of Sport Medicine
Clinical Neurology and Neurosurgery
Clinical Orthopaedics and Related Research
Foot & Ankle International
Injury
Journal of Bone and Joint Surgery (American)
Journal of Clinical Endocrinology & Metabolism
Journal of Hand Surgery (American)
Journal of Hand Therapy
Journal of Neurosurgery Spine
Journal of Orthopaedic and Sports Physical Therapy
Journal of Orthopaedic Research
Journal of Orthopaedic Trauma
Journal of Plastic, Reconstructive & Aesthetic Surgery
Journal of Trauma and Acute Care Surgery
Journal of Vascular Surgery
Journal of the American Academy of Orthopaedic Surgeons
Lancet
Metabolism
Orthopedics
Pediatric Emergency Care
Radiology
Sarcoma
Skeletal Radiology
Spine
Spine Journal
Sports Medicine
Thrombosis Research

STANDARD ABBREVIATIONS

The following terms are abbreviated in this edition: acquired immunodeficiency syndrome (AIDS), anterior cruciate ligament (ACL), anteroposterior (AP), avascular necrosis (AVN), cardiopulmonary resuscitation (CPR), central nervous system (CNS), cerebrospinal fluid (CSF), computed tomography (CT), deoxyribonucleic acid (DNA), electrocardiography (ECG), health maintenance organization (HMO), human immunodeficiency virus (HIV), intensive care unit (ICU), intramuscular (IM), intravenous (IV), magnetic resonance (MR) imaging (MRI), range of motion (ROM), ribonucleic acid (RNA), total hip arthroplasty (THA), total knee arthroplasty (TKA), ultrasound (US), and ultraviolet (UV).

NOTE

The YEAR BOOK OF ORTHOPEDICS® is a literature survey service providing abstracts of articles published in the professional literature. Every effort is made to assure the accuracy of the information presented in these pages. Neither the editors nor the publisher of the YEAR BOOK OF ORTHOPEDICS® can be responsible for errors in the original materials. The editors' comments are their own opinions. Mention of specific products within this publication does not constitute endorsement.

To facilitate the use of the YEAR BOOK OF ORTHOPEDICS® as a reference tool, all illustrations and tables included in this publication are now identified as they appear in the original article. This change is meant to help the reader recognize that any illustration or table appearing in the YEAR BOOK OF ORTHOPEDICS® may be only one of many in the original article. For this reason, figure and table numbers will often appear to be out of sequence within the YEAR BOOK OF ORTHOPEDICS®.

Introduction

The literature review for this year's YEAR BOOK OF ORTHOPEDICS continues to demonstrate the changing face of orthopedic clinical research. In the sections that I personally reviewed, as well as those my colleagues reviewed, I was impressed with the tendency to identify analytical reviews and summary-type articles, as well as the information obtained from studying large national databases as a "source of truth." As I reviewed my own selections and contrasted them with the YEAR BOOK reviews in the past, I was struck by the relatively few case series that we have elected to include in this year's volume. This, of course, is reflective of a growing awareness of the value of evidence-based research. The reality that is well known to all orthopedic surgeons has, however, become obvious; specifically, there is a relative dearth of high-quality, randomized, controlled trials investigating orthopedic issues. For this reason, I consider the next best opportunity to provide relevant insight into problematic issues in our discipline to be the identification of high-quality literature reviews. However, rather than a simple regurgitation of what has been published, I have specifically tried to identify those in which there is a level of interpretation to the findings. In addition, I have attempted to identify those reviews that focus on what I at least consider to be of most clinical relevance.

It is recognized that with the ever-changing landscape of orthopedic knowledge, there is an even more rapidly changing process and pace as to how the orthopedic surgeon identifies and assimilates knowledge. It is my hope that this year's YEAR BOOK OF ORTHOPEDICS will continue to be a useful source of a broad spectrum of valid information to the orthopedic surgeon, particularly the orthopedic surgeon who engages in a more general practice of our specialty. As always, I consider it an honor to be the editor of this volume, and I hope it is of some value to my colleagues.

Bernard F. Morrey, MD

1 Basic Science

Introduction

The selections in Basic Science this year, as in the past, have been designed to provide basic investigative insight into issues that are clinically relevant. However, the selections are also intended to reflect the ever-changing refinements of methodologies being applied to musculoskeletal research. Hence, there are several articles that attempt to provide insight into the pathophysiology of tendinopathy, as well as the biological solutions for treating musculoskeletal diseases. The application of basic investigations to clinically relevant issues, such as that of metal ion concentrations after metal-on-metal articulations, has been an important topic in the past and continues to be reviewed in this year's selections. Overall, the hope is that the reader will find this section to be relevant and useful in the care of our patients.

Bernard F. Morrey, MD

Inhibition of 5-LOX, COX-1, and COX-2 Increases Tendon Healing and Reduces Muscle Fibrosis and Lipid Accumulation After Rotator Cuff Repair
Oak NR, Gumucio JP, Flood MD, et al (Univ of Michigan Med School, Ann Arbor)
Am J Sports Med 42:2860-2868, 2014

Background.—The repair and restoration of function after chronic rotator cuff tears are often complicated by muscle atrophy, fibrosis, and fatty degeneration of the diseased muscle. The inflammatory response has been implicated in the development of fatty degeneration after cuff injuries. Licofelone is a novel anti-inflammatory drug that inhibits 5-lipoxygenase (5-LOX), as well as cyclooxygenase (COX)—1 and COX-2 enzymes, which play important roles in inducing inflammation after injuries. While previous studies have demonstrated that nonsteroidal anti-inflammatory drugs and selective inhibitors of COX-2 (coxibs) may prevent the proper healing of muscles and tendons, studies about bone and cartilage have demonstrated that drugs that inhibit 5-LOX concurrently with COX-1 and COX-2 may enhance tissue regeneration.

Hypothesis.—After the repair of a chronic rotator cuff tear in rats, lico-felone would increase the load to failure of repaired tendons and increase the force production of muscle fibers.

Study Design.—Controlled laboratory study.

Methods.—Rats underwent supraspinatus release followed by repair 28 days later. After repair, rats began a treatment regimen of either licofe-lone or a vehicle for 14 days, at which time animals were euthanized. Supraspinatus muscles and tendons were then subjected to contractile, mechanical, histological, and biochemical analyses.

Results.—Compared with controls, licofelone-treated rats had a grossly apparent decrease in inflammation and increased fibrocartilage formation at the enthesis, along with a 62% increase in the maximum load to failure and a 51% increase in peak stress to failure. Licofelone resulted in a marked reduction in fibrosis and lipid content in supraspinatus muscles as well as reduced expression of several genes involved in fatty infiltration. Despite the decline in fibrosis and fat accumulation, muscle fiber specific force production was reduced by 23%.

Conclusion.—The postoperative treatment of cuff repair with licofelone may reduce fatty degeneration and enhance the development of a stable bone-tendon interface, although decreases in muscle fiber specific force production were observed, and force production in fact declined.

Clinical Relevance.—This study demonstrates that the inhibition of 5-LOX, COX-1, and COX-2 modulates the healing process of repaired rotator cuff tendons. Although further studies are necessary, the treatment of patients with licofelone after cuff repair may improve the development of a stable enthesis and enhance postoperative outcomes.

▶ This well-conceived and executed study is important because it takes us a step closer to defining medical adjuncts to surgical management. That Cox inhibition is associated with less inflammation and hence less fibrosis and less fatty degen-eration is an important observation. This experiment also revealed increased strength to failure with this treatment. This could lead to a valuable medical com-plement to surgical management of some rotator cuff tears.

As an aside, the Mayo Clinic is also investigating this line of research with similar encouraging results.

B. F. Morrey, MD

Glucocorticoids induce specific ion-channel-mediated toxicity in human rotator cuff tendon: a mechanism underpinning the ultimately deleterious effect of steroid injection in tendinopathy?
Dean BJF, Franklin SL, Murphy RJ, et al (Nuffield Orthopaedic Centre, Oxford, UK)
Br J Sports Med 48:1620-1626, 2014

Background.—Glucocorticoid injection (GCI) and surgical rotator cuff repair are two widely used treatments for rotator cuff tendinopathy. Little is known about the way in which medical and surgical treatments affect the human rotator cuff tendon in vivo. We assessed the histological and immunohistochemical effects of these common treatments on the rotator cuff tendon.

Study Design.—Controlled laboratory study.

Methods.—Supraspinatus tendon biopsies were taken before and after treatment from 12 patients undergoing GCI and 8 patients undergoing surgical rotator cuff repair. All patients were symptomatic and none of the patients undergoing local GCI had full thickness tears of the rotator cuff. The tendon tissue was then analysed using histological techniques and immunohistochemistry.

Results.—There was a significant increase in nuclei count and vascularity after rotator cuff repair and not after GCI (both $p = 0.008$). Hypoxia inducible factor 1α (HIF-1α) and cell proliferation were only increased after rotator cuff repair (both $p = 0.03$) and not GCI. The ionotropic N-methyl-D-aspartate receptor 1 (NMDAR1) glutamate receptor was only increased after GCI and not rotator cuff repair ($p = 0.016$). An increase in glutamate was seen in both groups following treatment (both $p = 0.04$), while an increase in the receptor metabotropic glutamate receptor 7 (mGluR7) was only seen after rotator cuff repair ($p = 0.016$).

Conclusions.—The increases in cell proliferation, vascularity and HIF-1α after surgical rotator cuff repair appear consistent with a proliferative healing response, and these features are not seen after GCI. The increase in the glutamate receptor NMDAR1 after GCI raises concerns about the potential excitotoxic tendon damage that may result from this common treatment.

▶ This is a useful basic investigation to help understand an important clinical question. The well-designed study assesses this issue before and after cuff repair as well as the use of glucocorticoids in the face of a torn rotator cuff. Several analyses clearly document the positive effect of rotator cuff surgery to promote a healing response featured by cell proliferation and increased vascularity. In contrast, this study helps explain the ever-increasing concern regarding the use of steroids. Glucocorticoids were demonstrated to generate potentially cytotoxic tendon changes after administration to a nonrepaired tendon.

B. F. Morrey, MD

Distinct Effects of Platelet-Rich Plasma and BMP13 on Rotator Cuff Tendon Injury Healing in a Rat Model
Lamplot JD, Angeline M, Angeles J, et al (The Univ of Chicago Med Ctr, IL)
Am J Sports Med 42:2877-2887, 2014

Background.—Although platelet-rich plasma (PRP) is used clinically to augment tendon healing, bone morphogenetic protein—13 (BMP13) may provide a better therapeutic avenue to improve early tendon healing and repair.

Hypothesis.—Exogenous expression of BMP13 in tenocytes will up-regulate genes involved in tendon healing. Direct delivery of adenovirus-mediated BMP13 (AdBMP13) into the injured rat supraspinatus tendon will increase biomechanical properties.

Study Design.—Controlled laboratory study.

Methods.—Exogenous expression of BMP13 and the major growth factors in PRP (transforming growth factor—β1 [TGF-β1], vascular endothelial growth factor—A [VEGF-A], and platelet-derived growth factor—BB [PDGF-BB]) was accomplished by using recombinant adenoviral vectors. The expression of tendon- and matrix-associated genes in growth factor—treated tenocytes was analyzed by use of semiquantitative reverse-transcription polymerase chain reaction. A total of 32 rats with supraspinatus defect were divided into 4 groups and injected with adenovirus-containing green fluorescent protein (AdGFP; negative control), PRP, AdBMP13, or PRP+AdBMP13. All rats were sacrificed at 2 weeks after surgery, and tendons were harvested for biomechanical testing and histologic analysis.

Results.—BMP13 up-regulated type III collagen expression compared with AdGFP control and PRP growth factors ($P < .01$). BMP13 and PRP

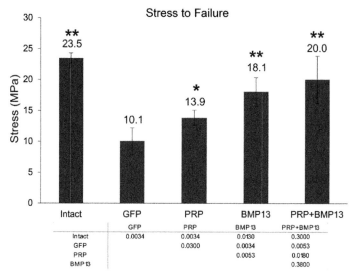

	GFP	PRP	BMP13	PRP+BMP13
Intact	0.0034	0.0034	0.0130	0.3000
GFP		0.0300	0.0034	0.0053
PRP			0.0053	0.0180
BMP13				0.3800

FIGURE 5.—Bone morphogenetic protein—13 (BMP13) increases biomechanical properties of supraspinatus tendon compared with platelet-rich plasma (PRP) and control. (A) The mean stress to failure was significantly higher in the intact, untreated tendons compared with green fluorescent protein (GFP) control, BMP13, and PRP but not BMP13+PRP. Compared with the GFP control, the mean stress to failure was significantly higher in BMP13, PRP, and BMP131+PRP. Compared with the PRP alone, the mean stress to failure was significantly higher in the BMP13 and BMP131+PRP. Graphs represent the mean for each group, and error bars represent ± 1 SD. *$P < .05$; **$P < .01$. (Reprinted from Lamplot JD, Angeline M, Angeles J, et al. Distinct effects of platelet-rich plasma and BMP13 on rotator cuff tendon injury healing in a rat model. *Am J Sports Med.* 2014;42:2877-2887, with permission from The Author(s).)

growth factors each up-regulated fibronectin expression ($P < .01$). There was an increase in stress to failure in each of the 3 treatment groups ($P < .05$ for PRP; $P < .01$ for AdBMP13 or PRP+AdBMP13) compared with AdGFP control. AdBMP13 demonstrated higher stress to failure than did the PRPs ($P < .01$). The addition of PRP did not increase the BMP13-enhanced stress to failure or stiffness. The biomechanical results were further supported by histologic analysis of the retrieved samples.

Conclusion.—Exogenous expression of BMP13 enhances tendon healing more effectively than PRP as assessed by tendon- and matrix-associated gene expression, biomechanical testing, and histologic analysis.

Clinical Relevance.—While PRP is used in the clinical setting, BMP13 may be explored as a superior biofactor to improve rotator cuff tendon healing and reduce the incidence of retears (Fig 5A).

▶ Clinically, the value of platelet-rich plasma (PRP) continues to be used and assessed. The complexity of the formulation adds to the complexity of the question of the efficacy of PRP in various settings. One of the most difficult features of the question is the multitude of bioactive factors included in the PRP preparation, which varies according to the method and technique used to process the therapeutic agent. These investigators clearly demonstrate the value of a single bone morphogenic protein, 13, as being superior to the PRP in promoting the healing of the rotator cuff in a rat model (Fig 5A). One implication of this research, rather than the obvious, is the potential to refine the PRP preparation according to the factors contained therein that have been shown to be most effective in different experimental clinical states.

B. F. Morrey, MD

Fluoroquinolones Impair Tendon Healing in a Rat Rotator Cuff Repair Model: A Preliminary Study

Fox AJS, Schär MO, Wanivenhaus F, et al (Hosp for Special Surgery, NY)
Am J Sports Med 42:2851-2859, 2014

Background.—Recent studies suggest that fluoroquinolone antibiotics predispose tendons to tendinopathy and/or rupture. However, no investigations on the reparative capacity of tendons exposed to fluoroquinolones have been conducted.

Hypothesis.—Fluoroquinolone-treated animals will have inferior biochemical, histological, and biomechanical properties at the healing tendon-bone enthesis compared with controls.

Study Design.—Controlled laboratory study.

Methods.—Ninety-two rats underwent rotator cuff repair and were randomly assigned to 1 of 4 groups: (1) preoperative (Preop), whereby animals received fleroxacin for 1 week preoperatively; (2) pre- and postoperative (Pre/Postop), whereby animals received fleroxacin for 1 week preoperatively and for 2 weeks postoperatively; (3) postoperative (Postop), whereby animals received fleroxacin for 2 weeks postoperatively; and (4) control, whereby animals received vehicle for 1 week preoperatively and for 2 weeks postoperatively. Rats were euthanized at 2 weeks postoperatively for biochemical, histological, and biomechanical analysis. All data were expressed as mean ± standard error of the mean (SEM). Statistical comparisons were performed using either 1-way or 2-way ANOVA, with $P < .05$ considered significant.

Results.—Reverse transcriptase quantitative polymerase chain reaction (RTqPCR) analysis revealed a 30-fold increase in expression of matrix metalloproteinase (MMP)-3, a 7-fold increase in MMP-13, and a 4-fold increase in tissue inhibitor of metalloproteinases (TIMP)-1 in the Pre/Postop group compared with the other groups. The appearance of the healing enthesis in all treated animals was qualitatively different than that in controls. The tendons were friable and atrophic. All 3 treated groups showed significantly less fibrocartilage and poorly organized collagen at the healing enthesis compared with control animals. There was a significant difference in the mode of failure, with treated animals demonstrating an intrasubstance failure of the supraspinatus tendon during testing. In contrast, only 1 of 10 control samples failed within the tendon substance. The healing enthesis of the Pre/Postop group displayed

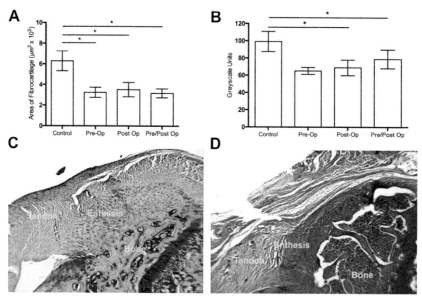

FIGURE 2.—Histological results. (A) Area of fibrocartilage: All 3 fluoroquinolone (FQ)-treated groups showed significantly less fibrocartilage compared with control rats. (B) Collagen organization: All 3 FQ-treated groups showed significantly less organized collagen at the healing enthesis compared with control rats. Safranin-O staining of the (C) control and (D) Pre/Postop groups. There was a significantly reduced area of fibrocartilage in the Pre/Postop group compared with control rats (×40). All data expressed as mean ± standard error of the mean (SEM) (error bars). *$P < .05$. (Reprinted from Fox AJS, Schär MO, Wanivenhaus F, et al. Fluoroquinolones impair tendon healing in a rat rotator cuff repair model: a preliminary study. *Am J Sports Med.* 2014;42:2851-2859, with permission from The Author(s).)

significantly reduced ultimate load to failure compared with the Preop, Postop, and control groups. There was no significant difference in load to failure in the Preop group compared with the Postop group. Pre/ Postop animals demonstrated significantly reduced cross-sectional area compared with the Postop and control groups. There was also a significant reduction in area between the Preop and control groups.

Conclusion.—In this preliminary study, fluoroquinolone treatment negatively influenced tendon healing.

Clinical Relevance.—These findings indicate that there was an active but inadequate repair response that has potential clinical implications for patients who are exposed to fluoroquinolones before tendon repair surgery (Fig 2).

▶ This important basic investigation was reviewed primarily to emphasize its clinical implication. The literature is replete with data that fluoroquinolones (FQ) are associated with generalized tendinopathy in some patients. Although the incidence is relatively small at about 1% or less, it is enough of a problem to prompt the Food and Drug Administration to issue a black box warning of this association. Numerous studies have implicated various abnormalities of tendon metabolism involving the cellular matrix.

This study reveals clear abnormalities of the tendon fibroblast as well as disorganization of healing collagen (Fig 2). The process clinically appears to be dose-dependent with considerable host variation. The message? Avoid FQ medication, if possible. I personally have found that surgical treatment of these tendinopathies does not provide satisfying results in many patients.

B. F. Morrey, MD

A Myofibroblast—Mast Cell—Neuropeptide Axis of Fibrosis in Post-Traumatic Joint Contractures: An In Vitro Analysis of Mechanistic Components

Hildebrand KA, Zhang M, Befus AD, et al (Univ of Calgary, Alberta, Canada; Univ of Alberta, Edmonton, Canada)
J Orthop Res 32:1290-1296, 2014

Previous studies have implicated a myofibroblast—mast cell—neuropeptide axis of fibrosis in pathologic joint capsules from post-traumatic contractures. The hypothesis to be tested is that joint capsule cells (JC) from human elbows with post-traumatic contractures and their interactions with mast cells (MC) and neuropeptides in the microenvironment underlie the pathogenesis of contractures. The hypothesis was tested using an in vitro collagen gel contraction model. The JC were isolated from human elbow capsules and mixed with neutralized PureCol collagen I. The gels were treated in various ways, including addition of MC (HMC-1), the neuropeptide substance P (SP), an NK_1 receptor (SP receptor) antagonist RP67580 and the mast cell stabilizer ketotifen fumarate (KF). The collagen gels were released from the wells and gel size (contraction) was measured optically at multiple time points. The JC contracted collagen gels in a dose-dependent manner. This was enhanced in the presence of MC and increased further with SP. Increasing concentrations of the SP receptor antagonist, RP67580 or the mast cell stabilizer, KF decreased the magnitude of contraction. These observations identify putative mechanistic components of a myofibroblast–mast cell–neuropeptide axis of fibrosis in the joint capsules in post-traumatic contractures and potential prophylactic or therapeutic interventions (Fig 1).

▶ Frankly, this contribution was selected in part because it aligns with our own research interests. But more importantly, it demonstrates a level of investigation to better understand one of the most perverse responses of injury to the musculoskeletal system, arthrofibrosis. The authors demonstrate a direct relationship

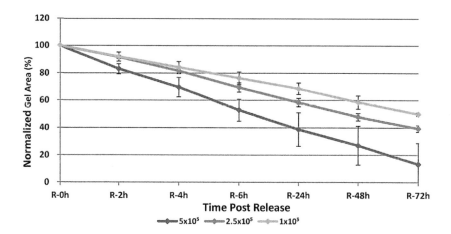

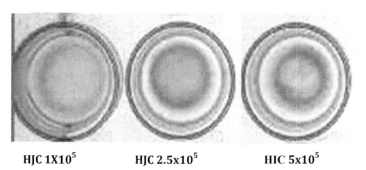

HJC 1X10⁵   **HJC 2.5x10⁵**   **HIC 5x10⁵**

FIGURE 1.—Collagen gel contraction at three different JC densities. Photographs of the wells at 24 h post release. (Reprinted from Hildebrand KA, Zhang M, Befus AD, et al. A myofibroblast-mast cell-neuropeptide axis of fibrosis in post-traumatic joint contractures: an in vitro analysis of mechanistic components. *J Orthop Res.* 2014;32:1290-1296, with permission from Journal of Orthopaedic Research and John Wiley and Sons, www.interscience.wiley.com.)

between the presence of mast cells and neuropeptides in the development of a joint contracture as portrayed with contracture of a gel medium containing a human joint capsule. Although I have some reservations regarding the methodology, the authors do demonstrate a clear relationship (Fig 1). This may give insight as to possible pharmacological methods to prevent joint contracture by inhibiting mast cell function in the posttraumatic environment.

B. F. Morrey, MD

Association Between Metabolic Syndrome, Radiographic Knee Osteoarthritis, and Intensity of Knee Pain: Results of a National Survey
Shin D (Seoul Natl Univ Hosp, South Korea)
J Clin Endocrinol Metab 99:3177-3183, 2014

Context.—Although osteoarthritis (OA) has been suggested as another component of metabolic syndrome (MetS), weight-independent associations between MetS and knee OA or intensity of arthritic knee pain remain unclear.

Objective.—The objective of the study was to evaluate the above associations and suggest possible mechanisms.

Design and Setting.—This was a cross-sectional study using the fifth Korean National Health and Nutrition Examination Survey (2010).

Participants.—A total of 2363 adults ($\geq$50 y of age) who had completed both laboratory examinations and an evaluation for radiographic knee OA participated in the study.

Main Outcome and Measures.—Radiographic knee OA was defined as a Kellgren/Lawrence grade of 2 or greater, and the intensity of arthritic knee pain was assessed using a self-reported numeric rating scale. MetS was diagnosed based on National Cholesterol Education Program-Adult Treatment Panel III criteria, and insulin resistance was evaluated using the homeostasis model assessment-estimated insulin resistance index.

Results.—In a multivariable logistic regression analysis, MetS was associated with radiographic knee OA (adjusted odds ratio 1.49; 95% confidence interval 1.23–1.79; $P < .001$). This association was not changed significantly after further adjusting for homeostasis model assessment-estimated insulin resistance but became nonsignificant after adjusting for weight or body mass index. Age-, sex-, and weight (or body mass index)-adjusted mean score of knee pain was significantly higher in subjects with more components of MetS (P for trend $= .010$ or .035, respectively).

Conclusions.—The association between MetS and radiographic knee OA can be largely explained by an excessive weight but not by insulin resistance, a key pathophysiology of MetS. Because accumulation of MetS components appears to be associated with a higher intensity of

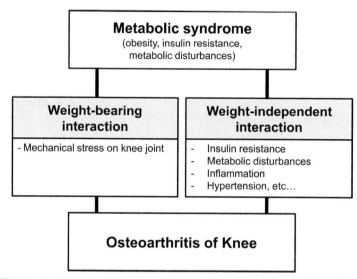

FIGURE 2.—Basic concept of the association between MetS and OA. (Reprinted from Shin D. Association between metabolic syndrome, radiographic knee osteoarthritis, and intensity of knee pain: results of a national survey. *J Clin Endocrinol Metab.* 2014;99:3177-3183, Copyright © 2014, with permission from the Author[s] and The Endocrine Society.)

knee pain, independently of weight, appropriate treatment for MetS may be helpful for subjects with knee pain (Fig 2).

▶ This interesting article from Korea was selected to introduce the concept of metabolic syndrome to the orthopedic, if he or she is not already familiar with this concept. The components of metabolic syndrome consist of insulin resistance, central obesity, hypertension, and hyperlipidemia.

The complexity of the question is obvious, as elements of any one of these conditions are implicated as a cause or effect of the other. However, these investigators were able to show a correlation of not only osteoarthritis with metabolic syndrome, but also, independently, of central obesity (Fig 2). Although the practical implication of these findings may not be obvious, as mentioned, it is important to appreciate the existence of the syndrome and that it does have some effect on the development of arthritis, independent of body weight.

B. F. Morrey, MD

A Lexicon for Wear of Metal-on-Metal Hip Prostheses
McKellop HA, Hart A, Park S-H, et al (UCLA & Orthopaedic Inst for Children; Univ College London & Royal Natl Orthopaedic Hosp, Middlesex-Stanmore, UK)
J Orthop Res 32:1221-1233, 2014

Research on metal-on-metal (MoM) hip bearings has generated an extensive vocabulary to describe the wear processes and resultant surface

TABLE 1.—Wear Modes

	Wear Mode	Examples
Mode 1	Bearing surface vs. bearing surface	Ball is articulating fully within the socket
Mode 2	Bearing surface vs. non-bearing surface	Ball vs. edge of contact zone, or rim of socket (e.g., due to micro-separation or complete dislocation)
Mode 3	Bearing surface vs. bearing surface with 3rd body particles between them	Entrapped particles broken away from a porous coating; fragments of PMMA cement
Mode 4	Non-bearing surface vs. non-bearing surface	Backside wear of an acetabular shell; fretting at the Morse taper junction

Reprinted from McKellop HA, Hart A, Park S-H, et al. A Lexicon for Wear of Metal-on-Metal Hip Prostheses. *J Orthop Res.* 2014;32:1221-1233, with permission from Journal of Orthopaedic Research and John Wiley and Sons, www.interscience.wiley.com.

TABLE 2.—Types of Wear Mechanisms

Wear Mechanism	Types of Damage Produced
Adhesive	Local bonding between two surfaces pulls out a fragment of one surface; can lead to pitting, scratching and formation of 3rd body abrasive particles
Abrasive	Asperities on one surface (or 3rd body fragments) cut and plow the opposing surface; large scale causes scratching, very small scale causes polishing
Fatigue	Repetitive loading initiates cracks in the surface or subsurface, which can coalesce, leading to pitting or delamination
Tribochemical	Tribochemical reaction layers

Reprinted from McKellop HA, Hart A, Park S-H, et al. A Lexicon for Wear of Metal-on-Metal Hip Prostheses. *J Orthop Res.* 2014;32:1221-1233, with permission from Journal of Orthopaedic Research and John Wiley and Sons, www.interscience.wiley.com.

damage. However, a lack of consistency and some redundancy exist in the current terminology. To facilitate the understanding of MoM tribology and to enhance communication of results among researchers and clinicians, we propose four categories of wear terminology: wear *modes* refer to the in vivo conditions under which the wear occurred; wear *mechanisms* refer to fundamental wear processes (adhesion, abrasion, fatigue, and tribochemical reactions); wear *damage* refers to the resultant changes in the morphology and/or composition of the surfaces; and wear *features* refer to the specific wear phenomena that are described in terms of the relevant modes, mechanisms, and damage. Clarifying examples are presented, but it is expected that terms will be added to the lexicon as new mechanisms and types of damage are identified. *Corrosion* refers to electrochemical processes that can remove or add material and thus also generate damage. Corrosion can act alone or may interact with mechanical wear. Examples of corrosion damage are also presented. However, an

TABLE 4.—Types of Damage Described in Prior Analyses of Retrieved MoM Hip Arthroplasties

Study	Scratches or Scratching	Polishing	Gouges	Pits or Pitting	Etching	Surface Films	Surface Deposits	Embedded 3rd Body Particles	Tribochemical Reaction Layers
Present study	Y	Y	Y	Y	Y	Y	Y	Y	Y
Walker and Gold[21]	Y	"Run in"							
Semlitsch et al.[22]	Y	Y		Y					
Täger[23]	Y		"Eruptions"			"Dried organic substance"	"Dark oxide coatings" "Thin fibrinoid deposits"		
McKellop et al.[24]	Y	Y	"Dents"	"Casting pores"			"Adherent coatings or precipitates"		
Rieker et al.[25]	Y			"Micro-pits"					
Park et al.[26]	Y	Y		"Carbide craters" & "micropits"			"Deposits of calcium phosphate-based ppt."		
Willert and Buchhorn[27]	Y	Y							
Reinisch et al.[28]	Y	Y					"Organic deposits"	"Al₂O₃"	
Milosev et al.[29]	Y	Y					"Organic deposits"		
Matthies et al.[30]	Y	Y							
Braunstein et al.[31]	Y						Y "thin" and "thick"		Y
Currier et al., AAOS[32]	Y		Y			Y			
Wimmer et al.[20]	Y					Y	Y		Y

A "Y" indicates that that type of damage was described in the publication. In some cases, the actual terminology used by the authors is given.

Editor's Note: Please refer to original journal article for full references.

Reprinted from McKellop HA, Hart A, Park S-H, et al. A Lexicon for Wear of Metal-on-Metal Hip Prostheses. *J Orthop Res.* 2014;32:1221-1233, with permission from Journal of Orthopaedic Research and John Wiley and Sons, www.interscience.wiley.com.

in-depth discussion of the many types of corrosion and their effects is beyond the scope of the present wear lexicon (Tables 1, 2 and 4).

▶ This is an uncommon type of article to place in the YEAR BOOK. However, because the issue of wear dominates the concern over the long-term effectiveness of arthroplasty in general, this offers a nice summary of the terminology of which we might become familiar. The essence of the message resides in the concepts of 4 distinct modes of wear (Table 1). The result is a wear that can be further characterized into 4 types or mechanisms (Table 2). Finally, each of these discrete but overlapping patterns result in 4 expressions of pathology or damage (Table 4). It is thought that summarizing these concepts will help understand the issues and the basis of the debate. Ultimately, this may help with the selection of the bearing surface of choice in one's practice.

B. F. Morrey, MD

Characterization of Macrophage Polarizing Cytokines in the Aseptic Loosening of Total Hip Replacements
Jämsen E, Kouri V-P, Olkkonen J, et al (Univ of Helsinki, Finland; et al)
J Orthop Res 32:1241-1246, 2014

Aseptic loosening of hip replacements is driven by the macrophage reaction to wear particles. The extent of particle-induced macrophage activation is dependent on the state of macrophage polarization, which is dictated by the local cytokine microenvironment. The aim of the study was to characterize cytokine microenvironment surrounding failed, loose hip replacements with an emphasis on identification of cytokines that regulate macrophage polarization. Using qRT-PCR, the expression of interferon gamma (IFN-γ), interleukin-4 (IL-4), granulocyte—macrophage colony-stimulating factor (GM-CSF), IL-13, and IL-17A was low and similar to the expression in control synovial tissues of patients undergoing primary hip replacement. Using immunostaining, no definite source of IFN-γ or IL-4 could be identified. IL-17A positive cells, identified as mast cells by double staining, were detected but their number was significantly reduced in interface tissues compared to the controls. Significant up-regulation of IL-10, M-CSF, IL-8, CCL2-4, CXCL9-10, CCL22, TRAP, cathepsin K, and down regulation of OPG was seen in the interface tissues, while expression of TNF-α, IL-1β, and CD206 were similar between the conditions. It is concluded that at the time of the revision surgery the peri-implant macrophage phenotype has both M1 and M2 characteristics and that the phenotype is regulated by other local and systemic factors than traditional macrophage polarizing cytokines.

▶ Understanding the precise mechanism of implant loosening is a critical issue. The relationship of wear particles is well appreciated, but the mechanism through which these particles actually cause loosening and bone resorption remains unclear. This assessment furthers our knowledge by demonstrating that cytokines that control macrophage polarization is a key function controlling this process. It would also appear, given the marked individual variation exhibited in this study, that there is considerable host variation that controls or at least influences this process. This is consistent with the clinical observation of the marked tolerance or sensitivity to the influence of wear debris among different patients.

B. F. Morrey, MD

Are Harris Hip Scores and Gait Mechanics Related Before and After THA?
Behery OA, Foucher KC (Rush Univ Med Ctr, Chicago, IL; Univ of Illinois at Chicago)
Clin Orthop Relat Res 472:3452-3461, 2014

Background.—Discordance between subjective and objective functional measures hinders the development of new ways to improve THA outcomes.

Questions/Purposes.—We asked if (1) any kinematic or kinetic gait variables are correlated with preoperative Harris hip scores (HHS), (2) any kinematic or kinetic gait variables are correlated with postoperative HHS, and (3) pre- to postoperative changes in any kinematic or kinetic gait variables are associated with the change in HHS?

Methods.—For this retrospective study, an institutional review board-approved data repository that included all individuals who participated in motion analysis research studies was used to identify subjects evaluated before ($n = 161$) and at least 6 months after primary unilateral THA ($n = 156$). Selected kinematic (sagittal plane dynamic hip ROM) and kinetic (peak external moments about the hip in the sagittal, frontal, and transverse planes) gait variables were collected at subjects' self-selected normal walking speeds. We used first-order partial correlations to identify relationships between HHS and gait variables, controlling for the influence of speed.

Results.—Preoperative HHS correlated with hip ROM ($R_{|speed} = 0.260$ $p < 0.001$) and the peak extension moment ($R_{|speed} = 0.164$ $p = 0.038$), postoperative HHS correlated with the peak internal rotation moment ($R_{|speed} = 0.178$ $p = 0.034$), and change in HHS correlated with change in hip ROM ($R_{|speed} = 0.288$ $p = 0.001$) and peak external rotation moment ($R_{|speed} = 0.291$ $p = 0.002$). Similar associations were seen when the HHS pain and function were analyzed separately.

Conclusions.—This study identified relationships between a common clinical outcome measure and specific, modifiable gait adaptations that can persist after THA—ROM and transverse plane gait moments. Addressing these aspects of gait dysfunction through focused rehabilitation could be a new strategy for improving clinical outcomes. Prospective studies are needed to evaluate this concept.

Level of Evidence.—Level III, diagnostic study. See the Instructions for Authors for a complete description of levels of evidence.

▶ It is well known that the Harris Hip Score (HHS) is a universally used but also a somewhat insensitive outcome tool. Similarly, the value of biomechanically measured gait parameters before or after hip replacement is often not considered clinically relevant. Hence the demonstration of these correlations are of some interest. Preoperative HHS did correlate to range of motion (ROM) and extension strength. Furthermore, ROM as well as internal and external strength were correlated after surgery. As the authors suggest, these correlations may help direct physical therapy focus in selected patients.

B. F. Morrey, MD

2   General Orthopedics

Introduction

I enjoy selecting articles for the General Orthopedics section as much as any of the other sections that I review. This gives me a chance to personally maintain a broad-based understanding of current issues and solutions in our specialty. In this section, therefore, I picked some articles that discuss hip and knee replacement as a group, but some topics are also relevant to orthopedic surgeons in general, such as thrombophlebitis. We have also found interest in social and more general questions that arise in the orthopedic practice. Implications of cost-effectiveness and outcomes are also included in this section. These trends continue to be strongly investigated in our profession and thus are reflected here.

Bernard F. Morrey, MD

Clinical Practice Guidelines: Their Use, Misuse and Future Directions
Sanders JO, Bozic KJ, Glassman SD, et al (Univ of Rochester, NY; Univ of California, San Francisco; Univ of Louisville, KY; et al)
J Am Acad Orthop Surg 22:135-144, 2014

Evidence-based clinical practice guidelines (CPGs) have the potential to bring the best-quality evidence to orthopaedic surgeons and their patients. CPGs can improve quality by decreasing the variability in orthopaedic care, but they can also be misused through inappropriate development or application. The quality of a CPG is dependent on the strength of its evidence base, which is often deficient in orthopaedic publications. In addition, many surgeons express concern about legal liability associated with CPGs. Specific processes in CPG development and implementation can counter these potential problems. Other evidence tools, such as appropriate use criteria, also can help in the application of the proper treatment of patients by identifying those who are appropriate for specific procedures. Because payers, patients, and surgeons need access to the best evidence, CPGs will continue to be developed, and orthopaedic surgeons have the opportunity to ensure their proper development and implementation by understanding and participating in the process.

▶ This is a reasonable review article for surgeons who are confused by the interpretation and formulation of clinical practice guidelines in orthopedic surgery. These are becoming more common as different groups seek to standardize the evidence behind orthopedic surgery procedures. This is a reasonable article to acquaint physicians with the history of the development of these and their limitations. The interaction of clinical practice guidelines with insurers and other payors is discussed, as is the mechanism through which these are formulated. Appropriate use criteria, a related topic, are also addressed.

Many of these have been developed by the Academy and by other professional organizations. As these become more common, the understanding of how they apply to clinical practice and how they can be implemented is important for surgeons to understand.

P. S. Rose, MD

Evaluation of the First-Generation AAOS Clinical Guidelines on the Prophylaxis of Venous Thromboembolic Events in Patients Undergoing Total Joint Arthroplasty: Experience with 3289 Patients from a Single Institution

Lewis CG, Inneh IA, Schutzer SF, et al (Orthopedic Associates of Hartford, Farmington, CT; Saint Francis Hosp and Med Ctr, Farmington, CT)
J Bone Joint Surg Am 96:1327-1332, 2014

Background.—Patients undergoing total hip or total knee arthroplasty have risks that include venous thromboembolism. The American Academy of Orthopaedic Surgeons has promulgated guidelines for the preoperative assessment of patients with the primary objective of preventing pulmonary embolism. We aimed to evaluate and establish the utility of the first-generation American Academy of Orthopaedic Surgeons guidelines for the prophylaxis of venous thromboembolism in patients undergoing total joint arthroplasty at a single institution.

Methods.—A prospective analysis of 3289 consecutive patients managed with total hip or total knee arthroplasty at the Connecticut Joint Replacement Institute between June 1, 2009, and April 30, 2011, was conducted. Data on age, sex, body mass index, American Society of Anesthesiologists classification, and a personal or family history of blood clots requiring long-term warfarin use were analyzed, as were data on a personal history of a malignant tumor, a bleeding disorder, gastrointestinal bleeding, or a hemorrhagic cerebrovascular accident. All patients were managed prophylactically with a specific algorithm based on the American Academy of Orthopaedic Surgeons guidelines. All of the patients were mobilized on postoperative day one, and pneumatic foot-pump compression was used for the duration of the hospitalization.

Results.—Thirty-six major venous thromboembolic events were documented with Doppler ultrasound or computed tomography angiography, for a ninety-day incidence of 1.1% (95% confidence interval, 0.8% to 1.5%). A personal history of blood clots was significantly associated with a blood clot in the proximal part of the thigh or a pulmonary embolism, but a family history of blood clots and a personal history of a malignant tumor did not show a significant relationship with venous thromboembolism. The ninety-day incidence of venous thromboembolism was significantly different between total hip arthroplasty patients (0.56%; 95% confidence interval, 0.30% to 1.15%) and total knee arthroplasty patients (1.46%; 95% confidence interval, 1.01% to 2.10%). The risk was greater in high-risk total knee arthroplasty patients compared with high-risk total hip arthroplasty patients despite comparable prophylaxis with enoxaparin sodium for twenty-eight days.

Conclusions.—The prospective use of the first-generation American Academy of Orthopaedic Surgeons guidelines resulted in a low incidence of clinically important thromboembolic events in total hip and total knee arthroplasty patients. When properly used in these patients, the guidelines to minimize adverse outcomes are executable and effective.

Level of Evidence.—Therapeutic Level IV. See Instructions for Authors for a complete description of levels of evidence (Table 2).

▶ It is encouraging to see the question of practical or measurable usefulness of clinical guidelines being studied. I commend the authors for this effort. The

TABLE 2.—Presence of Risk Factors and Risk Categorizations*

Risk Factors	All Patients (N = 3289)	Total Hip Arthroplasty Patients (N = 1366)	Total Knee Arthroplasty Patients (N = 1923)
Family history (%)			
Blood clots	190 (5.8)	76 (5.6)	114 (5.9)
Personal history (%)			
Blood clots	185 (5.6)	73 (5.3)	112 (5.8)
Bleeding disorder	23 (0.7)	7 (0.5)	16 (0.8)
Gastrointestinal bleeding	127 (3.9)	47 (3.4)	80 (4.2)
Hemorrhagic cerebrovascular accident	12 (0.4)	6 (0.4)	6 (0.3)
Malignant tumor (active or in remission)	452 (13.7)	162 (11.9)	290 (15.1)
Risk (%)			
Standard[†]	1966 (59.8)	920 (67.3)	1046 (54.4)
High[‡]	610 (18.5)	203 (14.9)	407 (21.2)

*Data are expressed as the frequency with the percentages in parentheses.

[†]Patients were considered to be at standard risk if they had no personal or family history of blood clots requiring long-term warfarin use or no personal history of a malignant tumor (and no current tumor), bleeding disorder, gastrointestinal bleeding, or hemorrhagic cerebrovascular accident.

[‡]Patients were considered to be at high risk if they had a personal or family history of blood clots requiring long-term warfarin use or a personal history of a malignant tumor (active or in remission), bleeding disorder, gastrointestinal bleeding, or hemorrhagic cerebrovascular accident.

Reprinted from Lewis CG, Inneh IA, Schutzer SF, et al. Evaluation of the First-Generation AAOS Clinical Guidelines on the Prophylaxis of Venous Thromboembolic Events in Patients Undergoing Total Joint Arthroplasty: Experience with 3289 Patients from a Single Institution. *J Bone Joint Surg Am.* 2014;96:1327–1332. http://jbjs.org/.

findings of the investigation into the question of high risk for thromboembolic events are shown in Table 2. The observations are not unique to this study. It is known that a higher risk of this complication exists for knee compared with hip replacement. It is also known that a personal history of a clotting or bleeding disorder places the patient at an increased risk for these complications after surgery. The first-generation guidelines recognize these risks. What is not completely clear is whether specifically following the guidelines improved the results compared with current practice, which does recognize these risk features.

B. F. Morrey, MD

Occupational Hazards for Pregnant or Lactating Women in the Orthopaedic Operating Room
Downes J, Rauk PN, Vanheest AE (Univ of Minnesota, Minneapolis)
J Am Acad Orthop Surg 22:326-332, 2014

Pregnant or lactating staff working in the orthopaedic operating room may be at risk of occupational exposure to several hazards, including blood-borne pathogens, anesthetic gases, methylmethacrylate, physical stress, and radiation. Because the use of proper personal protective equipment is mandatory, the risk of contamination with blood-borne pathogens such as hepatitis B, hepatitis C, and HIV is low. Moreover, effective postexposure prophylactic regimens are available for hepatitis B and HIV. In the 1960s, concerns were raised about occupational exposure to harmful chemicals in the operating room such as anesthetic gases and methylmethacrylate. Guidelines on safe levels of exposure to these chemicals and the use of personal protective equipment have helped to minimize the risks to pregnant or lactating staff. Short periods of moderate physical activity are beneficial for pregnant women, but prolonged strenuous activity can lead to increased pregnancy complications. The risk of prenatal radiation exposure during orthopaedic procedures is of concern, as well. However, proper lead protection and contamination control can minimize the risk of occupational exposure to radiation.

▶ The common practice of orthopedic surgery can potentially expose pregnant or lactating women to occupational hazards while carrying out their duties in the operating room. This exposure includes surgeons and other personnel who are in the operating suite caring for patients. This article outlines risks in several categories (blood-borne pathogens, anesthetic gases, methyl methacrylate vapor exposure, physical stress, and radiation exposure) and reviews the available evidence for what is and is not safe exposure and protective adaptations for pregnant and lactating women. This is a reasonable article for all surgeons, as many of the personnel in and around the operating room may be pregnant or lactating and are at risk for these exposures. Although the subject has received limited study, reasonable evidence is present for a number of issues raised to guide clinical practice and safe conduct of surgery.

P. S. Rose, MD

ACGME Duty Hour Requirements: Perceptions and Impact on Resident Training and Patient Care
Levine WN, Spang RC III (Columbia Univ Med Ctr, NY)
J Am Acad Orthop Surg 22:535-544, 2014

In 2003, the Accreditation Council for Graduate Medical Education (ACGME) created national guidelines for resident work hours to promote safe care and high-quality learning. However, some reports suggested that the 2003 rules did not reduce resident fatigue or improve patient care. Since July 2011, further restrictions have been in effect. The changes have been the source of much controversy regarding their impact on resident education and patient safety. We reviewed existing literature on the effects of the new and old rules, with a focus on the field of orthopaedics. In addition, we conducted a national survey of orthopaedic residents and residency directors to assess the general opinions of the orthopaedic community. Overall, only 19.7% of all respondents were satisfied with the new 2011 regulations, whereas 58.9% believe the 80-hour work week averaged over 4 weeks is appropriate. The results will inform discussions and decisions related to changing residency education in the future.

▶ Surgeons who work with residents and fellows are becoming increasingly aware of the Accreditation Council for Graduate Medical Education duty hour requirements. These were initially created in 2003 in an attempt to optimize the learning environment and quality of care for patients and have since been expanded with further restrictions in 2011. Controversy exists as to whether these duty hour restrictions have achieved their goals and whether they are having a beneficial impact on education and patient care. This article outlines the nature of these regulations for physicians who may have heard of them only anecdotally as well as what initial data are present on their effect. As such, this is a valuable subject for clinicians who work in or around residents or fellows to be familiar with. Although many surgeons do not agree with these, the consequences for violating them are significant for residents, fellows, and training programs.

P. S. Rose, MD

Availability of Consumer Prices for Bunion Surgery

Willey JC, Reuter LS, Belatti DA, et al (Univ of Iowa)
Foot Ankle Int 35:1309-1315, 2014

Background.—Today, insurance insulates most patients from the true costs of the health care services they consume. Economists believe that the absence of price signals incentivizes patients to pursue more extensive care than they would otherwise. Reformers propose restoring price consciousness to patients as a way to tame the soaring costs of American health care. To test this idea, we decided to gauge the availability and variability of price quotes for a common elective surgery—bunion repair.

Methods.—Orthopedic clinics were sorted by state and randomly selected from an online directory maintained by the American Orthopaedic Foot and Ankle Society. Each selected clinic was contacted up to 3 times in an attempt to get a full, bundled price quote using a standardized patient script. If this was unavailable, an isolated quote for the physician fee alone was solicited.

Results.—Of the 141 clinics contacted, 56 (39.7%) could provide a physician price estimate and 12 (8.5%) could give a complete bundled estimate, including hospital fees. The overall mean bundled price quoted was $18 332, while the overall mean physician fee quoted was $2487. There was no statistically significant difference in the mean price quoted by academic and private clinics, nor was regional variation observed.

Conclusion.—We found low price availability for elective bunion procedures.

Clinical Relevance.—However, the wide variation observed in the prices that were quoted suggests that a very determined patient may be able to spend substantially less on an elective surgery if they were willing to select a provider carefully (Tables 1 and 2).

▶ I really liked this study—or more to the point, I liked the question being addressed. It is amazing that institutions do not really know the cost, especially the "true" cost, of procedures (Table 1). This is going to have to change. Also, the assessment found little regional variation is surprising, based on other cost-of-service studies. Although there was no statistical difference between

TABLE 1.—Price Availability by Clinic Type

Variable	Academic (n = 39)	Private (n = 102)	P Value[a]
Complete bundled price	10 (4)	8 (8)	.737
Physician price only	28 (11)	44 (45)	.123
Unable to provide any price	62 (24)	48 (49)	.188

Values are percentages, with n in parentheses.
[a]Fischer's exact test.

TABLE 2.—Price Variability by Clinic Type

Variable	Academic (n = 39)		Private (n = 102)		P Value
	Range	Mean (SD)	Range	Mean (SD)	
Bundled price	11 706-19 009	14 442 (3165)	3542-52 207	22 222 (17 606)	.261[a]
Physician price	1200-6900	2728 (1467)	800-7834	2246 (1206)	.211[b]

[a]Welch's *t* test.
[b]Student's *t* test.

academic and private costs, this is deceiving because of the wide variation of the data. There is a real difference in the mean charges of $14 400 for academic providers versus $22 200 for private providers (Table 2).

I found it interesting that a cost in excess of $18 000 for a bunion procedure was considered reasonable. Where will this all end?

B. F. Morrey, MD

American Medical Society for Sports Medicine Position Statement: Interventional Musculoskeletal Ultrasound in Sports Medicine

Finnoff JT, Hall MM, Adams E, et al (Univ of California Davis School of Medicine, Sacramento; Univ of Iowa Sports Medicine; Midwest Sports Medicine Inst, Middleton, WI; et al)
Clin J Sport Med 25:6-22, 2015

The use of diagnostic and interventional ultrasound has significantly increased over the past decade. A majority of the increased utilization is by nonradiologists. In sports medicine, ultrasound is often used to guide interventions such as aspirations, diagnostic or therapeutic injections, tenotomies, releases, and hydrodissections. This American Medical Society for Sports Medicine (AMSSM) position statement critically reviews the literature and evaluates the accuracy, efficacy, and cost-effectiveness of ultrasound-guided injections in major, intermediate, and small joints, and soft tissues, all of which are commonly performed in sports medicine. New ultrasound-guided procedures and future trends are also briefly discussed. Based on the evidence, the official AMSSM position relevant to each subject is made.

▶ This is an excellent paper that exhaustively assesses the utility of ultrasound-guided injections for musculoskeletal disorders. The authors employed 124 carefully selected papers to construct 13 tables comparing both the accuracy and efficacy of ultrasound-guided injections (USGI) compared with landmark-guided injections (LMGI). The interpretation of numerous stratifications of the material and citing 168 references provide 3 reliable conclusions: (1) there is level A evidence indicating superior accuracy; (2) level B evidence for the efficacy of USGI; and (3) of additional importance is the demonstration of level B evidence for the cost-effectiveness of USGI. This is definitive, in my opinion.

B. F. Morrey, MD

Approach to Pain Management in Chronic Opioid Users Undergoing Orthopaedic Surgery

Devin CJ, Lee DS, Armaghani SJ, et al (Vanderbilt Univ Med Ctr, Nashville, TN)

J Am Acad Orthop Surg 22:614-622, 2014

Opioids are commonly used for the management of pain in patients with musculoskeletal disorders; however, national attention has highlighted the

---

TABLE 3.—Approach to Managing Varying Degrees of Preoperative Opioid Use in the Orthopaedic Patient[a]

Low (0-30 mg/d)	Moderate (30-60 mg/d)	High (>60 mg/d)
Preoperative Visit Set goal of gradually eliminating opioid intake prior to surgical date Provide non-opioid alternatives as appropriate Clearly delineate amount of postoperative opioid prescriptions to be dispensed Reinforce weaning of opioids during additional preoperative visits	**Preoperative Visit** Set goal of decreasing opioid intake to mutually agreed on amount prior to surgical date Discuss pain-related beliefs and provide non-opioid alternatives as appropriate Clearly delineate amount of postoperative opioid prescriptions to be dispensed Reinforce target opioid intake goal	**Preoperative Visit** Educate patient regarding implications of high opioid intake Offer and recommend addiction specialist consultation Determine need for additional measures (eg, detoxification, counseling) as guided by addiction specialist consultation
Surgery Consider regional anesthesia as appropriate Judicious opioid administration in perioperative period	**Surgery** Consider regional anesthesia as appropriate Consider additional multimodal measures with anesthesia provider (preemptive analgesia, NSAIDS/ketorolac, acetaminophen, anticonvulsants, ketamine) Judicious opioid administration in perioperative period	**Surgery** Consider regional anesthesia as appropriate Implement additional multimodal measures with anesthesia provider (preemptive analgesia, NSAIDS/ketorolac, acetaminophen, anticonvulsants, ketamine) Judicious opioid administration in perioperative period
Postoperative Visits Assess opioid intake at each postoperative visit Encourage and facilitate opioid independence	**Postoperative Visits** Assess opioid intake at each postoperative visit Encourage and facilitate opioid independence	**Postoperative Visits** Assess opioid intake at each postoperative visit Ensure continued follow-up with addiction specialist Agree on single provider to dispense additional opioid prescriptions Encourage and facilitate opioid independence

[a]Assessment and management that includes a patient history and physical examination, followed by opioid use quantification (daily morphine equivalent).

Reprinted from Devin CJ, Lee DS, Armaghani SJ, et al. Approach to Pain Management in Chronic Opioid Users Undergoing Orthopaedic Surgery. *J Am Acad Orthop Surg.* 2014;22:614-622.

potential adverse effects of the use of opioid analgesia in this and other nonmalignant pain settings. Chronic opioid users undergoing orthopaedic surgery represent a particularly challenging patient population in regard to their perioperative pain control and outcomes. Preoperative evaluation provides an opportunity to estimate a patient's preoperative opioid intake, discuss pain-related fears, and identify potential psychiatric comorbidities. Patients using high levels of opioids may also require referral to an addiction specialist. Various regional blockade and pharmaceutical options are available to help control perioperative pain, and a multimodal pain management approach may be of particular benefit in chronic opioid users undergoing orthopaedic surgery (Table 3).

▶ For better or for worse, opioid pain medications are increasingly prescribed for chronic pain management by other than pain management specialists. Many patients may be managed with opioids chronically for musculoskeletal conditions that come to surgical intervention. As such, being familiar with the management of pain medications and the impact on patient care that preoperative chronic opioid use has is important for physicians to understand.

This is a practical article that contains information on preoperative evaluation, perioperative pain control, and postoperative visits in patients with varying degrees of opioid use preoperatively. It includes data on morphine equivalence to allow conversion between different outpatient opioid preparations and potential inpatient parenteral treatment regimens (Table 3). As such, it is a helpful reference for physicians to have as they treat and evaluate these patients.

P. S. Rose, MD

A systematic review and meta-analysis of the topical administration of tranexamic acid in total hip and knee replacement

Alshryda S, Sukeik M, Sarda P, et al (Central Manchester Univ Hosps, UK; Univ College London Hosp, UK; Medway Maritime Hosp, Gillingham, UK; et al)
Bone Joint J 96-B:1005-1015, 2014

Intravenous tranexamic acid (TXA) has been shown to be effective in reducing blood loss and the need for transfusion after joint replacement. Recently, there has been interest in applying it topically before the closure of surgical wounds. This has the advantages of ease of application, maximum concentration at the site of bleeding, minimising its systemic absorption and, consequently, concerns about possible side-effects.

We conducted a systematic review and meta-analysis which included 14 randomised controlled trials (11 in knee replacement, two in hip replacement and one in both) which investigated the effect of topical TXA on blood loss and rates of transfusion. Topical TXA significantly reduced the rate of blood transfusion (total knee replacement: risk ratio (RR) 4.51; 95% confidence interval (CI): 3.02 to 6.72; $p < 0.001$ (nine trials, $I^2 = 0\%$); total hip replacement: RR 2.56; 95% CI: 1.32 to 4.97,

Study or subgroup	Control Events	Total	Topical TXA Events	Total	Weight	Risk ratio M-H, Fixed, 95% CI	Risk ratio M-H, Fixed, 95% CI
Canata et al[38] 2012	2	32	1	32	4.4%	2.00 [0.19 to 20.97]	
Wong et al[11] 2010	5	35	4	64	12.4%	2.29 [0.66 to 7.97]	
Ishida et al[36] 2011	1	50	0	50	2.2%	3.00 [0.13 to 71.92]	
Sa-Ngasoongsong et al[36] 2011	10	45	6	90	17.5%	3.33 [1.29 to 8.59]	
Roy et al[31] 2012	7	25	2	25	8.8%	3.50 [0.80 to 15.23]	
Seo et al[34] 2012	47	50	10	50	43.8%	4.70 [2.69 to 8.22]	
Sa-Ngasoongsong et al[37] 2013	8	24	1	24	4.4%	8.00 [1.08 to 59.13]	
Georgiadis et al[33] 2013	4	51	0	50	2.2%	8.83 [0.49 to 159.80]	
Alshryda et al[38] 2013 (TRANX-K)	13	78	1	79	4.4%	13.17 [1.76 to 98.24]	
Total (95% CI)		390		464	100.0%	4.51 [3.02 to 6.72]	
Total events	97		25				

Heterogeneity: Chi² = 3.80, df = 8 (P = 0.87); I² = 0%
Test for overall effect: Z = 7.38 (P < 0.001)

0.001 0.1 1 10 1000
Favours control Favours topical TXA

FIGURE 2.—Trials of topical tranexamic acid (TXA) *vs* placebo: Forest plot of blood transfusion rate. CI, confidence intervals, M-H, Mantel-Haenszel. *Editor's Note:* Please refer to original journal article for full references. (Reprinted from Alshryda S, Sukeik M, Sarda P, et al. A systematic review and meta-analysis of the topical administration of tranexamic acid in total hip and knee replacement. *Bone Joint J.* 2014;96-B:1005-1015, with permission from The British Editorial Society of Bone & Joint Surgery.)

$p = 0.004$ (one trial)). The rate of thromboembolic events with topical TXA were similar to those found with a placebo. Indirect comparison of placebo-controlled trials of topical and intravenous TXA indicates that topical administration is superior to the intravenous route.

In conclusion, topical TXA is an effective and safe method of reducing the need for blood transfusion after total knee and hip replacement. Further research is required to find its optimum dose for topical use (Fig 2).

▶ This is a must read. It demonstrates the increasing use of a refined literature search methodology to address a difficult question. A major reason for including it is to acquaint readers with the tremendous value of tranexamic acid to reduce postoperative blood loss. Initially introduced as an intravenous medication, this study clearly demonstrates its value when applied topically. The results demonstrate a clear value over a control, usually normal saline (Fig 2). Furthermore, there was no evidence of an increased incidence of deep vein thrombosis. The use of tranexamic acid is now a standard practice with hip and knee replacements at the Mayo Clinic.

B. F. Morrey, MD

Can Therapy Dogs Improve Pain and Satisfaction After Total Joint Arthroplasty? A Randomized Controlled Trial

Harper CM, Dong Y, Thornhill TS, et al (Harvard Med School, Boston, MA; Dept of Orthopaedic Surgery, Boston, MA)
Clin Orthop Relat Res 473:372-379, 2014

Background.—The use of animals to augment traditional medical therapies was reported as early as the 9th century but to our knowledge has not been studied in an orthopaedic patient population. The purpose of this study was to evaluate the role of animal-assisted therapy using therapy dogs in the postoperative recovery of patients after THA and TKA.

Questions/Purposes.—We asked: (1) Do therapy dogs have an effect on patients' perception of pain after total joint arthroplasty as measured by the VAS? (3) Do therapy dogs have an effect on patients' satisfaction with their hospital stay after total joint arthroplasty as measured by the Hospital Consumer Assessment of Healthcare Providers and Systems (HCAHPS)?

Methods.—A randomized controlled trial of 72 patients undergoing primary unilateral THA or TKA was conducted. Patients were randomized to a 15 minute visitation with a therapy dog before physical therapy or standard postoperative physical therapy regimens. Both groups had similar demographic characteristics. Reduction in pain was assessed using the VAS after each physical therapy session, beginning on postoperative Day 1 and continuing for three consecutive sessions. To ascertain patient satisfaction, the proportion of patients selecting top-category ratings in each subsection of the HCAHPS was compared.

Results.—Patients in the treatment group had lower VAS scores after each physical therapy session with a final VAS score difference of 2.4 units (animal-assisted therapy VAS, 1.7; SD, 0.97 [95% CI, 1.4–2.0] versus control VAS, 4.1; SD, 0.97 [95% CI, 3.8–4.4], $p < 0.001$) after the third physical therapy session. Patients in the treatment group had a higher proportion of top-box HCAHPS scores in the following fields: nursing communication (33 of 36, 92% [95% CI, 78%–98%] versus 69%, 25 of 36 [95% CI, 52%–84%], $p = 0.035$; risk ratio, 1.3 [95% CI of risk ratio, 1.0–1.7]; risk difference, 23% [95% CI of risk difference, 5%–40%]), pain management (34 of 36, 94% [95% CI, 81%–99%], versus 26 of 36, 72% [95% CI, 55%–86%], $p = 0.024$; risk ratio, 1.3 [95% CI of risk ratio, 1.1–1.6]; risk difference, 18% [95% CI of risk difference, 5%–39%]). The overall hospital rating also was greater in the treatment group (0–10 scale) (9.6; SD, 0.7 [95% CI, 9.3–9.8] versus 8.6, SD, 0.9 [95% CI, 8.3–8.9], $p < 0.001$).

Conclusions.—The use of therapy dogs has a positive effect on patients' pain level and satisfaction with hospital stay after total joint replacement. Surgeons are encouraged to inquire about the status of volunteer-based animal-assisted therapy programs in their hospital as this may provide a means to improve the immediate postoperative recovery for a select group of patients having total joint arthroplasty.

Level of Evidence.—Level II, randomized controlled study. See Instructions for Authors for a complete description of levels of evidence (Fig 3).

▶ The message of this unusual study is straightforward. I am amazed that 3 visits from therapy dogs of 15 minutes each over a course of traditional therapy would have such a profound impact on rehabilitation, as reflected by the impressive visual analog scale scores (Fig 3). The authors are from Harvard, and thus we expect a high level of science; this is accordingly a well done controlled study. One might question, with the impressive patient care

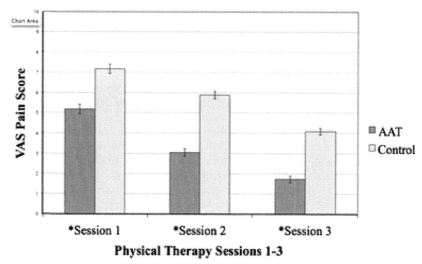

Physical Therapy Sessions 1-3

FIGURE 3.—The VAS for the animal-assisted therapy group after physical therapy was significantly lower than that of the control group at three times *Session 1: 5.2 ± 1.5 versus 7.1 ± 1.3, $p < 0.001$; *Session 2: 3.05 ± 1.3 versus 5.8 ± 0.74, $p < 0.001$; *Session 3: 1.71 ± 0.88 versus 4.07 ± 1.05, $p < 0.001$. The bars indicate standard error. AAT =animal-assisted therapy. (With kind permission from Springer Science+Business Media: Harper CM, Dong Y, Thornhill TS, et al. Can therapy dogs improve pain and satisfaction after total joint arthroplasty? A randomized controlled trial. *Clin Orthop Relat Res.* 2014;473:372-379, with permission from The Association of Bone and Joint Surgeons.)

results exhibited by the therapy dog, whether we should start interviewing retrievers for our residency programs; the effect of the patient interaction is clearly superior to that of some residents we have observed!

B. F. Morrey, MD

Evaluation of Malnutrition in Orthopaedic Surgery
Cross MB, Yi PH, Thomas CF, et al (Rush Univ Med Ctr, Chicago, IL)
J Am Acad Orthop Surg 22:193-199, 2014

Malnutrition can increase the risk of surgical site infection in both elective spine surgery and total joint arthroplasty. Obesity and diabetes are common comorbid conditions in patients who are malnourished. Despite the relatively high incidence of nutritional disorders among patients undergoing elective orthopaedic surgery, the evaluation and management of malnutrition is not generally well understood by practicing orthopaedic surgeons. Serologic parameters such as total lymphocyte count, albumin level, prealbumin level, and transferrin level have all been used as markers for nutrition status. In addition, anthropometric measurements, such as calf and arm muscle circumference or triceps skinfold, and standardized scoring systems, such as the Rainey-MacDonald nutritional index, the Mini Nutritional Assessment, and institution-specific nutritional scoring tools, are useful to define malnutrition. Preoperative nutrition assessment and optimization of nutritional parameters, including tight glucose control, normalization of serum albumin, and safe weight loss, may reduce the risk of perioperative complications, including infection.

▶ Many patients encountered in clinical practice may have a degree of clinical or subclinical malnutrition. When evaluating patients for elective surgical procedures, recognizing these patients ahead of time can likely decrease complications and optimize patient outcomes. Malnutrition is associated with an increase in risk of infection and other adverse outcomes after surgery.

This review article is aimed at the practicing orthopedic surgeon to help identify patients who are malnourished. Although there are some basic treatment guidelines, a busy surgeon will probably not undertake such treatment on his or her own. However, the main value of an article of this nature is to highlight aspects of the patient's presentation that may cause a surgeon to recognize malnutrition so that surgery can be delayed until such a time as it is corrected.

P. S. Rose, MD

"When can I Return to driving?": a review of the current literature on returning to driving after lower limb injury or arthroplasty
MacLeod K, Lingham A, Chatha H, et al (Royal Natl Orthopaedic Hosp Stanmore, Brockley Hill, UK; School of Medicine, London, UK; Orthopaedics Trainee Univ Hosp, Aintree, UK; et al)
Bone Joint J 95-B:290-294, 2013

Clinicians are often asked by patients, "When can I drive again?" after lower limb injury or surgery. This question is difficult to answer in the absence of any guidelines. This review aims to collate the currently available evidence and discuss the factors that influence the decision to allow a patient to return to driving. Medline, Web of Science, Scopus, and EMBASE were searched using the following terms: 'brake reaction time', 'brake response time', 'braking force', 'brake pedal force', 'resume driving', 'rate of application of force', 'driving after injury', 'joint replacement and driving', and 'fracture and driving'. Of the relevant literature identified, most studies used the brake reaction time and total brake time as the outcome measures. Varying recovery periods were proposed based on the type and severity of injury or surgery. Surveys of the Driver and Vehicle Licensing Agency, the Police, insurance companies in the United Kingdom and Orthopaedic Surgeons offered a variety of opinions.

There is currently insufficient evidence for any authoritative body to determine fitness to drive. The lack of guidance could result in patients being withheld from driving for longer than is necessary, or returning to driving while still unsafe (Table 1).

▶ This is a very important topic because the question being addressed occurs across the spectrum of lower extremity trauma and elective surgery. Although

TABLE 1.—Summary of the Literature

Authors	Sample (n)	Indication*	Method	Safe to drive
Dalury et al[4]	29	TKR	Brake reaction time	4 weeks
Egol et al [5]	31	Ankle fracture	Reaction time	9 weeks
Egol et al[6]	22 right leg	Complex lower trauma	Reaction time	6 weeks
	35 left leg			
Ganz et al[7]	90	THR	Reaction time	4 to 6 weeks
Gotlin et al[8]	12	ACL repair	Reaction time	4 to 6 weeks
Hau et al [9]	30	Knee arthroscopy	Reaction time, clinical test	1 week
Holt et al[10]	28	First metatarsal osteotomy	Reaction time	6 weeks
Kane et al[11]	25	Ankle fracture	Reaction time	4 weeks post-operative; 2 weeks plaster
Liebensteiner et al [12]	62	TKR	Brake reaction time	Maximum 2-week wait
MacDonald and Owen[13]	25	THR	Reaction time, brake force	8 weeks
Marques et al[14]	24	Left TKR	Brake reaction time	10 days
Marques et al[15]	21	Right TKR	Brake reaction time	30 days
Nguyen et al[16]	72	ACL repair	Reaction time, clinical test	Left: 2 weeks. Right: 6 weeks
Nunn et al[17]	-	Below-knee cast	Driving ability	Left: safe in automatic cars. Right: unsafe
Orr et al[18]	35	Immobilisation	Total brake time	Right leg: unsafe
Pierson et al[19]	31	TKR	Reaction time	6 weeks
Spalding et al[2]	20 control	TKR	Reaction time, brake force	Left: no effect. Right: 8 weeks
	40 patients			
Tremblay et al[3]	48	Different casts: Walking Cast; Aircast Walker	Reaction time, brake force	Increases brake reaction time and total braking time

Editor's Note: Please refer to original journal article for full references.

*TKR, total knee replacement; THR, total hip replacement; ACL, anterior cruciate ligament.

Reprinted from MacLeod K, Lingham A, Chatha H, et al. "When can I Return to driving?": a review of the current literature on returning to driving after lower limb injury or arthroplasty. *Bone Joint J*. 2013;95-B:290-294.

the conclusion that there is no consensus and no guidance to answer the question is disappointing, it is no less true. In a word, there is no country that has provided any real guidance to answer the question of when it is safe to drive. If one were to consider what is in the literature and that brake reaction time is the standard on which a decision is made, then Table 1 does offer some valuable insight. In general, it would seem 6 weeks is a safe interval for one to return to driving after surgery on the extremity used to brake a vehicle, and a couple of weeks less for the opposite extremity. Also, a longer time, up to 9 weeks, might be best for those with ankle fracture requiring open reduction and internal fixation. In the final analysis, it's up to the surgeon, but one should have some basis for the recommendation such as the information found in Table 1.

B. F. Morrey, MD

Obesity, Orthopaedics and Outcomes

Mihalko WM, Bergin PF, Kelly FB, et al (Univ of Tennessee-Campbell Clinic, Memphis; Univ of Mississippi Med Ctr, Jackson; Forsyth Street Orthopaedics, Macon, GA)
J Am Acad Orthop Surg 22:683-690, 2014

Obesity, one of the most common health conditions, affects an ever-increasing percentage of orthopaedic patients. Obesity is also associated with other medical conditions, including diabetes, cardiovascular disease, pulmonary disease, metabolic syndrome, and obstructive sleep apnea. These comorbidities require specific preoperative and postoperative measures to improve outcomes in this patient population. Patients who are obese are at risk for increased perioperative complications; however, orthopaedic procedures may still offer notable pain relief and improved quality of life.

▶ Physicians are all too familiar with the growing prevalence of obesity in patients. This article, directed at the practicing orthopedic surgeon, outlines the specific medical conditions that surgeons must be concerned about as they evaluate and care for obese patients. The article includes specific aspects about anesthetic considerations, as well as postoperative considerations and data on the differential outcomes that may be seen from common orthopedic procedures in obese patients. It is a worthwhile read for all of us who take care of patients in this current era to be certain that we do not make errors in case preparation, medication dosing, and patient outcome counseling in dealing with obese patients.

P. S. Rose, MD

1-year follow-up of 920 hip and knee arthroplasty patients after implementing fast-track: Good outcomes in a Norwegian university hospital

Winther SB, Foss OA, Wik TS, et al (Trondheim Univ Hosp, Norway; et al)
Acta Orthop 86:78-85, 2015

Background.—Fast-track has become a well-known concept resulting in improved patient satisfaction and postoperative results. Concerns have been raised about whether increased efficiency could compromise safety, and whether early hospital discharge might result in an increased number of complications. We present 1-year follow-up results after implementing fast-track in a Norwegian university hospital.

Methods.—This was a register-based study of 1,069 consecutive fast-track hip and knee arthroplasty patients who were operated on between September 2010 and December 2012. Patients were followed up until 1 year after surgery.

Results.—987 primary and 82 revision hip or knee arthroplasty patients were included. 869 primary and 51 revision hip or knee patients attended 1-year follow-up. Mean patient satisfaction was 9.3 out of a maximum of 10. Mean length of stay was 3.1 days for primary patients. It was 4.2 days in the revision hip patients and 3.9 in the revision knee patients. Revision rates until 1-year follow-up were 2.9% and 3.3% for primary hip and knee patients, and 3.7% and 7.1% for revision hip and knee patients. Function scores and patient-reported outcome scores were improved in all groups.

Interpretation.—We found reduced length of stay, a high level of patient satisfaction, and low revision rates, together with improved health-related

TABLE 3.—Complications Within 1 Year of Primary Total Hip Arthroplasty or Primary Total Knee Arthroplasty

	Primary THA			Primary TKA		
	n	RR[a]	95% CI	n	RR[a]	95% CI
Total	619			368		
Re-admissions	35	5.7	4.3−7.0	37	10.0	8.4−12
Revisions	18	2.9	2.0−3.9	12	3.3	2.3−4.3
Infection	10	1.6	0.9−2.3	5	1.4	0.7−2.0
Dislocation	6	1.0	0.4−1.5	−	−	−
Impaired mobility	−	−	−	1	0.3	0.0−0.6
Fracture	1	0.2	−0.1−0.4	−	−	−
Mechanical causes	1	0.2	−0.1−0.4	5	1.4	0.7−2.0
Reoperations	7	1.1	0.5−1.7	12	3.3	2.3−4.3
Dislocation	5	0.8	0.3−1.3	3	0.8	0.3−1.3
Gluteal insufficiency	1	0.2	−0.1−0.4	−	−	−
Quadriceps rupture	−	−	−	1	0.3	0.0−0.6
Impaired mobility	−	−	−	6	1.6	0.9−2.3
Fracture	1	0.2	−0.1−0.4	1	0.3	0.0−0.6
Other causes	−	−	−	1	0.3	0.0−0.6
Other causes	10	1.6	0.9−2.6	13	3.5	2.5−4.6
DVT	1	0.2	−0.1−0.4	−	−	−
Hematoma	1	0.2	−0.1−0.4	−	−	−
Stroke	1	0.2	−0.1−0.4	−	−	−
Ileus	1	0.2	−0.1−0.4	−	−	−
Superficial infection	−	−	−	1	0.3	0.0−0.6
Peroneus palsy	−	−	−	1	0.3	0.0−0.6
Quadriceps rupture	−	−	−	1	0.3	0.0−0.6
Urinary infection	−	−	−	1	0.3	0.0−0.6
Gluteal insufficiency	2	0.3	0.0−0.6	−	−	−
Other causes	4	0.6	0.2−1.1	9	2.4	1.6−3.3
Leg length difference (> 2 cm)	3	0.5	0.1−0.9	1	0.3	0.0−0.6
Superficial infection	13	2.1	1.3−2.9	15	4.1	3.0−5.2
Urinary infection	27	4.4	3.2−5.5	22	6.0	4.6−7.3
Pneumonia	2	0.3	0.0−0.6	−	−	−
Impaired mobility	−	−	−	12	3.3	2.3−4.3
Peroneus palsy	−	−	−	1	0.3	0.0−0.6
Gluteal insufficiency	2	0.3	0.0−0.6	−	−	−
Other causes	15	2.4	1.6−3.3	11	3.0	2.0−4.0

[a]Relative risk, %.

Reprinted from Winther SB, Foss OA, Wik TS, et al. 1-year follow-up of 920 hip and knee arthroplasty patients after implementing fast-track: Good outcomes in a Norwegian university hospital. *Acta Orthop.* 2015;86:78-85, reprinted by permission of Taylor & Francis Ltd, http://www.informaworld.com.

quality of life and functionality, when we introduced fast-track into an orthopedic department in a Norwegian university hospital (Table 3).

▶ This is an important article that provides useful information not only about an emerging trend in joint replacement surgery, but also relevant information in terms of the full spectrum of reconstructive surgery. Simply stated, fast track is associated with a high frequency of patient satisfaction: 85% for the hip and 73% after knee replacement. What is important to realize is that 80% of patients returned home after an average of 3 days of hospitalization for primary procedures, and 4 days later after revisions. The other important data relate to readmissions and complications. As expected, these relate to infection for both, stiffness for the knee and dislocation for the hip (Table 3). The one thing that is lacking in the article is comparison of the pre-fast track data and the current information. We did do this assessment at Mayo 15 years ago and found that the fast track had no additional complications or higher readmission rates. This is our future practice.

B. F. Morrey, MD

Do Patients With Insulin-dependent and Noninsulin-dependent Diabetes Have Different Risks for Complications After Arthroplasty?
Lovecchio F, Beal M, Kwasny M, et al (Univ Feinberg School of Medicine, Chicago, IL)
Clin Orthop Relat Res 472:3570-3575, 2014

Background.—Patients with diabetes are known to be at greater risk for complications after arthroplasty than are patients without diabetes. However, we do not know whether there are important differences in the risk of perioperative complications between patients with diabetes who are insulin-dependent (Type 1 or 2) and those who are not insulin-dependent.

Questions/Purposes.—The purpose of our study was to compare (1) medical complications (including death), (2) surgical complications, and (3) readmissions within 30 days between patients with insulin-dependent and noninsulin dependent diabetes, and with patients who do not have diabetes.

Methods.—A total of 43,299 patients undergoing THA or TKA between 2005 and 2011 were selected from the American College of Surgeon's National Surgical Quality Improvement Program's (ACS-NSQIP®) database. Generalized linear models were used to assess the relationship between diabetes status and outcomes (no diabetes [n = 36,574], insulin dependent [n = 1552], and noninsulin dependent [n = 5173]). Multivariate models were established adjusting for confounders including age, sex, race, BMI, smoking, steroid use, hypertension, chronic obstructive pulmonary disease, and anesthesia type. Post hoc comparisons between patient groups were made using a Bonferroni correction.

Results.—Patients who were insulin dependent had increased odds of experiencing a medical complication (OR, 1.6 95% CI, 1.2–2.0

$p < 0.001$), as did patients who were noninsulin dependent (OR, 1.2 95% CI, 1.1−1.4 $p < 0.001$). An increased likelihood of 30 day mortality was found only for patients who were insulin dependent (OR, 3.74 95% CI, 1.6−8.5 $p = 0.007$). However, neither diabetic state was associated with surgical complications. Finally, readmission was found to be independently associated with insulin-dependent diabetes (OR, 1.6 95% CI, 1.1−2.1 $p = 0.023$).

Conclusions.—Patients with insulin-dependent diabetes are most likely to have a medical complication or be readmitted within 30 days after total joint replacement. However, patients who are insulin dependent or noninsulin dependent are no more likely than patients without diabetes to have a surgical complication. Physicians and hospitals should keep these issues in mind when counseling patients and generating risk-adjusted outcome reports.

Level of Evidence.—Level III, therapeutic study. See the Instructions for Authors for a complete description of levels of evidence.

▶ This question has been asked and answered in the past, and thus this study was accepted to reinforce what is already known, but this is based on a large national database. The findings that diabetes, independent of insulin dependency, increases medical complications in those having a hip or knee replacement is well known. That insulin dependency increases the 30-day mortality and the likelihood of an unplanned readmission is worth noting. Unfortunately, the database has no A1c data. Hence, the statement that diabetes does not increase surgical complications is not accurate because this has been shown to be correlated to the control of the disease as expressed by A1c levels.

B. F. Morrey, MD

Diagnosis and Management of Soft-tissue Masses
Mayerson JL, Scharschmidt TJ, Lewis VO, et al (The Ohio State Univ, Columbus; Anderson Cancer Ctr, Houston, TX; et al)
J Am Acad Orthop Surg 22:742-750, 2014

Soft-tissue masses of the extremities are common entities encountered by nearly all providers of musculoskeletal patient care. Proper management of these lesions requires a specific process of evaluation. A detailed history and physical examination must be performed. Appropriate imaging studies must be obtained based on clinical indications. MRI is the imaging modality of choice for diagnosis of soft-tissue masses, with CT and ultrasonography used as secondary options. These modalities aid the clinician in developing an appropriate differential diagnosis and treatment plan. When the initial evaluation is inconclusive, biopsy must be performed. A diagnosis must be established before definitive treatment with surgical excision or, in rare cases, radiation therapy is performed. Clinicians without significant experience in treating soft-tissue masses should

TABLE 1.—Characteristics of Select Soft-tissue Tumors and Appropriate Diagnostic Imaging

			Appropriate Diagnostic Imaging			
Mass	Pain	Multifocal	Plain Radiography	Ultrasonography	CT	MRI
Lipoma	No	Sometimes				×
Hemangioma/lymphangioma	Sometimes	Sometimes	×	×		×
Abscess	Yes	Rarely		×		×
Myositis ossificans	Sometimes	No	×		×	
Ganglion cyst	Sometimes	Rarely		×		×
Schwannoma	Sometimes	Rarely				×
Desmoid	Sometimes	Rarely				×
Pigmented villonodular synovitis	Yes	No				×
Sarcoma	No	No			×	×

Reprinted from Mayerson JL, Scharschmidt TJ, Lewis VO, et al. Diagnosis and Management of Soft-tissue Masses. *J Am Acad Orthop Surg.* 2014;22:742-750.

consider referral to a musculoskeletal oncologist for specialized care when a definitive diagnosis of a benign lesion cannot be made. Several studies have shown that multidisciplinary care in specialized referral centers optimizes outcomes and diminishes comorbid complications (Table 1).

▶ This article from an instructional course lecture at the American Academy of Orthopaedic Surgeons meeting outlines the common clinical scenario of the patient with a soft-tissue lump or bump that needs evaluation to determine whether it is benign or malignant in etiology. Benign soft tissue masses outnumber malignant by more than 100 to 1. This practical article outlines the evaluation of patients presenting with soft-tissue masses to the general orthopedic surgeon. Although it does delve into aspects of biopsy, this is probably best reserved for tumor surgeons who would be involved in the treatment of the specific lesion. However, the bulk of the text deals with the evaluation and pre-biopsy diagnostic modalities, which are important for all surgeons to be familiar with (Table 1).

P. S. Rose, MD

Oncologic Conditions That Simulate Common Sports Injuries
Krych A, Odland A, Rose P, et al (Mayo Clinic, Rochester, MN)
J Am Acad Orthop Surg 22:223-234, 2014

Primary bone and soft-tissue tumors that mimic common sports injuries are relatively rare and are not often encountered by most orthopaedists. Prompt and accurate diagnosis of these tumors is crucial to maximize the clinical outcome. Many bone and soft-tissue tumors present disproportionately in young and active patients who are often involved in athletic activities. Thus, the clinician may misdiagnose these rare tumors as more common sports injuries. Symptoms that should raise suspicion for a neoplastic process include pain unrelated to activity and a clinical course that does not follow the typically expected recovery for a common sports injury. An awareness of the salient features of several bone and soft-tissue tumors as well as nononcologic processes that may simulate sports injuries can aid clinicians in the prompt diagnosis and clinical decision making of these rare tumors.

▶ Athletic injuries are a staple of orthopedic practice. However, many primary malignancies may arise in adolescents and young adults who are active in athletic competition. These malignancies often present with pain or other functional limitation that may mimic an orthopedic sports injury. Clinicians should be cognizant of this as they evaluate a patient population that is otherwise generally regarded as healthy and active.

This article outlines aspects of patient presentation, including history and physical examination, imaging evaluation, and other aspects that may highlight the presence of a neoplastic condition in a young, athletic patient. This article is useful for trainees as they evaluate patients. Clinicians must remain vigilant to identify the few patients who may present with one of these serious conditions in a population of otherwise healthy and conventionally injured patients.

P. S. Rose, MD

Anterior knee pain caused by patellofemoral pain syndrome can be relieved by Botulinum toxin type A injection
Chen JT-N, Tang AC-W, Lin S-C, et al (Veterans General Hosp, Taipei, Taiwan; Chang Gung Memorial Hosp, Linkou, Taiwan; et al)
Clin Neurol Neurosurg 129:S27-S29, 2015

Objective.—To investigate the therapeutic effects of Botulinum toxin type A (BTA) for anterior knee pain caused by patellofemoral pain syndrome (PFPS).

Design.—Prospective case control study for intervention.

Setting.—A tertiary hospital rehabilitation center.

Participants.—Twelve bilateral PFPS patients with anterior knee pain were recruited. The worse pain knee was selected for injection, and the counterpart was left untreated.

Intervention.—Injection of BTA to vastus lateralis (VL) muscle.

Main Outcome Measures.—Western Ontario and McMaster Universities Osteoarthritis Index (WOMAC) was used to assess pain, stiffness, and functional status of the knee, and CYBEX isokinetic dynamometer to assess isokinetic muscle force before and after BTA application to VL.

Results.—Remarkable improvement after receiving BTA injection was obtained not only in the questionnaire of WOMAC ($p < 0.05$), but also in knee flexion torque ($p < 0.05$). No significant change of knee extension torque was noted ($p = 0.682$).

TABLE 1.—WOMAC Score (Mean ± Standard Deviation) of Experimental and Control Group

	Before	After 4 Weeks	After 4 8 Weeks	After 4 12 Weeks	p Value
Experimental group					
Pain	5.7 ± 3.2	4.7 ± 3.3	3.8 ± 3.1	3.9 ± 3.2	0.014*
Stiffness	2.5 ± 1.8	2.3 ± 2.1	1.9 ± 1.7	1.8 ± 1.8	0.147
Function	15.4 ± 11.0	13.7 ± 10.6	10.8 ± 7.4	8.8 ± 7.8	0.029*
Control group					
Pain	3.4 ± 4.1	3.6 ± 3.4	2.4 ± 3.0	2.5 ± 3.4	0.147
Stiffness	1.7 ± 2.1	1.7 ± 2.2	1.5 ± 1.9	1.1 ± 1.6	0.145
Function	10.0 ± 12.1	10.9 ± 12.0	7.5 ± 8.5	6.6 ± 8.7	0.319

*Significant at $p < 0.05$.
Reprinted from Chen JT-N, Tang AC-W, Lin S-C, et al. Anterior knee pain caused by patellofemoral pain syndrome can be relieved by Botulinum toxin type A injection. *Clin Neurol Neurosurg.* 2015;129:S27-S29.

Conclusion.—BTA injection is a good alternative treatment to improve anterior knee pain, knee function and isokinetic flexion torque (Table 1).

▶ Although this is a randomized controlled trial, it comprises a very small sample size. Yet as the authors state, the problem is ubiquitous, and thus its importance justifies sharing in the YEAR BOOK. I consider this a pilot study, but the effectiveness of Botulinum toxin injected in the vastus lateralis is dramatically effective in relieving pain and improving function (Table 1). Further, it does not weaken quadriceps function. The remaining questions are how to use this information in the long term because this study is of only 12 weeks' duration. One might speculate an aggressive rehabilitation program could be introduced while pain is controlled, whereas it may be less effective when the patient is more symptomatic. The information in this article is promising.

B. F. Morrey, MD

Incidence of Symptomatic and Asymptomatic Venous Thromboembolism After Elective Knee Arthroscopic Surgery: A Retrospective Study With Routinely Applied Venography
Sun Y, Chen D, Xu Z, et al (Drum Tower Hosp, Nanjing, China)
Arthroscopy 30:818-822, 2014

Purpose.—The purpose of this study was to assess the incidence of total venous thromboembolism (VTE) after knee arthroscopy with routinely applied venography.

Methods.—We reviewed 537 consecutive patients undergoing arthroscopic knee surgery from March 2012 to July 2013. The surgical procedure was categorized as simple anterior cruciate ligament reconstruction (ACLR), posterior cruciate ligament reconstruction (PCLR), or reconstruction of both cruciate ligaments. All patients having arthroscopy in our institution were routinely examined with venography on the third postoperative day. Clinical signs of DVT were checked and recorded before venography.

Results.—Eighty (14.9%) of 537 patients were diagnosed with VTE by venography. Of the 80 detected cases of VTE, only 20 (3.7%) patients presented with clinical signs of DVT, indicating that there were 60 (11.2%) asymptomatic cases. No patient died or presented with a clinically suspected pulmonary embolism (PE). Sex, body mass index (BMI), operative time, and duration of tourniquet application were not significant risk factors for DVT. Patient age ($P < .0001$) is a strongly significant risk factor for deep venous thrombosis (DVT). Compared with patients who underwent simple arthroscopic procedures, complex procedures—the reconstruction of 1 ($P < .005$) or both knee cruciate ligaments ($P < .0005$)—led to a significantly higher postoperative incidence of DVT.

Conclusions.—The total incidence of VTE diagnosed with venography after arthroscopic knee surgery was 14.9%, of which only 3.7% of cases were symptomatic, indicating 11.2% cases of silent VTE. Advanced age and complex arthroscopic surgery are strongly associated with VTE.

Level of Evidence.—Level IV, prognostic case series.

▶ This article caught my eye because the first patient of mine who developed a deep vein thrombosis (DVT) after arthroscopy was an attorney, of course. The study documents the 15% incidence of detectable DVT by venography, with less than 5% being clinically relevant. Thus, this is an objective set of data for what is known to be true clinically. What is less known, however, is that gender, tourniquet time, and body mass index were found not to be risk factors. The most important correlate to symptomatic DVT was a complex arthroscopic procedure. Regardless, there were, fortunately, no pulmonary emboli in this cohort.

B. F. Morrey, MD

Acetabular anteversion is associated with gluteal tendinopathy at MRI
Moulton KM, Aly A-R, Rajasekaran S, et al (Univ of Saskatchewan, Saskatoon, Canada; Health Pointe — Pain, Spine & Sport Medicine, Edmonton, Alberta, Canada)
Skeletal Radiol 44:47-54, 2015

Objective.—Gluteal tendinopathy and greater trochanteric pain syndrome (GTPS) remain incompletely understood despite their pervasiveness in clinical practice. To date, no study has analyzed the morphometric characteristics of the hip on magnetic resonance imaging (MRI) that may predispose to gluteal tendinopathy. This study aimed to evaluate whether acetabular anteversion (AA), femoral neck anteversion (FNA), and femoral neck-shaft angle (FNSA) are associated with MRI features of gluteal tendinopathy.

Materials and Methods.—A total of 203 MRI examinations of the hip met our inclusion and exclusion criteria. A single blinded investigator measured AA, FNA, and FNSA according to validated MRI techniques.

Two blinded subspecialty-trained musculoskeletal radiologists then independently evaluated the presence of gluteal tendinosis, trochanteric bursitis, and subgluteal bursitis. Statistical analysis was performed using a one-way analysis of variance (ANOVA; post-hoc Tukey's range test).

Results.—At MRI, 57 patients had gluteal tendinosis with or without bursitis, 26 had isolated trochanteric bursitis, and 11 had isolated subgluteal bursitis. AA was significantly ($p = 0.01$) increased in patients with MRI evidence of gluteal tendinosis with or without bursitis [mean: 18.4°, 95 % confidence interval (CI): 17.2°-19.6°] compared with normal controls (mean: 15.7°, 95 % CI: 14.7°-16.8°). Similarly, AA was significantly ($p = 0.04$) increased in patients with isolated trochanteric bursitis (mean: 18.8°, 95 % CI: 16.2°-21.6°). No association was found between FNA or FNSA and the presence of gluteal tendinopathy. Interobserver agreement for the presence and categorization of gluteal tendinopathy was very good (kappa = 0.859, 95 % CI: 0.815-0.903).

Conclusion.—Our MRI study suggests that there is an association between increased AA and gluteal tendinopathy, which supports a growing body of evidence implicating abnormal biomechanics in the development of this condition (Fig 2).

▶ This is a useful contribution to better understand the circumstances in which one might encounter gluteal tendinosis. We are increasingly diagnosing this condition and learning to distinguish it from trochanteric bursitis, which is

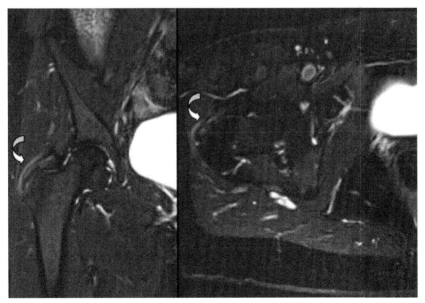

FIGURE 2.—Gluteus minimus tendinosis. Coronal and axial STIR images demonstrate hyperintensity and thickening of the gluteus minimus tendon (curved arrow). (With kind permission from Springer Science+Business Media: Moulton KM, Aly A-R, Rajasekaran S, et al. Acetabular anteversion is associated with gluteal tendinopathy at MRI. *Skeletal Radiol.* 2015;44:47-54, with permission from ISS.)

important because the tendinosis often does not respond to cortisone injections and can be quite debilitating. The article is straightforward. There is a direct correlation between both tendinosis and bursitis and acetabular anteversion (Fig 2). As a clinician, acetabular anteversion should be assessed when considering the diagnosis of gluteal tendinosis.

B. F. Morrey, MD

Evaluating the Quality of Internet Information for Femoroacetabular Impingement

Lee S, Shin JJ, Haro MS, et al (Rush Med College of Rush Univ, Chicago, IL)
Arthroscopy 30:1372-1379, 2014

Purpose.—The Internet has become a ubiquitous source of medical information for both the patient and the physician. However, the quality of this information is highly variable. We evaluated the quality of Internet information available for femoroacetabular impingement (FAI).

Methods.—Four popular search engines were used to collect 100 Web sites containing information on FAI. Web sites were evaluated based on authorship, various content criteria, and the presence of Health On the Net Code of Conduct (HONcode) certification. By use of a novel evaluation system for quality, Web sites were also classified as excellent, high, moderate, poor, or inadequate and were subsequently analyzed. Web sites were evaluated as a group, followed by authorship type, by HONcode certification, and by quality level.

Results.—Of the Web sites, 73 offered the ability to contact the author, 91 offered a considerable explanation of FAI, 54 provided surgical treatment options, 58 offered nonsurgical treatment options, 27 discussed possible complications, 11 discussed eligibility criteria, 31 discussed rehabilitation, 67 discussed a differential diagnosis, and 48 included peer-reviewed citations. We categorized 40 Web sites as academic, 33 as private, 9 as industry, 9 as public education, and 9 as blogs. Our novel quality evaluation system classified 16 Web sites as excellent, 18 as high, 17 as moderate, 18 as poor, and 31 as inadequate. Only 8% of all evaluated Web sites contained HONcode certification.

Conclusions.—We found that the quality of information available on the Internet about FAI was dramatically variable. A significantly large proportion of Web sites were from academic sources, but this did not necessarily indicate higher quality. Sites with HONcode certification showed as much variability in quality as noncertified sites.

Clinical Relevance.—This study increases clinician competence in the available Internet information about FAI and helps them to confidently guide patients to formulate appropriate medical decisions based on high-quality information.

▶ This interesting analysis was picked to reflect to the reader a sign of the times.

We all know the ever-increasing reliance of the public on the internet for information of all kinds. As expected, the range in quality is dramatic; this is expected. The encouraging point for me is that there are some high-quality internet sources of valid information about this important condition. The disappointing observation is that the best information is not always from academic sites, nor does the Health On the Net Code of Conduct correlate to higher quality information. So this leaves us with the knowledge that there are some good sites, but we don't know how to identify them in advance.

B. F. Morrey, MD

Factors Associated With the Failure of Surgical Treatment for Femoroacetabular Impingement: Review of the Literature

Saadat E, Martin SD, Thornhill TS, et al (Brigham and Women's Hosp, Boston, MA)
Am J Sports Med 42:1487-1495, 2014

Background.—With the recent increased recognition of femoroacetabular impingement (FAI) as a cause of hip pain and early osteoarthritis, surgical treatment has proliferated. There is a growing body of literature on outcomes of surgical intervention for FAI, but factors associated with inferior surgical outcomes have not been reviewed systematically.

Purpose.—To review the available literature and identify factors associated with the failure of open or arthroscopic surgery for FAI.

Study Design.—Systematic review.

Methods.—Using the PubMed database, we searched for relevant English-language articles published from January 1966 through August 2012. Inclusion criteria were a primary focus on the surgical treatment of FAI, measurement of functional or pain outcomes, identification of treatment failures, and statistical analysis of factors leading to failure. Exclusion criteria were review articles, technique-only articles, and studies of nonoperative management. Two definitions of failure were considered: (1) a lack of statistically significant improvement in validated measures of pain, function, or satisfaction postoperatively; and (2) revision surgery or conversion to hip arthroplasty because of persistent symptoms. The consistency of association between preoperative variables and clinical outcomes was reported across all studies.

Results.—Thirteen studies were included. Three were retrospective; there were no randomized controlled trials. Many studies had important methodological limitations. Preoperative cartilage damage or osteoarthritis had the strongest and most consistent relationship with conversion to hip arthroplasty and with a lack of improvement in pain or function. Greater age at the index operation, worse preoperative modified Harris Hip Score, and longer duration of symptoms preoperatively (>1.5 years) were associated with conversion to hip arthroplasty.

Conclusion.—Older age, presence of arthritic changes, longer duration of symptoms, and worse preoperative pain and functional scores are associated with poor outcomes of surgery for FAI. Incorporation of these data

TABLE 1.—Summary of Included Studies

Author (Year)	Study Design	Type of Surgery	Total No. of Hips	Mean Age of Participants, y	% Female
Naal et al[22] (2012)	Retrospective	Open	233	30	40
Cohen et al[16] (2012)	Prospective	Mini-open	47	32	35
Philippon et al[28] (2012)	Prospective	Arthroscopic	153	57	52
Larson et al[16] (2012)	Prospective	Arthroscopic	94	29	Not reported
Byrd and Jones[4] (2011)	Prospective	Arthroscopic	100	34	33
Larson et al[17] (2011)	Prospective	Arthroscopic	227	35	41
Gedouin et al[13] (2010)	Prospective multicenter	Arthroscopic	111	31	29
Horisberger et al[14] (2010)	Prospective	Arthroscopic	20	47.3	20
Peters et al[25] (2010)	Retrospective	Open	96	38	41
Ribas et al[29] (2010)	Prospective	Mini-open	117	37	36
Laude et al[19] (2009)	Retrospective	Arthroscopically assisted mini-open	100	33.4	48
Philippon et al[26] (2009)	Prospective	Arthroscopic	112	40.6	44
Beaule et al[1] (2007)	Not specified	Open	37	40.5	47

Editor's Note: Please refer to original journal article for full references.
Reprinted from Saadat E, Martin SD, Thornhill TS, et al. Factors Associated With the Failure of Surgical Treatment for Femoroacetabular Impingement: Review of the Literature. *Am J Sports Med.* 2014;42:1487-1495.

into discussions with patients may facilitate informed, shared decision making about the surgical treatment of FAI (Table 1).

▶ Femoroacetabular impingement (FAI) is a well-accepted condition that causes early-onset hip pain and early end-stage coxarthrosis. The key and ongoing question is whether the condition can be treated in a way that alters the natural history of the disease. Arthroscopic debridement and osteophyte removal is a common modality of treatment. Hence, the legitimacy of the question: Who does and who does not benefit? Reviewing 350 articles yielded 13 of value to answer the question (3%). The answer is actually simple: Older patients with more advanced, early arthritis do less well. It is of interest that although the condition has been recognized for more than 40 years, 10 of the 13 articles considered in the analysis were published since 2010, and all 13 have been published in the past 8 years (Table 1).

B. F. Morrey, MD

Arthroscopic surgery for degenerative tears of the meniscus: a systematic review and meta-analysis
Khan M, Evaniew N, Bedi A, et al (McMaster Univ, Hamilton, Ontario; Univ of Michigan, Ann Arbor)
CMAJ 186:1057-1064, 2014

Background.—Arthroscopic surgery for degenerative meniscal tears is a commonly performed procedure, yet the role of conservative treatment for these patients is unclear. This systematic review and meta-analysis evaluates the efficacy of arthroscopic meniscal débridement in patients with knee pain in the setting of mild or no concurrent osteoarthritis of the knee in comparison with nonoperative or sham treatments.

Methods.—We searched MEDLINE, Embase and the Cochrane databases for randomized controlled trials (RCTs) published from 1946 to Jan. 20, 2014. Two reviewers independently screened all titles and abstracts for eligibility. We assessed risk of bias for all included studies and pooled outcomes using a random- effects model. Outcomes (i.e., function and pain relief) were dichotomized to short-term (<6 mo) and long-term (<2 yr) data.

Results.—Seven RCTs (n = 805 patients) were included in this review. The pooled treatment effect of arthroscopic surgery did not show a significant or minimally important difference (MID) between treatment arms for long-term functional outcomes (standardized mean difference [SMD] 0.07, 95% confidence interval [CI] −0.10 to 0.23). Short-term functional outcomes between groups were significant but did not exceed the threshold for MID (SMD 0.25, 95% CI 0.02 to 0.48). Arthroscopic surgery did not result in a significant improvement in pain scores in the short term (mean difference [MD] 0.20, 95% CI −0.67 to 0.26) or in the long term (MD −0.06, 95% CI −0.28 to 0.15). Statistical heterogeneity was low to moderate for the outcomes.

Interpretation.—There is moderate evidence to suggest that there is no benefit to arthroscopic meniscal débridement for degenerative meniscal tears in comparison with nonoperative or sham treatments in middle-aged patients with mild or no concomitant osteoarthritis. A trial of nonoperative management should be the firstline treatment for such patients (Figs 3 and 4).

▶ Knee arthroscopy is one of, if not the most, commonly performed surgical procedure in the United States. Although it has been debated, it is generally

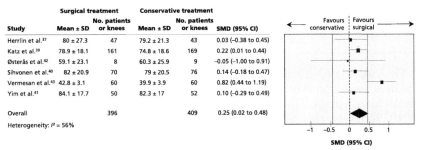

Study	Surgical treatment Mean ± SD	No. patients or knees	Conservative treatment Mean ± SD	No. patients or knees	SMD (95% CI)
Herrlin et al.[37]	80 ± 27.3	47	79.2 ± 21.3	43	0.03 (−0.38 to 0.45)
Katz et al.[39]	78.9 ± 18.1	161	74.8 ± 18.6	169	0.22 (0.01 to 0.44)
Østerås et al.[42]	59.1 ± 23.1	8	60.3 ± 25.9	9	−0.05 (−1.00 to 0.91)
Sihvonen et al.[40]	82 ± 20.9	70	79 ± 20.5	76	0.14 (−0.18 to 0.47)
Vermesan et al.[43]	42.8 ± 3.1	60	39.9 ± 3.9	60	0.82 (0.44 to 1.19)
Yim et al.[41]	84.1 ± 17.7	50	82.3 ± 17	52	0.10 (−0.29 to 0.49)
Overall		396		409	0.25 (0.02 to 0.48)
Heterogeneity: I² = 56%					

FIGURE 3.—Pooled short-term functional outcomes of conservative and surgical treatment. Red lines show a zone of clinical equivalence based on a minimal important difference of 10 on the Knee Injury and Osteoarthritis Outcome Score.[37,39,40−43] Note: CI = confidence interval, SD = standard deviation, SMD = standardized mean difference. *Editor's Note:* Please refer to original journal article for full references. (Reprinted from Khan M, Evaniew N, Bedi A, et al. Arthroscopic surgery for degenerative tears of the meniscus: a systematic review and meta-analysis. *CMAJ.* 2014;186:1057-1064, with permission from Canadian Medical Association.)

	Surgical treatment		Conservative treatment			
Study	Mean ± SD	No. patients or knees	Mean ± SD	No. patients or knees	SMD (95% CI)
Herrlin et al.[38]	93.5 ± 20	47	90 ± 11.9	49	0.21 (–0.19 to 0.61)
Katz et al.[39]	80.9 ± 17.8	161	80.7 ± 17.9	169	0.01 (–0.20 to 0.23)
Sihvonen et al.[40]	82.2 ± 16	70	83.4 ± 13.8	76	–0.08 (–0.40 to 0.24)
Vermesan et al.[43]	36.1 ± 3.6	60	34.7 ± 3.8	60	0.38 (0.01 to 0.74)
Yim et al.[41]	83.2 ± 12	50	84.3 ± 10.5	52	–0.10 (–0.49 to 0.29)
Overall		388		406	0.07 (–0.10 to 0.23)
Heterogeneity: I² = 20%					

FIGURE 4.—Pooled long-term functional outcomes of conservative and surgical treatment. Red lines show a zone of clinical equivalence based on a minimal important difference of 10 on the Knee Injury and Osteoarthritis Outcome Score.[38–41,43] Note: CI = confidence interval, SD = standard deviation, SMD = standardized mean difference. *Editor's Note:* Please refer to original journal article for full references. (Reprinted from Khan M, Evaniew N, Bedi A, et al. Arthroscopic surgery for degenerative tears of the meniscus: a systematic review and meta-analysis. *CMAJ.* 2014;186:1057-1064, with permission from Canadian Medical Association.)

accepted that the indication for arthroscopic debridement for a degenerative meniscus is the presence of mechanical symptoms, and concurrent degenerative changes lessens the likelihood of a successful outcome. The fact is, as this study reflects, the data from which to draw conclusions are meager at best. These authors included only 7 articles from a review of 944, providing just over 800 knees in which arthroscopic debridement and nonoperative management were compared. The conclusion is that there is moderate evidence that there is no advantage of arthroscopic intervention. Fig 4 certainly supports this conclusion for the longer follow-up period. However, there does appear to be a statistically insignificant, but definite advantage, in the short term (Fig 3). One is still left with the question of whether intervention is of value in those with mechanical symptoms, a question this study was unable to effectively address.

B. F. Morrey, MD

Cost analysis of fresh-frozen femoral head allografts: Is it worthwhile to run a bone bank?

Benninger E, Zingg PO, Kamath AF, et al (Univ of Zurich, Switzerland)
Bone Joint J 96-B:1307-1311, 2014

To assess the sustainability of our institutional bone bank, we calculated the final product cost of fresh-frozen femoral head allografts and compared these costs with the use of commercial alternatives. Between 2007 and 2010 all quantifiable costs associated with allograft donor screening, harvesting, storage, and administration of femoral head allografts retrieved from patients undergoing elective hip replacement were analysed.

From 290 femoral head allografts harvested and stored as full (complete) head specimens or as two halves, 101 had to be withdrawn. In total, 104 full and 75 half heads were implanted in 152 recipients. The calculated final product costs were 1367 per full head. Compared with the use of commercially available processed allografts, a saving of at least 43 119 was realised over four-years (10 780 per year) resulting in a cost-effective intervention at our institution. Assuming a price of between 1672 and 2149 per commercially purchased allograft, breakeven analysis revealed that implanting between 34 and 63 allografts per year equated to the total cost of bone banking.

▶ To me, this is a "concept" type of contribution. Although the specific information regarding the break-even point for a self-contained bone bank is of value, I feel there is equal merit in considering the question of a break-even point to begin with. Of course, there are also less objective factors, such as quality and convenience issues, to be considered. To the extent that our processes lend themselves to such an analysis, we must begin to perform more of these types of assessments if we hope to control the spiraling cost of our care.

B. F. Morrey, MD

3 Forearm, Wrist, and Hand

Introduction

The selections for the Forearm, Wrist, and Hand section this year were chosen as a counterbalance to the onslaught of submissions to the literature about open reduction with internal fixation and volar plating of distal radius fractures, which has been the predominate subject of the past several years. I was trying to make certain that this section does not become synonymous with distal radius, but that is very hard to avoid given the number of submissions on this subject each year. Although refinements in surgical management of distal radius fractures and important outcome data have been included this year, some new information regarding bone health in older men and methods for rehabilitation should, I think, provide readers with clinically relevant information. Also in the trauma realm, I have selected articles on arthroscopic treatment of acute scaphoid fractures and late treatment of scaphoid fracture nonunions, along with a nice article on return to football following repair of thumb metacarpophalangeal joint ulnar collateral ligament repair.

I have also included an excellent, up-to-date article on burns of the hand, which should serve as a current concepts review. I have also selected several articles on prognostic factors and outcomes for treatment of nerve injuries and disorders, which I hope readers will find to be important in their practices. All in all, a nice balance of articles round out this section for 2015.

Stephen D. Trigg, MD

Evaluation and Diagnosis

Distal Radial Fractures in Older Men: A Missed Opportunity?

Harper CM, Fitzpatrick SK, Zurakowski D, et al (Harvard Combined Orthopaedic Residency, Boston, MA; Harvard Med School, Boston, MA; Children's Hosp Boston, MA)
J Bone Joint Surg Am 96:1820-1827, 2014

Background.—Fractures of the distal aspect of the radius are common, yet little is known about this type of fracture among older men. The purpose of this study was to compare fracture characteristics, treatment, and osteoporosis evaluation among men and women who had sustained a distal radial fracture. We hypothesized that the men would have similar patterns of injury and lower rates of evaluation for osteoporosis.

Methods.—We retrospectively reviewed the medical records of ninety-five men and 344 women over the age of fifty years who were treated for a distal radial fracture at a single institution over a five-year period. We assessed whether the patients had received a dual x-ray absorptiometry (DXA) scan and osteoporosis treatment within six months following the injury. Multivariate analysis identified independent predictors of bone mineral density (BMD) testing and osteoporosis treatment.

Results.—Men had less severe fractures than women (a Type-C fracture rate of 20% for men compared with 40% for women; $p = 0.014$). While 184 (53%) of the women had a DXA scan after injury, only seventeen (18%) of the men were evaluated ($p < 0.001$). Among the patients who underwent DXA scan, nine men (9% of men overall) and sixty-five women (19% of women overall) had a diagnosis of osteoporosis ($p = 0.01$). Male sex was an independent predictor of failure to undergo BMD testing as well as receive subsequent treatment with calcium and vitamin D or bisphosphonates ($p < 0.001$).

Conclusions.—Significantly fewer men received evaluation for osteoporosis following a distal radial fracture, with rates of evaluation unacceptably low according to published guidelines.

▶ Over the past decade, the evaluation and treatment of fragility fractures secondary to age-related osteoporosis has become a major public health care initiative worldwide. Commensurate with a rise in an aging population in the next 2 decades, there is an expectation that there will be an increase in fragility fractures. Importantly, distal radius fractures have been shown to be an independent predictor of future hip fractures. To date, the heath care initiatives to increase awareness in evaluation, prevention, and treatment of fragility fractures have largely targeted postmenopausal women. This is an important study that significantly adds to our knowledge base and exposes the gap in the evaluation and treatment of distal radius fractures in elderly men compared with recent advances in the care of postmenopausal women with a similar injury.

S. D. Trigg, MD

Effect of Anxiety and Catastrophic Pain Ideation on Early Recovery After Surgery for Distal Radius Fractures

Roh YH, Lee BK, Noh JH, et al (Gachon Univ School of Medicine, Incheon, South Korea; Kangwon Natl Univ Hosp, Gangwon-do, South Korea; Seoul Natl Univ College of Medicine, Seoul, South Korea)

J Hand Surg Am 39:2258-2264, 2014

Purpose.—To evaluate the effects of preoperative anxiety and catastrophic pain ideation on perceived disability and objective measures after distal radius fracture surgery.

Methods.—A total of 121 patients with distal radius fractures treated with volar plate fixation were enrolled. The wrist range of motion (ROM), grip strength, and perceived disability as measured by the Michigan Hand Questionnaire (MHQ) score were assessed 4, 12, and 24 weeks after surgery. To evaluate psychological factors related to pain, catastrophic pain ideation was measured using the Pain Catastrophizing Scale (PCS) and pain anxiety was measured using the Pain Anxiety Symptom Scale (PASS). Then relative contributions of pain anxiety and catastrophic pain ideation and other clinical parameters to functional recovery in terms of grip strength, ROM, and MHQ score were assessed.

Results.—An increase in the PCS score was associated with the wrist ROM and grip strength only at week 4, whereas an increase in the PASS score was associated with the wrist ROM at week 4 and grip strength at weeks 4 and 12. According to a multivariate regression analysis, an increase in the PCS score was associated with a decrease in grip strength, ROM, and MHQ score at week 4; and an increase in the PASS score was associated with a decrease in grip strength, ROM, and MHQ score at week 4 and grip strength and MHQ score at week 12. At week 24, only age and fracture severity were associated with the MHQ score. In addition, age was associated with grip strength and fracture type was associated with ROM.

Conclusions.—Preoperative PCS and PASS were significantly associated with delayed recovery as evidenced by scores on both objective and subjective measures of function. Given these relationships, it becomes important to assess preoperative PCS and PASS and address issues for patients at risk with brief psychosocial intervention early in the recovery process.

Type of Study/Level of Evidence.—Prognostic II.

▶ Performing surgery correctly is all too often only half the battle in obtaining a favorable clinical result. Although functional outcomes and pain scoring analysis has been reported extensively in studies of volar locking plate fixation of distal radius fractures, the inclusion of psychometric testing data has not received much attention. This is unfortunate because psychological factors have been shown elsewhere to have predictive validity in surgical outcomes and variations in disabilities in both the short and long term. This prospective study provides us with important information that I hope will provide insight into identifying patients at risk for psychological issues that may impede their recovery and the need for referral for counseling.

S. D. Trigg, MD

Does the CT improve inter- and intra-observer agreement for the AO, Fernandez and Universal classification systems for distal radius fractures?
Arealis G, Galanopoulos I, Nikolaou VS, et al (Queen's Hosp, Burton on Trent, UK; Athens Univ, Greece; 401 Military Hosp, Athens, Greece)
Injury 45:1579-1584, 2014

Introduction.—Distal radius fractures are very common upper limb injuries irrespective of the patient's age. The aim of our study is to evaluate the reliability of the three systems that are often used for their classification (AO — Arbeitsgemeinschaft für Osteosynthesefragen/Association for the Study of Internal Fixation, Fernandez and Universal) and to assess the need for computed tomography (CT) scan to improve inter- and intra-observer agreement.

Materials and Methods.—Five orthopaedic surgeons and two hand surgeons classified radiographs and CT scans of 26 patients using the Fernandez, AO and Universal systems. All data were recorded using MS Excel and Kappa statistics were performed to determine inter- and intra-observer agreement and to evaluate the role of CT scan.

Results.—Fair-to-moderate inter-observer agreement was noted with the use of X-rays for all classification systems. Intra-observer reproducibility did not improve with the addition of CT scans, especially for the senior hand surgeons.

Conclusions.—The agreement rates observed in the present study show that currently there is no classification system that is fully reproducible. Adequate experience is required for the assessment and treatment of these injuries. CT scan should be requested only by experienced hand surgeons in order to help guide treatment, as it does not significantly improve inter- and intra-observer agreement for all classification systems.

▶ Wilhelm Roentgen discovered the X-ray in 1895. Interestingly, one of his first images was of his wife's hand and wrist. Within a year of Roentgen's discovery, surgeons were using the technology to locate bullets in the bodies of wounded soldiers. Arguably, the rapid and widespread use of X-rays is one of the sentinel events in the development of orthopedics into a surgical subspecialty. With permanent X-rays as a blueprint, we have been classifying fractures and musculoskeletal conditions ever since. Interestingly, despite the fact that fractures of the distal radius are among the most common of all fractures in both children and adults, we have yet to come to some sort of agreement on a universally accepted unifying and reproducible fracture classification system. More recently, as CT scanning and MRI have become more accessible, these imaging modalities have become commonplace in current practice. CT scans have been increasingly used to provide more complete imaging of complex fractures but are costly and expose our patients to greater levels of radiation. Given that we currently have no universally accepted gold standard classification system to describe the distal radius and in acknowledgment of the trait of humans that we will endeavor to use or find uses for new technology, this article takes on a worthy investigation. The authors' findings and conclusions are deserving of your review.

S. D. Trigg, MD

The Influence of Vitamin C on the Outcome of Distal Radial Fractures: A Double-Blind, Randomized Controlled Trial
Ekrol I, Duckworth AD, Ralston SH, et al (Royal Infirmary of Edinburgh, UK; Univ of Edinburgh, UK)
J Bone Joint Surg Am 96:1451-1459, 2014

Background.—Vitamin C has been proposed to improve outcomes after a distal radial fracture by promotion of bone and soft-tissue healing and reduction of the prevalence of complex regional pain syndrome (CRPS). Our primary aim was to examine the effect of vitamin C on functional outcome after a distal radial fracture.

Methods.—A total of 336 adult patients with an acute fracture of the distal aspect of the radius were recruited over a one year period and randomized to receive 500 mg of vitamin C or placebo daily for fifty days after the fracture. The primary outcomes were the DASH (Disabilities of the Arm, Shoulder and Hand) score at six weeks and at one year. Secondary variables included complications, wrist and finger motion, grip and pinch strength, pain, and a CRPS score.

Results.—There were no significant differences in patient or fracture characteristics between the treatment groups. There was no significant effect of vitamin C on the DASH score throughout the study period. At six weeks, patients in the vitamin C group with a nondisplaced fracture had a significantly greater wrist flexion deficit ($p = 0.008$) and pinch strength deficit ($p = 0.020$) and a greater rate of CRPS ($p = 0.022$), but there was no difference in the CRPS rate at any other time point. At twenty-six weeks, there was a higher rate of complications ($p = 0.043$) and greater pain with use ($p = 0.045$) in the patients with a displaced fracture treated with vitamin C. There was no significant difference in the time to fracture-healing.

Conclusions.—This study demonstrated no significant difference at one year in the DASH score, other functional outcomes, the rate of CRPS, or osseous healing of nondisplaced or displaced distal radial fractures treated with vitamin C compared with placebo. We conclude that administration of vitamin C confers no benefit to patients with a displaced or nondisplaced fracture of the distal aspect of the radius.

Level of Evidence.—Therapeutic Level II. See Instructions for Authors for a complete description of levels of evidence.

▶ The American Academy of Orthopedic Surgery (AAOS) develops evidence-based clinical practice guidelines to aid its member surgeons on recommended treatment methods and alternatives and complications of various orthopedic injuries and conditions. In 2009, the AAOS recommended the use of 500 mg of oral vitamin C daily for 50 days for patients who sustained a distal radius fracture to reduce or prevent the occurrence of complex regional pain syndrome (CRPS). CRPS is one of the most perplexing, costly, and disabling complications after distal radius fractures. The AAOS recommendation for the use of vitamin C was based on available evidence from several randomized studies showing efficacy weighed against the ready availability, low cost, and lack of adverse side effects from this dosage of vitamin C but that further study was recommended. Vitamin C has been shown to reduce free radicals (which have been implicated in the pathogenesis CRPS) and to improve fracture callous formation. The finding of this prospective randomized study demonstrated no benefit from administration of vitamin C in objective functional outcomes, time to fracture healing, or reduction of the rate of CRPS following treatment of patients who had sustained a distal radius fracture. Clearly, these data are somewhat deflating given the relative innocuous use vitamin C as a promising therapeutic adjunct in lowering the rate of a most dreaded complications in the treatment of distal radius fractures.

S. D. Trigg, MD

Forearm and Wrist

Arthroscopic Management of Chronic Unstable Scaphoid Nonunions: Effects on Restoration of Carpal Alignment and Recovery of Wrist Function
Kim JP, Seo JB, Yoo JY, et al (Dankook Univ College of Medicine, Cheonan, Republic of Korea)
Arthroscopy 31:460-469, 2015

Purpose.—The purpose of this study was to assess the effects of arthroscopically assisted reduction and osteosynthesis on restoration of carpal alignment and recovery of clinical wrist function in patients with unstable scaphoid nonunion.

Methods.—Thirty-six patients who underwent arthroscopically assisted osteosynthesis with or without bone grafting for unstable scaphoid nonunion between July 2006 and January 2012 were enrolled. The average time from injury to surgery was 51 ± 78.3 months. Radiographic and clinical evaluations were assessed on preoperative and postoperative days, and follow-up evaluation took place at a minimum of 24 months.

Results.—Union was achieved in 86% (31 of 36) of patients at a mean of 11 ± 2.7 weeks. Scaphoid axial length (SAL), lateral intrascaphoid angle (ISA), scapholunate angle (SLA), and reversed carpal height ratio (CHR) was significantly improved after surgery, and those correction ratios

averaged   66% ± 46.8%,   74% ± 58.2%,   81% ± 59.8%,   and
94% ± 46%, respectively. The range of wrist motion was unchanged
after surgery, but the grip strength improved from 74% ± 22.1% preoperatively to 89% ± 13.7% postoperatively compared with the contralateral
side ($P =.042$). Mean Disabilities of the Arm, Shoulder, and Hand (DASH)
and Patient-Related Wrist Evaluation (PRWE) scores improved significantly ($P < .001$) from 44 and 51 preoperatively to 13 and 23 postoperatively, respectively. The radiological parameters of the scaphoid and
carpal alignment in patients who achieved bony union did not correlate
with clinical wrist function.

Conclusions.—Arthroscopic reduction and osteosynthesis of chronic
unstable scaphoid nonunion is limited for restoration of normal carpal
alignment but has positive effects on the recovery of clinical wrist
function.

Level of Evidence.—Level IV, therapeutic case series.

▶ The contributions to the literature on arthroscopic-assisted reduction and
internal fixation of acute and subacute fractures of the scaphoid are limited,
but the advantages of direct visualization of reduction, along with the minimal
invasive aspects of this technique, are intriguing on several levels. The investigators of this article have pushed the envelope, so to speak, by applying this technology toward treatment of chronic unstable scaphoid nonunions, and their
results and experience are, I think, important.

S. D. Trigg, MD

**Does osteoporosis have a negative effect on the functional outcome of an
osteoporotic distal radial fracture treated with a volar locking plate?**
Choi W-S, Lee HJ, Kim D-Y, et al (Ajou Univ Hosp, Suwon, Korea; Hanyang
Univ, Seoul, Korea; et al)
Bone Joint J 97-B:229-234, 2015

We performed a retrospective study to determine the effect of osteoporosis on the functional outcome of osteoporotic distal radial fractures treated
with a volar locking plate. Between 2009 and 2012 a total of 90 postmenopausal women with an unstable fracture of the distal radius treated with a
volar locking plate were studied. Changes in the radiological parameters of
51 patients with osteoporosis (group 1, mean age 66.9, mean T-score −3.16
(SD 0.56)) were not significantly different from those in 39 patients without
osteoporosis (group 2, mean age 61.1, mean T-score −1.72 (SD 0.57)). The
mean Disabilities of the Arm, Shoulder and Hand (DASH) score at final
follow-up was 11.5 (SD 12.2) in group 1 and 10.5 (SD 13.25) in group 2.
The mean modified Mayo wrist score at final follow-up was 79.0 (SD
14.04) in group 1 and 82.6 (SD 13.1) in group 2. However, this difference
was not statistically significant ($p = 0.35$ for DASH score, $p = 0.2$ for modified Mayo wrist score). Univariable and multivariable logistic regression

analysis showed that only the step-off of the radiocarpal joint was related to both a poor DASH and modified Mayo wrist score. Pearson's correlation coefficient showed a weak negative relationship only between the T-score and the change in volar tilt (intraclass coefficient -0.26, $p = 0.02$).

We found that osteoporosis does not have a negative effect on the functional outcome and additional analysis did not show a correlation between T-score and outcome.

▶ The surge toward treatment of adult displaced unstable distal radius fractures with volar locking plates supplanting all other operative methods is now in its second decade and shows no sign of abatement. Osteoporosis is well recognized as a risk factor for sustaining more severe patterns of distal radius fractures and has been shown to be associated with an increased incidence of loss of reduction after cast immobilization, both of which are factors necessitating operative intervention (and as noted increasingly with volar locking plate fixation). Several studies investigating functional outcomes comparing osteoporotic and nonosteoporotic patients after volar plate fixation suggested that osteoporotic patients had comparatively poorer outcomes despite similar radiographic measurements. The authors of this study raise an interesting query as to why osteoporosis alone, independent of any other factors, would yield poorer functional outcomes because it is an asymptomatic condition. Their findings and analytical study methods are worthy of your review.

S. D. Trigg, MD

The Effect of Brachioradialis Release During Distal Radius Fracture Fixation on Elbow Flexion Strength and Wrist Function

Kim JK, Park JS, Shin SJ, et al (Ewha Woman Univ, Seoul, South Korea)
J Hand Surg Am 39:2246-2250, 2014

Purpose.—To identify whether brachioradialis (BR) release during volar plate fixation for a distal radius fracture affects elbow flexion strength and wrist function.

Methods.—A total of 42 consecutive patients who were treated by open reduction volar plate fixation for unstable distal radius fractures were enrolled in this study. The BR was not released in 20 of 42 patients (BR preserved group) and was released in 22 patients (BR released group). The primary outcome variable was isokinetic strength and endurance testing of elbow flexion measured by the Cybex isokinetic system 3 months after surgery. Measured at the same time, secondary outcome variables were grip strength, a visual analog scale score for wrist pain, Disabilities of the Arm, Shoulder, and Hand score, and radiographic parameters. We used Manne—Whitney U tests to compare these variables between groups.

Results.—Neither elbow flexion strength and endurance nor any of the secondary outcome variables differed significantly between groups.

Conclusions.—Release of the BR during a volar approach for a distal radius fracture did not adversely affect elbow flexion strength and wrist function.
Type of Study/Level of Evidence.—Prognostic III.

▶ The findings of this study deliver clinically practical information. The distal Henry surgical approach is the most commonly recommended approach for volar plate fixation of distal radius fractures. As most of you who perform this procedure have recognized, the brachioradialis (BR) can be a deforming structure to the fracture reduction, particularly in intra-articular fractures or those that are addressed in a subacute timeframe. Early on in the development of the technique of surgical management of distal radius fractures with volar fixed angle-locking plates, the pioneering investigators recommended incising the BR tendon to facilitate fracture fragment reduction. Many advocated repairing the tendon with the intent on preserving the action of the BR as an elbow flexor, and others did not. My own practice has been to z-cut the tendon and then attempt to repair the BR when closing. I have to admit that the repair is often pretty darn tenuous depending on the bulk of the native tendon. This prospectively designed but nonrandomized study brings forth new functional outcome information on the BR tendon release, and the data are relevant to anyone who performs this procedure.

S. D. Trigg, MD

Reduction and Association of the Scaphoid and Lunate Procedure: Short-Term Clinical and Radiographic Outcomes
Larson TB, Stern PJ (Univ of Cincinnati College of Medicine, OH)
J Hand Surg Am 39:2168-2174, 2014

Purpose.—To evaluate the success of reduction and association of the scaphoid and lunate with a fibrous union in an effort to evaluate the technique's validity and reproducibility.
Methods.—A retrospective review was performed on 7 patients (8 wrists) with an average follow-up of 38 months. Static and grip radiographs were examined in the preoperative, immediate postoperative, and final follow-up settings to evaluate scapholunate (SL) diastasis, SL angle, hardware position, and complications. At final follow-up, grip strength and wrist range of motion were recorded, and patients completed the Disabilities of the Arm, Shoulder, and Hand and the Patient-Rated Wrist Evaluation outcome questionnaires.
Results.—Radiographic success, defined by maintenance of corrected SL diastasis, absence of dorsal intercalated segmental instability, and no progression of SL advanced collapse was achieved in 3 of the 8 wrists. One wrist developed radioscaphoid arthritis. No patients required a salvage procedure. Despite the loss of reduction that occurred in all patients, the

patients' disability remained minimal as detected by the scores on the outcome measures.

Conclusions.—The procedure was ineffective in providing stability about the SL interval. With a majority of patients experiencing early radiographic failure of the procedure in the short term, our experience suggests that the reduction and association of the scaphoid and lunate procedure should be abandoned despite the relatively low outcomes measures scores, which may be reflective of the short follow-up duration for this series.

Type of Study/Level of Evidence.—Therapeutic IV.

▶ The treatment of subacute or chronic scapholunate (SL) dissociation with resultant carpal instability where direct or augmented repair is not possible remains an unresolved problem because no procedure has been proven to be superior. Many methods of capsulodesis, SL ligament reconstruction tenodesis, and limited intercarpal arthrodesis procedures have been advocated. Many of these are technically complicated, which no doubt raised the interest for many treating surgeons (myself included) for the reduction and association of the scaphoid and lunate procedure as developed by Rosenwasser et al in 1997. The attractiveness of the procedure is that a stable reduced SL association could be restored through the placement of a headless compression screw through the scaphoid and lunate without the need for further soft tissue augmentation. The findings of this limited retrospective study are sobering and do not mirror the original reports of the innovator of the procedure. My own reason for abandoning this procedure was not that the fixation failed but that postoperative wrist range of motion was unacceptable compared with several soft-tissue reconstructive procedures that I have tried.

S. D. Trigg, MD

Application of 3-Dimensional Printing in Hand Surgery for Production of a Novel Bone Reduction Clamp
Fuller SM, Butz DR, Vevang CB, et al (Univ of Chicago Medicine, IL; Univ of Illinois at Chicago)
J Hand Surg Am 39:1840-1845, 2014

Three-dimensional printing is being rapidly incorporated in the medical field to produce external prosthetics for improved cosmesis and fabricated molds to aid in presurgical planning. Biomedically engineered products from 3-dimensional printers are also utilized as implantable devices for knee arthroplasty, airway orthoses, and other surgical procedures. Although at first expensive and conceptually difficult to construct, 3-dimensional printing is now becoming more affordable and widely accessible. In hand surgery, like many other specialties, new or customized instruments would be desirable; however, the overall production cost restricts their development. We are presenting our step-by-step experience in creating a bone reduction clamp for finger fractures using 3-dimensional printing technology. Using free, downloadable software, a 3-dimensional model of a bone reduction clamp for hand fractures was created based on the senior author's (M.V.M.) specific design, previous experience, and preferences for fracture fixation. Once deemed satisfactory, the computer files were sent to a 3-dimensional printing company for the production of the prototypes. Multiple plastic prototypes were made and adjusted, affording a fast, low-cost working model of the proposed clamp. Once a workable design was obtained, a printing company produced the surgical clamp prototype directly from the 3-dimensional model represented in the computer files. This prototype was used in the operating room, meeting the expectations of the surgeon. Three-dimensional printing is affordable and offers the benefits of reducing production time and nurturing innovations in hand surgery. This article presents a step-by-step description of our design process using online software programs and 3-dimensional printing services. As medical technology advances, it is important that hand surgeons remain aware of available resources, are knowledgeable about how the process works, and are able to take advantage of opportunities in order to advance the field.

▶ This article speaks for itself. Three-dimensional printing of devices applicable to hand surgery and orthopedics is in its infancy, but the science and technology of this process is rapidly expanding in other fields of medicine and the manufacturing industry as a whole. No doubt the capability to create even a novel surgical device such as that described here might seem incredible today, but the future of biomedically engineered 3-dimensional printed devices will certainly eclipse what we can mentally process or imagine at this point. This article is written in a stepwise and logical fashion that mirrors both the creative process from the idea of the need for an improved reduction clamp to completion using this technology. The authors are clearly inviting us to step aboard and learn something about this exiting technology. The future looks interesting indeed.

S. D. Trigg, MD

Accelerated Rehabilitation Compared with a Standard Protocol After Distal Radial Fractures Treated with Volar Open Reduction and Internal Fixation: A Prospective, Randomized, Controlled Study

Brehmer JL, Husband JB (Univ of Minnesota, Minneapolis; Univ of Minnesota, Bloomington)
J Bone Joint Surg Am 96:1621-1630, 2014

Background.—There are relatively few studies in the literature that specifically evaluate accelerated rehabilitation protocols for distal radial fractures treated with open reduction and internal fixation (ORIF). The purpose of this study was to compare the early postoperative outcomes (at zero to twelve weeks postoperatively) of patients enrolled in an accelerated rehabilitation protocol with those of patients enrolled in a standard rehabilitation protocol following ORIF for a distal radial fracture. We hypothesized that patients with accelerated rehabilitation after volar ORIF for a distal radial fracture would have an earlier return to function compared with patients who followed a standard protocol.

Methods.—From November 2007 to November 2010, eighty-one patients with an unstable distal radial fracture were prospectively randomized to follow either an accelerated or a standard rehabilitation protocol after undergoing ORIF with a volar plate for a distal radial fracture. Both groups began with gentle active range of motion at three to five days postoperatively. At two weeks, the accelerated group initiated wrist/forearm passive range of motion and strengthening exercises, whereas the standard group initiated passive range of motion and strengthening at six weeks postoperatively. Patients were assessed at three to five days, two weeks, three weeks, four weeks, six weeks, eight weeks, twelve weeks, and six months postoperatively. Outcomes included Disabilities of the Arm, Shoulder and Hand (DASH) scores (primary outcome) and measurements of wrist flexion/extension, supination, pronation, grip strength, and palmar pinch.

Results.—The patients in the accelerated group had better mobility, strength, and DASH scores at the early postoperative time points (zero to eight weeks postoperatively) compared with the patients in the standard rehabilitation group. The difference between the groups was both clinically relevant and statistically significant.

Conclusions.—Patients who follow an accelerated rehabilitation protocol that emphasizes motion immediately postoperatively and initiates strengthening at two weeks after volar ORIF of a distal radial fracture have an earlier return to function than patients who follow a more standard rehabilitation protocol.

Level of Evidence.—Therapeutic Level I. See Instructions for Authors for a complete description of levels of evidence.

▶ Arguably, stable internal fixation of adult unstable, malangulated, or displaced fractures with volar locking plates is perhaps the single most important advancement in the treatment of these common injuries since the implementation of plaster casts and the common use of X-rays. Clearly, among the major benefits from use of these implants is that "early" postoperative range of motion therapy can be initiated, resulting in accelerated and improved functional outcomes. The weight of submissions to the literature on plate design, surgical techniques, and complications has dwarfed the amount of relevant study data on variations and improvements in postoperative rehabilitation of patients following these procedures. This prospective study brings forth new information that may guide you to review or modify your postoperative management.

S. D. Trigg, MD

Distal Scaphoid Resection for Degenerative Arthritis Secondary to Scaphoid Nonunion: A 20-Year Experience

Malerich MM, Catalano LW III, Weidner ZD, et al (St. Luke's-Roosevelt Hosp, NY)
J Hand Surg Am 39:1669-1676, 2014

Purpose.—To evaluate the long-term results of distal scaphoid excision for degenerative arthritis secondary to scaphoid nonunion and compare them with our original results published in 1999.

Methods.—Nineteen patients who were treated by distal scaphoid resection arthroplasty from 1987 through 2010 were included. The mean follow-up was 15 years (range, 10—25 y) vs 4 years in the previous study. Clinical evaluation included measurement of the visual analog pain scale, wrist range of motion, and grip strength. Radiographs were taken at follow-up to assess for signs of arthritis and wrist collapse.

Results.—The outcomes of this procedure include increased grip strength and total arc of motion, a small decrease in revised carpal height ratio, and a small increase in radiolunate angle. Two patients failed distal scaphoid resection arthroplasty necessitating proximal row carpectomy (1) and wrist arthrodesis (1) for recalcitrant pain. More than half of the remaining patients developed midcarpal arthritis on radiographs that was asymptomatic. No patients developed radiolunate arthritis.

Conclusions.—This study showed that distal scaphoid resection arthroplasty produced favorable, long-term clinical results and did not result in noteworthy wrist collapse. Midcarpal arthritis, which may develop after the procedure, did not cause appreciable deterioration in patient outcomes. This procedure also did not eliminate the option of using additional, more conventional reconstructive procedures if needed.

Type of Study/Level of Evidence.—Therapeutic IV.

▶ The optimal surgical procedure to reduce the pain and improve wrist range of motion from chronic scaphoid fracture nonunions with advanced carpal collapse remains unclear. Several salvage procedures have been proposed, including radial styloidectomy, proximal row carpectomy, and scaphoid excision with intercarpal arthrodesis. Each of these procedures has been studied over the long term, resulting in varying functional and patient-reported outcome data but with no clear winner emerging. Less commonly recommended is distal scaphoid excision. In the few reported short-term studies (including an earlier report on these patients) on outcomes after distal scaphoid excision, the early results would suggest that the procedure is generally comparable to the other methods. It is not clear why the procedure has not gained wider acceptance given the relative technical simplicity of the procedure along with a shorter period of postoperative immobilization and return to unrestricted activities. The authors' explanation for why the high rate of development of midcarpal arthritis did not significantly affect patient outcomes is speculative and deserves further study.

S. D. Trigg, MD

Biomechanical Comparison of Bicortical Locking Versus Unicortical Far-Cortex–Abutting Locking Screw-Plate Fixation for Comminuted Radial Shaft Fractures

Overturf SJ, Morris RP, Gugala Z, et al (Univ of Texas Med Branch, Galveston)
J Hand Surg Am 39:1907-1913, 2014

Purpose.—To provide comparative biomechanical evaluation of bicortical locking versus unicortical-abutting locking screw-plate fixation in a comminuted radius fracture model.

Methods.—A validated synthetic substitute of the adult human radius with a 1.5-cm-long segmental mid-diaphyseal defect was used in the study to simulate a comminuted fracture. Stabilization was achieved with an 8-hole locking plate and either bicortical screws or unicortical-abutting screws. The specimens were tested using nondestructive cyclical loading in 4-point bending, axial compression, and torsion to determine stiffness and displacement and subsequently in 4-point bending to assess load to failure.

Results.—There were no statistically significant differences between bicortical versus unicortical-abutting locking screw fixation in nondestructive 4-point bending, axial compression, and torsion. Both locking screw constructs also demonstrated comparable 4-point bending loads to failure.

Conclusion.—The biomechanical equivalence between bicortical locking versus unicortical abutting locking screw-plate fixation suggests that adequate locking plate fixation can be achieved without perforation of the far cortex. The abutment of the screw tip within the far cortex enhances the unicortical screw positional stability and thereby effectively opposes the

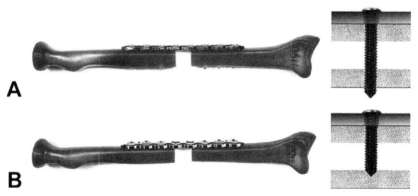

FIGURE 1.—Validated synthetic adult human radii with simulated unstable comminuted fractures were stabilized using 8-hole 3.5-mm titanium locking plate and bicortical locking screws **A** or unicortical abutting locking screws **B**. The unicortical screw abutment was achieved consistently at 2-mm depth within the inner aspect of the far cortex. (Reprinted from The Journal of Hand Surgery. Overturf SJ, Morris RP, Gugala Z, et al. Biomechanical comparison of bicortical locking versus unicortical far-cortex–abutting locking screw-plate fixation for comminuted radial shaft fractures. *J Hand Surg Am.* 2014;39:1907-1913, Copyright 2014, with permission from the American Society for Surgery of the Hand.)

displacement of the screw when subjected to bending or axial or rotational loads.

Clinical Relevance.—Unicortical-abutting screws potentially offer several clinical advantages. They eliminate the need for drilling through the far cortex and thereby a risk of adjacent neurovascular injury or soft tissue structure compromise. They eliminate the issues associated with symptomatic screw prominence. They can decrease risk of refracture after screw-plate removal. In case of revision plating, they permit conversion to bicortical locking screws through the same near-cortex screw holes, which eliminates the need for a longer or repositioned plate (Fig 1).

▶ This is an interesting study that should have important clinical relevance in upper extremity fracture management where far cortex screw tip protrusion in bicortical locking plate-screw fixation constructs may risk injury to nearby neurovascular, tendinous, and articular structures. The authors' development of a modified unicortical-abutting locking screw placement, which achieves near biomechanical testing equivalence to standard bicortical locking plate-screw fixation, is novel and deserves your review.

S. D. Trigg, MD

Hand

Return to Football and Long-Term Clinical Outcomes After Thumb Ulnar Collateral Ligament Suture Anchor Repair in Collegiate Athletes

Werner BC, Hadeed MM, Lyons ML, et al (Univ of Virginia Health System, Charlottesville)
J Hand Surg Am 39:1992-1998, 2014

Purpose.—To evaluate return to play after complete thumb ulnar collateral ligament (UCL) injury treated with suture anchor repair for both skill position and non—skill position collegiate football athletes and report minimum 2-year clinical outcomes in this population.

Methods.—For this retrospective study, inclusion criteria were complete rupture of the thumb UCL and suture anchor repair in a collegiate football athlete performed by a single surgeon who used an identical technique for all patients. Data collection included chart review, determination of return to play, and Quick Disabilities of the Arm, Shoulder, and Hand (*Quick*-DASH) outcomes.

Results.—A total of 18 collegiate football athletes were identified, all of whom were evaluated for follow-up by telephone, e-mail, or regular mail at an average 6-year follow-up. Nine were skill position players; the remaining 9 played in nonskill positions. All players returned to at least the same level of play. The average *Quick*DASH score for the entire cohort was 1 out of 100; *Quick*DASH work score, 0 out of 100; and sport score, 1 out of 100. Average time to surgery for skill position players was 12 days compared with 43 for non—skill position players. Average return to play for skill position players was 7 weeks postoperatively compared with

4 weeks for non—skill position players. There was no difference in average *Quick*DASH overall scores or subgroup scores between cohorts.

Conclusions.—Collegiate football athletes treated for thumb UCL injuries with suture anchor repair had quick return to play, reliable return to the same level of activity, and excellent long-term clinical outcomes. Skill position players had surgery sooner after injury and returned to play later than non—skill position players, with no differences in final level of play or clinical outcomes. Management of thumb UCL injuries in collegiate football athletes can be safely and effectively tailored according to the demands of the player's football position.

Type of Study/Level of Evidence.—Therapeutic IV.

▶ I found this article to be interesting and clinically relevant. Anyone who has taken care of collegiate or professional football players can attest to the commonality of thumb injuries during the course of a season. Frequently, injury to the thumb metacarpophalangeal joint is involved, drawing concerns for a diagnosis of a complete rupture of the ulnar collateral ligament. Complete ruptures of the ulnar collateral ligament will often disable the function of the hand to the extent that the player cannot compete. The author of this study correctly points out the special case of college athletes who have at most a 4- or 5-year career, which then puts pressure on the treating surgeon to get the player back on the field as quickly as possible and to perform a durable repair that will allow the athlete to do so. There is not a lot written on this subject in the hand surgery literature, making the judgment of timing to return to play an individually based decision. The authors' protocol for altering the postsurgical rehabilitation and time to return to practice between skilled and nonskilled position players is instructive. I would draw readers' attention to the authors' use of 2 suture anchors for the repair, which may be considered as a topic for future study.

S. D. Trigg, MD

Acute Surgical Management of Hand Burns
Richards WT, Vergara E, Dalaly DG, et al (Univ of Florida, Gainesville; Shands Med Ctr, Gainesville)
J Hand Surg Am 39:2075-2085, 2014

A hand represents 3% of the total body surface area. The hands are involved in close to 80% of all burns. The potential morbidity associated with hand burns can be substantial. Imagine a patient carrying a pan of flaming cooking oil to the doorway or someone lighting a room-sized pile of leaves and branches doused with gasoline. It is clear how the hands are at risk in these common scenarios. Not all burn injuries will require surgical intervention. Recognizing the need for surgery is paramount to achieving good functional outcomes for the burned hand. The gray area between second- and third-degree burns tests the skill and experience of every burn/hand surgeon. Skin anatomy and the size of injury dictate the surgical technique used to close the burn wound. In addition to meticulous surgical technique, preoperative and postoperative hand therapy for the burned hand is essential for a good functional outcome. Recognizing the burn depth is paramount to developing the appropriate treatment plan for any burn injury. This skill requires experience and practice. In this article, we present an approach to second- and third-degree hand burns.

▶ I generally do not select surgical technique articles for this section. However, this article is particularly concise, up to date, and supported with excellent clinical photographs. Moreover, the authors stress with clarity the critical importance of recognizing the clinical distinctions between deep second-degree burns and third-degree burns. Owing to the networks of burn treatment centers that are available in most developed countries, most surgeons will not be faced with the necessity of providing secondary surgical treatment for more serious burn injuries. That said, a working knowledge of the information put forth in this article should be known by anyone who provides emergent treatment of musculoskeletal injuries of the extremities.

S. D. Trigg, MD

Rigid versus semi-rigid orthotic use following TMC arthroplasty: A randomized controlled trial

Prosser R, Hancock MJ, Nicholson L, et al (Sydney Hand Therapy & Rehabilitation Centre, Sydney, Australia; Univ of Sydney, Australia; et al)
J Hand Ther 27:265-271, 2014

Introduction.—The trapeziometacarpal (TMC) joint of the human thumb is the second most common joint in the hand affected by osteoarthritis. TMC arthroplasty is a common procedure used to alleviate symptoms. No randomized controlled trials have been published on the efficacy of different postoperative orthotic regimes.

Method.—Fifty six participants who underwent TMC arthroplasty were allocated to either rigid orthotic or semi-rigid orthotic groups. Both groups started an identical exercise program at two weeks following surgery. Outcome measures were assessed by an assessor blinded to group allocation. The primary outcome was the Patient Rated Wrist and Hand Evaluation (PRWHE) and secondary outcomes included the Michigan Hand Questionnaire (MHQ), thumb palmar abduction, first metacarpophalangeal extension and three point pinch grip. Measures were taken pre-operatively, at six weeks, three months and one year post-operatively. Between-group differences were analyzed with linear regression.

Results.—Both groups performed equally well. There was no significant between-group difference for PRWHE scores (0.47, CI -11.5 to 12.4), including subscales for pain and function, or for any of the secondary outcomes at one year follow-up.

Conclusion.—We found no difference in outcomes between using a rigid or semi-rigid orthosis after TMC arthroplasty. Patient comfort, cost and availability may determine choice between orthoses in clinical practice.
Level of Evidence.—1b RCT.

▶ Trapezium resection ligament reconstruction tendon interposition (LRTI) surgery is one of the most frequently performed hand reconstructive arthroplasty procedures. The bulk of the contributions to the literature on LRTI focuses on outcomes from a particular surgical technique or comparison among several. Logically, one would assume that functional outcomes from LRTI surgery are dependent to some degree on the duration and type of postoperative immobilization and subsequent hand therapy protocol, or do they? One would have difficulty coming to a consensus to select an optimal postoperative hand therapy program for LRTI surgery because reports in the literature vary so widely. That is why prospective randomized comparative studies such as this that consider the differences in costs associated with hand splinting and frequency of therapy weighed against measured length of disability before return to work or desired level of function are so important.

S. D. Trigg, MD

Comparison of Arthroplasties With or Without Bone Tunnel Creation for Thumb Basal Joint Arthritis: A Randomized Controlled Trial
Vermeulen GM, Spekreijse KR, Slijper H, et al (Diakonessenhuis Utrecht, The Netherlands; Erasmus MC Univ Med Ctr, Rotterdam, The Netherlands; Dept of Rehabilitation Medicine, Rotterdam; et al)
J Hand Surg Am 39:1692-1698, 2014

Purpose.—To compare the results for treatment of basal thumb osteoarthritis with and without the use of a bone tunnel at the base of the first metacarpal.

Methods.—Women aged 40 years or older with stage IV osteoarthritis were randomized to 1 of 2 treatments. Patients were evaluated preoperatively and postoperatively at 3 and 12 months by assessing pain, outcome function measures, range of motion, strength, time to return to work or activities, satisfaction with the results, and complication rate.

Results.—A total of 79 patients were enrolled in this study. Three months after surgery, Patient-Rated Wrist and Hand Evaluation pain and total scores were significantly improved in the bone tunnel group compared with the tunnel-free group. At 12 months, however, we found no significant differences for all outcome scores between groups. In addition, we observed no significant differences between groups in strength, duration to return to work or activities, patient satisfaction, and complication rates.

Conclusions.—After the bone tunnel technique, patients have better function and less pain 3 months after surgery than do those in the non—bone tunnel group, which indicates faster recovery. However, 12 months after surgery, the functional outcome was similar. Because of faster recovery, we prefer the bone tunnel technique in the treatment of stage IV osteoarthritis.

Type of Study/Level of Evidence.—Therapeutic I.

▶ Trapezium resection and ligament reconstruction with tendon interposition (LRTI) is one of the most frequently performed arthritis reconstructive arthroplasty procedures in hand surgery. The 2 LRTI procedures compared in this study are among the most frequently reported methods but have not been extensively compared head to head. The Weilby technique for harvesting the flexor carpi radialis (FCR) tendon as described here is generally accurate to the original description. The Burton-Pellegrini technique has been reported elsewhere as harvesting the entire FCR tendon, whereas in this report only half of the tendon was harvested as tendon graft, similar to the Weilby technique. Whether this has any bearing on outcomes is a matter for future study. That said, I was surprised by the outcome data of this study, as I abandoned the Burton-Pellegrini technique more than a decade ago in favor of the Weilby technique specifically because in my experience the Weilby procedure resulted in less pain and faster recovery for the patient. Although the optimal method for trapezium resection LRTI is not certain and will no doubt be hotly debated going forward, this randomized study furthers the knowledge base, which may result in a healthy reappraisal of one's current choice of technique.

S. D. Trigg, MD

Nerve

Prognostic factors for outcome after median, ulnar, and combined median−ulnar nerve injuries: A prospective study

Hundepool CA, Ultee J, Nijhuis THJ, et al (Univ Med Ctr, Rotterdam, The Netherlands; et al)
J Plast Reconstr Aesthet Surg 68:1-8, 2015

Background.—A major problem in the surgical treatment of peripheral nerve injuries of the upper extremities is the unpredictable final outcome. More insight and understanding of the prognostic factors is necessary to improve functional outcome after repair of the peripheral nerves. The objective of this study was to identify prognostic factors for the functional recovery of peripheral nerve injury of the forearm and their independent contribution in the outcome in the first year after reconstruction.

Methods.—A multicentered prospective study in the Netherlands resulted in the inclusion of 61 patients with a median, ulnar, or combined median−ulnar nerve injury. The age, level of injury, type of nerve injury, number of damaged structures, number of damaged arteries, education, smoking, and posttraumatic stress were analyzed as prognostic factors for functional outcome after repair of the peripheral nerves. The outcome parameters were sensory recovery (Semmes−Weinstein monofilament test) and motor recovery (Medical Research Council (MRC) score, power grip, and pinch grip) and the ability to perform daily activities.

Results.—Gender, age, level of education, number of injured arteries and structures, damaged nerve, location of the injury, type of the nerve injury, and posttraumatic stress at 1 and 3 months after repair of the peripheral nerve injury were found to be predictors of functional recovery.

Conclusions.—Our prospective analysis of prognostic factors shows several factors to be predictive for the functional recovery after peripheral nerve injuries of the median and/or ulnar nerve of the forearm. Sensibility of the hand, power grip, and DASH score (DASH, Disabilities of Arm, Shoulder and Hand) have proven to be the three best prognostic factors in this study. Of these prognostic factors, only posttraumatic stress can be influenced to optimize functional outcome.

▶ Despite significant technical advancements in the surgical treatment of peripheral nerve injuries in recent years, we still have difficulty predicting outcomes; thus, what we discuss with our patients about what they might expect or how to plan for their future (eg, return to previous employment status) is individually variable. There remain sparse data on which patient factors are independent predictors of functional outcome after surgical repair of median and/or ulnar nerve injuries. This prospective study provides us with important prognostic information that may help in discussions with patients who sustain these injuries.

S. D. Trigg, MD

The anatomical relationship of the superficial radial nerve and the lateral antebrachial cutaneous nerve: A possible factor in persistent neuropathic pain

Poublon AR, Walbeehm ET, Duraku LS, et al (Erasmus MC, Rotterdam, The Netherlands; RadboudUMC, Nijmegen, The Netherlands)
J Plast Reconstr Aesthet Surg 68:237-242, 2015

The superficial branch of the radial nerve (SBRN) is known for developing neuropathic pain syndromes after trauma. These pain syndromes can be hard to treat due to the involvement of other nerves in the forearm. When a nerve is cut, the Schwann cells, and also other cells in the distal segment of the transected nerve, produce the nerve growth factor (NGF) in the entire distal segment. If two nerves overlap anatomically, similar to the lateral antebrachial cutaneous nerve (LACN) and SBRN, the increase in secretion of NGF, which is mediated by the injured nerve, results in binding to the high-affinity NGF receptor, tyrosine kinase A (TrkA). This in turn leads to possible sprouting and morphological changes of uninjured fibers, which ultimately causes neuropathic pain. The aim of this study was to map the level of overlap between the SBRN and LACN.

Twenty arms (five left and 15 right) were thoroughly dissected. Using a new analysis tool called CASAM (Computer Assisted Surgical Anatomy Mapping), the course of the SBRN and LACN could be compared visually. The distance between both nerves was measured at 5- mm increments, and the number of times they intersected was documented.

In 81% of measurements, the distance between the nerves was >10 mm, and in 49% the distance was even <5 mm. In 95% of the dissected arms, the SBRN and LACN intersected. On average, they intersected 2.25 times.

The close (anatomical) relationship between the LACN and the SBRN can be seen as a factor in the explanation of persistent neuropathic pain in patients with traumatic or iatrogenic lesion of the SBRN or the LACN.

▶ Anyone who has any experience in treating neuropathic pain after injury to the superficial branch of the radial nerve has learned first and foremost that achieving favorable patient-reported pain outcomes is exceedingly difficult and that a given successful treatment for one patient may not prove successful for others with a similar injury. As a result, many patients are abandoned after an initial treatment surgical procedure or are readily referred to pain specialist without considering further treatment alternatives. Although it is known that the lateral antebrachial cutaneous nerve (LACN) and the superficial branch of the radial nerve (SBRN) lie in close anatomic proximity along the lateral forearm and wrist, this study is one of the few that accurately describes this. The authors postulate that neuropathic pain in the LACN distribution may be secondary to chemical mediators released by the adjacent injured SBRN, but this remains speculative. I chose this article for the methods and clarity of the anatomic cadaver dissections because it furthers our knowledge base as to why there is often a neuropathic pain overlap between both nerves, which will hopefully lead to a better understanding of how to sort this out.

S. D. Trigg, MD

An Outcomes Protocol for Carpal Tunnel Release: A Comparison of Outcomes in Patients With and Without Medical Comorbidities
Cagle PJ Jr, Reams M, Agel J, et al (Univ of Minnesota, Minneapolis; TRIA Orthopaedic Ctr, Bloomington, MN)
J Hand Surg Am 39:2175-2180, 2014

Purpose.—To prospectively report the outcomes of open carpal tunnel release with respect to patient age and medical comorbidities.

Methods.—Nine hundred fifty open carpal tunnel procedures in 826 patients (age range, 21–100 y) at a high-volume orthopedic surgery center were evaluated. Self-reported symptom severity and functional scores were collected using the validated Boston Carpal Tunnel Outcomes questionnaire preoperatively, and at 2 weeks, 6 weeks, and 12 weeks postoperatively.

Results.—Patients demonstrated a significant improvement in symptom severity scores at 2 weeks and functional severity scores at 6 weeks.

Documented patient medical comorbidities did not affect improvement after surgery. Patients with diabetes improved more slowly but were not significantly different at 6 weeks. Patients with workers' compensation insurance were significantly worse at baseline, 2 weeks, and 6 weeks but were not significantly different at 3 months. The risk of negative postoperative endpoints was slightly higher in patients with a medical comorbidity, though not statistically different.

Conclusions.—Significant improvements in symptom severity and hand function may be expected after open carpal tunnel release in the general population regardless of age, medical comorbidities, or workers' compensation status.

Type of Study/Level of Evidence.—Therapeutic III.

▶ This straightforward prospective study has practical clinical relevance. Many previously reported studies reporting outcome data after carpal tunnel release have excluded patients with medical comorbidities from their study populations. The study data derived from such exclusionary studies may not then fully answer what applicable outcome information a surgeon might reasonably expect in order to counsel their patients with 1 or more comorbidities, which is, in common practice, an all too frequent occurrence.

S. D. Trigg, MD

Outcomes of Revision Surgery for Cubital Tunnel Syndrome

Aleem AW, Krogue JD, Calfee RP (Washington Univ School of Medicine, St Louis, MO)
J Hand Surg Am 39:2141-2149, 2014

Purpose.—To compare both validated patient-rated and objective outcomes of patients following revision cubital tunnel surgery to a similar group of patients who underwent primary surgery.

Methods.—This case-control investigation enrolled 56 patients treated surgically for cubital tunnel syndrome (28 revision cases, 28 primary controls) at a tertiary center. Patients with a minimum of 2 years of follow-up were eligible. All patients completed an in-office study evaluation. Revision participants represented 55% of potential patients in our practice and controls (treated only with primary surgery) were chosen at random from our practice to reach a 1:1 case to control ratio. Preoperative McGowan grading was confirmed similar between the groups. Outcome measures included validated patient outcome questionnaires (Patient-Rated Elbow Evaluation, Levine-Katz questionnaire), symptoms, and physical examination findings. Statistical analyses were conducted to compare the patient groups.

Results.—Despite 79% of revision patients reporting symptomatic improvement, revision patients reported worse outcomes on all measured standardized questionnaires compared with primary patients. The Levine-Katz questionnaire indicated mild residual symptoms in the primary group

(1.6) versus moderate remaining symptoms following revision surgery (2.3). The Patient-Rated Elbow Evaluation also indicated superior results for the control group (9 ± 10) compared with the revision group (32 ± 22). Revision patients had a higher frequency of constant symptoms, elevated 2-point discrimination, and diminished pinch strength. McGowan grading improved after 25% of revision surgeries versus 64% of primary surgeries, and 21% of revision patients had deterioration of their McGowan grade.

Conclusions.—Subjective and objective outcomes of revision patients in this cohort were inferior to outcomes of similar patients following primary surgery. Revision surgery can be offered in the setting of persistent or recurrent symptoms that are unexplained by an alternative diagnosis, but patients should be counseled that complete resolution of symptoms is unlikely.

Type of Study/Level of Evidence.—Therapeutic III.

▶ Cubital tunnel syndrome is the second most common compressive neuropathy in the upper extremity. Despite the commonality of this condition, no primary surgical treatment method has been proven to be superior among several accepted methods of anterior transposition compared with decompression in situ. Moreover, in cases of persistent or recurrent ulnar neuropathic symptoms, it remains unclear what patient- or surgery-specific factors might be predictive of the need for revision surgery or what methods of revision surgery produce optimal improvement. The majority of information on outcomes from revision cubital tunnel surgery have been retrospective and lacking postoperative validated patient-rated and objective data. This study is among the few comparative studies to date that investigates revision cubital tunnel surgery with primary surgery. Their data provide us with new information worthy of your review.

S. D. Trigg, MD

4 Elbow

Introduction

Even though I am personally very interested in the elbow, this is appropriately the smallest section in this book. Most orthopedic surgeons deal with tennis elbow or elbow trauma rather than elbow replacement. For this reason, the articles in this section reflect what I consider to be the important topics for the practicing general orthopedic surgeon rather than the person who specializes in the upper extremity. The few articles that were selected deal with relevant topics and provide valid conclusions. Hence, I hope they will be of use to the orthopedic surgeon who does not deal with the elbow on a day-to-day basis.

Bernard F. Morrey, MD

Does Nonsurgical Treatment Improve Longitudinal Outcomes of Lateral Epicondylitis Over No Treatment? A Meta-analysis

Sayegh ET, Strauch RJ (Columbia Univ Med Ctr, NY)
Clin Orthop Relat Res 473:1093-1107, 2015

Background.—Lateral epicondylitis is a painful tendinopathy for which several nonsurgical treatment strategies are used. Superiority of these nonsurgical treatments over nontreatment has not been definitively established.

Questions/Purposes.—We asked whether nonsurgical treatment of lateral epicondylitis compared with observation only or placebo provides (1) better overall improvement, (2) less need for escape interventions, (3) better outcome scores, and (4) improved grip strength at intermediate-to long-term followup.

Methods.—The English language literature was searched using PubMed and the Cochrane Central Register of Controlled Trials. Randomized-controlled trials (RCTs) comparing any form of nonsurgical treatment with either observation only or placebo at followup of at least 6 months were included. Nonsurgical treatments included injections (corticosteroid, platelet-rich plasma, autologous blood, sodium hyaluronate, or glycosaminoglycan polysulfate), physiotherapy, shock wave therapy, laser, ultrasound, corticosteroid iontophoresis, topical glyceryl trinitrate, or oral naproxen.

Study or Subgroup	Treatment Events	Treatment Total	No Treatment Events	No Treatment Total	Weight	Risk Ratio M-H, Random, 95% CI	Risk Ratio M-H, Random, 95% CI
Bisset et al. [4]	103	128	56	62	14.0%	0.89 [0.79-1.00]	
Chesterton et al. [6]	84	121	79	120	11.0%	1.05 [0.89-1.26]	
Coombes et al. [7]	109	123	33	40	12.0%	1.07 [0.92-1.26]	
Haake et al. [10]	69	105	66	101	9.9%	1.01 [0.82-1.23]	
Haker and Lundeberg [11]	12	18	13	22	3.1%	1.13 [0.70-1.82]	
Haker and Lundeberg [13]	8	16	10	16	2.0%	0.80 [0.43-1.49]	
Haker and Lundeberg [14]	18	23	9	19	2.7%	1.65 [0.98-2.78]	
Hay et al. [15]	88	106	44	54	12.1%	1.02 [0.87-1.19]	
Mehra et al. [24]	10	13	1	11	0.2%	8.46 [1.28-56.14]	
Pettrone and McCall [28]	43	47	35	47	10.3%	1.23 [1.02-1.48]	
Rompe et al. [31]	24	38	16	40	3.4%	1.58 [1.01-2.48]	
Runeson and Haker [33]	16	20	18	21	6.8%	0.93 [0.71-1.24]	
Smidt et al. [35]	101	126	49	59	12.6%	0.97 [0.84-1.12]	
Total (95% CI)		884		612	100.0%	1.05 [0.96-1.15]	
Total events	685		429				

Heterogeneity: Tau^2 = 0.01; Chi^2 = 24.73, df = 12 (P = 0.02); I^2 = 51%
Test for overall effect: Z = 0.99 (P = 0.32)

0.1 0.2 0.5 1 2 5 10
Favors [no treatment] Favors [treatment]

FIGURE 3.—The forest plot shows the risk ratio of overall improvement. M-H = Mantel-Haenszel df = degrees of freedom. *Editor's Note:* Please refer to original journal article for full references. (With kind permission from Springer Science+Business Media: Sayegh ET, Strauch RJ. Does nonsurgical treatment improve longitudinal outcomes of lateral epicondylitis over no treatment? a meta-analysis. *Clin Orthop Relat Res.* 2015;473:1093-1107, with permission from The Association of Bone and Joint Surgeons.)

Methodologic quality was assessed with the Consolidated Standards of Reporting Trials (CONSORT) checklist, and 22 RCTs containing 2280 patients were included. Pooled analyses were performed to evaluate overall improvement requirement for escape interventions (treatment of any kind, outside consultation, and surgery) outcome scores (Patient-Rated Tennis Elbow Evaluation [PRTEE] DASH Pain-Free Function Index [PFFI] Euro-QoL [EQ]-5D and overall function) and maximum and pain-free grip strength. Sensitivity analyses were performed using only trials of excellent or good quality. Heterogeneity analyses were performed, and funnel plots were constructed to assess for publication bias.

Results.—Nonsurgical treatment was not favored over nontreatment based on overall improvement (risk ratio [RR] = 1.05 [0.96−1.15] $p = 0.32$), need for escape treatment (RR = 1.50 [0.84−2.70] $p = 0.17$), PRTEE scores (mean difference [MD] = 1.47, [0.68−2.26] $p < 0.001$), DASH scores (MD = −2.69, [−15.80 to 10.42] $p = 0.69$), PFFI scores (standardized mean difference [SMD] = 0.25, [−0.32 to 0.81] $p = 0.39$), overall function using change-from-baseline data (SMD = 0.11, [−0.14 to 0.36] $p = 0.37$) and final data (SMD = −0.16, [−0.79 to 0.47] $p = 0.61$), EQ-5D scores (SMD = 0.08, [−0.52 to 0.67] $p = 0.80$), maximum grip strength using change-from-baseline data (SMD = 0.12, [−0.11 to 0.35] $p = 0.31$) and final data (SMD = 4.37, [−0.65 to 9.38] $p = 0.09$), and pain-free grip strength using change-from-baseline data (SMD = −0.20, [−0.84 to 0.43] $p = 0.53$) and final data (SMD = −0.03, [−0.61 to 0.54] $p = 0.91$).

Conclusions.—Pooled data from RCTs indicate a lack of intermediate-to long-term clinical benefit after nonsurgical treatment of lateral epicondylitis compared with observation only or placebo.

Level of Evidence.—Level II, therapeutic study (Fig 3).

▶ I am drawn to meta-analyses, especially those that consider controversial questions. With growing concern about the use of cortisone injections being associated with poorer long-term outcomes, this study of the literature is particularly relevant. Despite individual articles touting the benefits of a host of non-operative treatments, this study of 22 randomized controlled trials found little advantage of various interventions to simple observation. The lack of statistical significance is reflected in the forest plot (Fig 3).

It should be noted, however, that this study does not suggest that all patients responded, just that there is no real difference to observation and the various interventions investigated.

B. F. Morrey, MD

Long-term Outcomes After Ulnar Collateral Ligament Reconstruction in Competitive Baseball Players: Minimum 10-Year Follow-up

Osbahr DC, Cain EL Jr, Raines BT, et al (Orlando Health Orthopedic Inst, FL; American Sports Medicine Inst, Birmingham, AL; Univ of Alabama at Birmingham School of Medicine)

Am J Sports Med 42:1333-1342, 2014

Background.—Ulnar collateral ligament reconstruction (UCLR) has afforded baseball players with excellent results; however, previous studies have described only short-term outcomes.

Purpose.—To evaluate long-term outcomes after UCLR in baseball players.

Study Design.—Case series; Level of evidence, 4.

Methods.—All UCLRs performed on competitive baseball players with a minimum 10-year follow-up were identified. Surgical data were collected prospectively and patients were surveyed by telephone follow-up, during which scoring systems were used to assess baseball career and post-baseball career outcomes.

Results.—Of 313 patients, 256 (82%) were contacted at an average of 12.6 years; 83% of these baseball players (90% pitchers) were able to return to the same or higher level of competition in less than 1 year, but results varied according to preoperative level of play. Baseball career longevity was 3.6 years in general and 2.9 years at the same or higher level of play, but major and minor league players returned for longer than did collegiate and high school players after surgery ($P < .001$). Baseball retirement typically occurred for reasons other than elbow problems (86%). Many players had shoulder problems (34%) or surgery (25%) during their baseball career, and these occurrences most often resulted in retirement attributable to shoulder problems ($P < .001$). For post—baseball career outcomes, 92% of patients were able to throw without pain, and 98% were still able to participate in throwing at least on a recreational level. The 10-year minimum follow-up scores (mean ± standard deviation) for the Disabilities of the Arm, Shoulder and Hand (DASH), DASH work module, and DASH sports module were 0.80 ± 4.43, 1.10 ± 6.90, and 2.88 ± 11.91, respectively. Overall, 93% of patients were satisfied, with few reports of persistent elbow pain (3%) or limitation of function (5%).

Conclusion.—Long-term follow-up of UCLRs in baseball players indicates that most patients were satisfied, with few reports of persistent elbow pain or limitation of function. During their baseball career, most of these athletes were able to return to the same or higher level of competition in less than 1 year, with acceptable career longevity and retirement typically for reasons other than the elbow. According to a standardized disability and outcome scale, patients also had excellent results after UCLR during daily, work, and sporting activities.

▶ I am pleased to see this report because it is the definitive word on this well-recognized condition. That more than 250 patients were followed for more than 10 years is an amazing accomplishment. As mentioned above, I would therefore consider these findings to be definitive. Although more than 80% of competitive players returned to the same level of competition, 90% of these were pitchers. Furthermore, new information is that the mean duration of the career is about 3 years, also very useful information when discussing with a potential candidate for the surgery. Finally, more than 90% were satisfied overall with the surgery, indicating that the problems with the ulnar nerve have largely been resolved.

B. F. Morrey, MD

Delayed-Onset Ulnar Neuritis After Release of Elbow Contractures: Clinical Presentation, Pathological Findings, and Treatment
Blonna D, Huffmann GR, O'Driscoll SW (Mayo Clinic, Rochester, MN)
Am J Sports Med 42:2113-2121, 2014

Background.—Little information exists regarding delayed-onset ulnar neuritis (DOUN) after arthroscopic release of elbow contractures.

Purpose.—To describe, in a large cohort of patients, the clinical presentation of and risk factors for developing DOUN after arthroscopic release of elbow contractures.

Study Design.—Case-control study; Level of evidence, 3.

Methods.—A retrospective study of 565 consecutive arthroscopic releases of elbow contractures was conducted. Essentially, DOUN was defined as ulnar neuritis or neuropathy, or worsening of pre-existing ulnar nerve symptoms, that developed postoperatively in patients with normal neurological examination findings immediately after surgery. After inclusion and exclusion criteria were met, 235 contracture releases in patients who had not undergone any ulnar nerve surgery remained and were used for the analysis of risk factors with a multivariate logistic regression analysis.

Results.—Twenty-six patients (11%) developed DOUN. The patients fell into 1 of 3 distinct groups. Fifteen (58%) presented with rapidly progressive DOUN, characterized by rapidly progressive sensorimotor ulnar neuropathy, increasing pain at the cubital tunnel during end-range flexion and/or extension, and rapidly deteriorating range of motion within the first week after surgery. Urgent ulnar subcutaneous nerve transposition

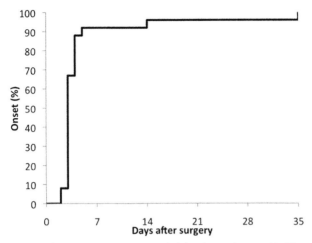

FIGURE 1.—Onset of symptoms in 23 patients with delayedonset ulnar neuritis. The graph does not include data of the 3 patients for whom the time of onset was not known. (Reprinted from Blonna D, Huffmann GR, O'Driscoll SW. Delayed-onset ulnar neuritis after release of elbow contractures: clinical presentation, pathological findings, and treatment. *Am J Sports Med.* 2014;42:2113-2121, with permission from The Author(s).)

was performed within 1 or 2 days of diagnosis. Eight (31%) presented with nonprogressive DOUN, characterized by mild sensory ulnar neuropathy, neither motor weakness nor substantial pain at the cubital tunnel, or loss of motion. Three (12%) presented with slowly progressive DOUN, characterized by the insidious onset of mild ulnar neuropathy. Significant risk factors for DOUN included a diagnosis of heterotopic ossification (odds ratio, 31; 95% CI, 5-191; $P < .001$), preoperative neurological symptoms (odds ratio, 6; 95% CI, 2-19; $P = .001$), and preoperative arc of motion (odds ratio, 0.97 per degree of motion; 95% CI, 0.96-0.99; $P = .02$).

Conclusion.—Delayed-onset ulnar neuritis is an important complication of arthroscopic release of elbow contractures. We recommend a high index of suspicion and monitoring patients with progressive loss of elbow motion and end-range pain for evidence of subclinical ulnar neuritis (Fig 1).

▶ The relevance of ulnar neuritis and treatment of stiff elbow has been known for some time. This in-depth assessment of arthroscopically treated patients provides objective insights into the circumstances that increase the likelihood of the occurrence of delayed ulnar neuritis and the implications of its development. The risk factors statistically demonstrated to be relevant are those with more limited preoperative arcs of motion, those with ulnar nerve symptoms preoperatively, and the presence of heterotopic bone. Most diagnoses are made between the third and fourth day after surgery (Fig 1). The authors document the value of early recognition and decompression. Currently, the recommendation is to release those with risk factors at the time of the capsular release.

B. F. Morrey, MD

Capitellar Fractures—Is Open Reduction and Internal Fixation Necessary?
Cutbush K, Andrews S, Siddiqui N, et al (Brisbane Hand and Upper Limb Research Inst, Australia)
J Orthop Trauma 29:50-53, 2015

Objective.—The purpose of this retrospective study was to evaluate the medium-term to longer-term results of type 1 displaced capitellar fractures treated with closed reduction.

Design.—Retrospective case series.

Patients.—Eight consecutive cases (7 adults; 1 child) with type 1 capitellar fractures.

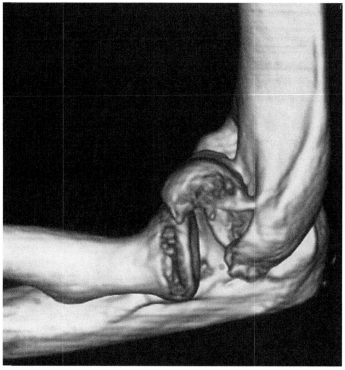

FIGURE 2.—Computed tomography of the same injury. *Editor's note:* A color image accompanies the online version of this article. (Reprinted from Cutbush K, Andrews S, Siddiqui N, et al. Capitellar fractures-is open reduction and internal fixation necessary? *J Orthop Trauma.* 2015;29:50-53, with permission from Lippincott Williams & Wilkins.)

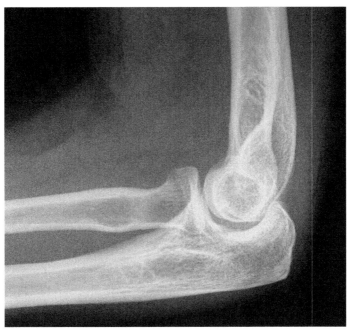

FIGURE 3.—Lateral radiograph 6 months after injury in the same patient showing complete union with no avascular necrosis or joint degeneration. (Reprinted from Cutbush K, Andrews S, Siddiqui N, et al. Capitellar fractures-is open reduction and internal fixation necessary? *J Orthop Trauma.* 2015;29:50-53, with permission from Lippincott Williams & Wilkins.)

Intervention.—Closed reduction of type 1 capitellar fractures and 4 weeks of postreduction immobilization.

Outcome Measures.—Complications (including radiographic), Disabilities of the Arm, Shoulder, and Hand Score, and active elbow range of motion.

Results.—Average follow-up was 41.6 months (range, 18–77 months). All 8 fractures were united. The patients obtained near full return of the range of motion when compared with the uninjured contralateral side. Mean average Disabilities of the Arm, Shoulder, and Hand Score scores were 4.36 (SD, 2.68; Range, 0–9). No complications were observed.

Conclusions.—This study demonstrated that type 1 capitellar fractures can be treated successfully with closed reduction and cast immobilization.

Level of Evidence.—Therapeutic Level IV. See Instructions for Authors for a complete description of levels of evidence (Figs 2 and 3).

▶ We don't review too many case series anymore, but this was selected because it counters the trend to open the Type I capitellar fracture. I was impressed the authors were able to reduce all 8 fractures by extending the elbow and exerting direct pressure on the anteriorly displaced fracture fragment (Figs 2 and 3). With 4 weeks' immobilization, an arc of motion lacking only about 10 degrees of extension was obtained with no evidence of arthritis or pain at an average of 3.5 years would certainly rival the open procedure. I think this does prompt surgeons to at least try the closed reduction. If it is not successful, then proceed to open reduction and internal fixation.

B. F. Morrey, MD

Can We Treat Select Terrible Triad Injuries Nonoperatively?
Chan K, MacDermid JC, Faber KJ, et al (McMaster Univ, Hamilton, Ontario; Univ of Western Ontario, London, Ontario)
Clin Orthop Relat Res 472:2092-2099, 2014

Background.—While the majority of terrible triad elbow injuries (ulnohumeral dislocation with radial head and coronoid fractures) are managed surgically, nonoperative treatment may be appropriate in selected patients, but results with this approach have been limited by very small studies.

Questions/Purposes.—We assessed (1) functional outcomes using two validated questionnaires, (2) elbow ROM, strength, and stability, (3) the presence of union and arthritis on radiographs, and (4) complications among a group of patients managed nonoperatively for terrible triad injuries.

Methods.—Between 2006 and 2012, we retrospectively identified 12 patients with terrible triad elbow injuries who were treated nonoperatively and met the following criteria: (1) a concentric joint reduction, (2) a radial head fracture that did not cause a mechanical block to rotation, (3) a smaller coronoid fracture (Regan-Morrey Type 1 or 2), and (4) a stable arc of motion to a minimum of 30° of extension to allow active motion within the first 10 days. Eleven patients were available for followup of at least 12 months after the injury (mean, 36 months; range, 12–90 months). Outcome measures included two patient-reported functional outcome measures (DASH, Mayo Elbow Performance Index [MEPI]), a standardized physical examination to record elbow ROM and stability, isometric strength measurements, and radiographic evidence of bony union and elbow arthrosis. Complications were also recorded.

Results.—At latest followup, mean ± SD DASH score was 8.0 ± 11.0 and mean MEPI score was 94 ± 9. Mean ROM of the affected elbow was 134° ± 5° flexion, 6° ± 8° extension, 87° ± 4° pronation, and 82° ± 10° supination. No instability was detected. Strength assessments demonstrated the following mean percentages of the contralateral, unaffected elbow: flexion 100%, extension 89%, pronation 79%, and supination 89%. Four patients had arthritic changes on radiographs that did not call for treatment as of latest followup. Complications included one patient who underwent surgical stabilization for early recurrent instability and another who underwent arthroscopic débridement for heterotopic bone.

Conclusions.—In selected patients, nonoperative treatment of terrible triad injuries is an option that can provide good function and restore stable elbow ROM. However, nonoperative management requires close clinical

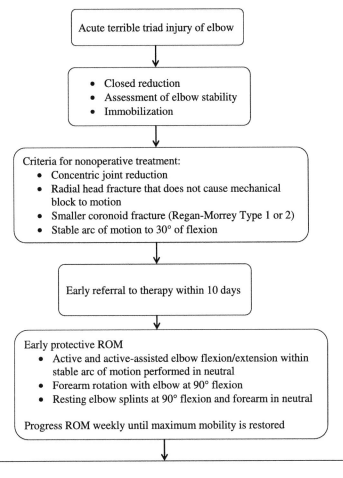

Acute terrible triad injury of elbow

- Closed reduction
- Assessment of elbow stability
- Immobilization

Criteria for nonoperative treatment:
- Concentric joint reduction
- Radial head fracture that does not cause mechanical block to motion
- Smaller coronoid fracture (Regan-Morrey Type 1 or 2)
- Stable arc of motion to 30° of flexion

Early referral to therapy within 10 days

Early protective ROM
- Active and active-assisted elbow flexion/extension within stable arc of motion performed in neutral
- Forearm rotation with elbow at 90° flexion
- Resting elbow splints at 90° flexion and forearm in neutral

Progress ROM weekly until maximum mobility is restored

After 6 weeks
- Static progressive extension splinting as required to manage flexion contractures
- Strengthening with sufficient soft tissue and bony healing

FIGURE 1.—The therapeutic algorithm for the nonoperative management of acute terrible triad elbow injuries is shown. (With kind permission from Springer Science+Business Media: Chan K, MacDermid JC, Faber KJ, et al. Can we treat select terrible triad injuries nonoperatively? *Clin Orthop Relat Res.* 2014;472:2092-2099, with permission from The Association of Bone and Joint Surgeons.)

and radiographic followup to monitor for any delayed elbow subluxation or fracture displacement.

Level of Evidence.—Level IV, therapeutic study. See Instructions for Authors for a complete description of levels of evidence (Fig 1).

▶ This is an important contribution because it offers objective data to reverse a misunderstanding of current treatment. Some have suggested that virtually every coronoid fracture, even the Regan-Morrey type 1, needs to be fixed. This is not borne out by the experience of many practitioners. The first key is to understand the features of the injury that justify nonoperative intervention (Fig 1) The second key is to appreciate the critical size of the coronoid fragment that may be consistent with a stable ulnohumeral joint, even if not fixed. This is a type II coronoid fracture or smaller.

B. F. Morrey, MD

Anconeus Interposition Arthroplasty: Mid- to Long-term Results
Baghdadi YMK, Morrey BF, Sanchez-Sotelo J (Mayo Clinic, Rochester, MN)
Clin Orthop Relat Res 472:2151-2161, 2014

Background.—Radiocapitellar arthritis and/or proximal radioulnar impingement can be difficult to treat. Interposition of the anconeus muscle has been described in the past as an alternative option in managing arthritis, but there are little published data about relief of pain and restoration of function over the long term in patients treated with this approach.

Questions/Purposes.—We sought (1) to determine whether interposition of the anconeus muscle in the radiocapitellar and/or proximal radioulnar joint relieves pain and restores elbow function; and (2) to identify complications and reoperations after anconeus interposition arthroplasty.

Methods.—Between 1992 and 2012, we surgically treated 39 patients having radiocapitellar arthritis and/or proximal radioulnar impingement with an anconeus interposition arthroplasty. These were performed for situations in which capitellar and/or radial head pathology was deemed not amenable to implant replacement. We had complete followup on 29 of them (74%) at a minimum of 1 year (mean, 10 years; range, 1–20 years). These 29 patients (21 males, eight females) had interposition of the anconeus muscle at the radiocapitellar joint (10 elbows), the proximal radioulnar joint (two elbows), or both (17 elbows). Their mean age at the time of surgery was 39 years (range, 14–58 years). The reasons for the previous determination or the indications included lateral-side elbow symptoms after radial head resection (eight elbows), failed internal fixation of radial head fracture (two elbows), failed radial head replacement with or without capitellar replacement (four elbows), osteoarthritis and Essex-Lopresti injury (six elbows), failed internal fixation of distal humeral fracture involving the capitellum (two elbows), posttraumatic osteoarthritis involving the lateral compartment (one elbow), lateral compartment osteoarthritis associated with chondropathies (three elbows), and primary osteoarthritis affecting the lateral compartment (three elbows). Patient-reported outcome tools included the quick-Disabilities of the Arm, Shoulder and Hand (quick-DASH) and the Mayo Elbow Performance Score (MEPS); we also performed a chart review for complications and reoperations.

Results.—During the followup duration, the mean MEPS was significantly improved from (mean ± SD) 64 ± 17 points before surgery to

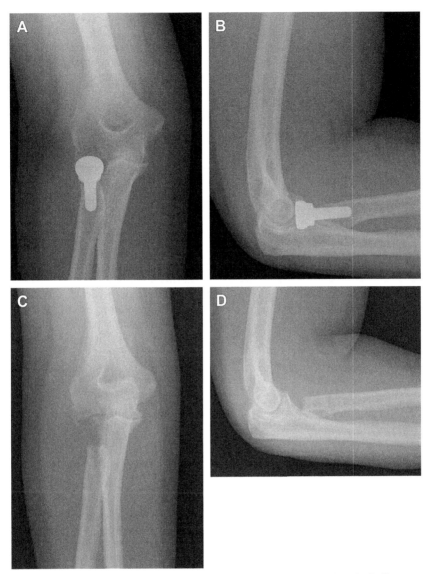

FIGURE 2.—(A) Preoperative AP and (B) lateral radiographs of a patient with lateral-side elbow pain and stiffness after radial head replacement with progressive capitellar erosion are shown. (C—D) Postoperative radiographs after contracture release, implant removal, and anconeus interposition showed no evidence of progressive valgus angulation, proximal radius migration, or progressive osteoarthritis. (With kind permission from Springer Science+Business Media: Baghdadi YM, Morrey BF, Sanchez-Sotelo J. Anconeus interposition arthroplasty: mid- to long-term results. *Clin Orthop Relat Res.* 2014;472:2151-2161, with permission from The Association of Bone and Joint Surgeons.)

82 ± 14 points after surgery ($p < 0.001$) with 21 elbows (72%) graded as excellent or good at most recent followup. The mean quick-DASH score was 24 ± 17 points (n = 25) at latest evaluation. Two patients (7%) had perioperative complications, including wound dehiscence (one elbow) and transient posterior interosseous nerve palsy (one elbow). Seven patients (24%) underwent additional surgery.

Conclusions.—Anconeus arthroplasty provides a reasonable surgical alternative in the armamentarium of procedures to address pathology at the radiocapitellar and/or proximal radioulnar joint. This procedure is especially attractive when other alternatives such as radial head replacement may be problematic secondary to capitellar erosion or marked proximal radius bone loss.

Level of Evidence.—Level IV, therapeutic study. See Guidelines for Authors for a complete description of levels of evidence (Fig 2).

▶ This contribution is included because it represents a reconstructive technique for the radiohumeral joint that can be performed by the well-prepared surgeon, even without formal training in elbow surgery. I personally elect not to replace the radial head unless this is the only option. However, there are few alternatives to prosthetic replacement for lateral elbow arthritis or laxity. This no-replacement option was studied over a 20-year period with a mean surveillance of 10 years. The 70% satisfactory outcomes would seem acceptable if this were to be considered a salvage reconstructive option, which is the way the authors view it (Fig 2a-d).

B. F. Morrey, MD

5 Shoulder

Introduction

Several years ago, I found upon review of my selections that almost the entire Shoulder section related to rotator cuff disease. I have, therefore, been very careful since then to try to limit the material dealing with the rotator cuff. However, this has not changed the fact that rotator cuff pathology and its treatment is probably the single most important topic for the general orthopedic surgeon, just as it is for the shoulder specialist. Therefore, this section includes what I consider to be relevant discussions of this topic. There is also an appropriate mix of contributions relating to other major issues, such as shoulder instability. Because shoulder replacement is typically reserved for those with special interest, there is relatively little on this topic. However, I have added a few articles in order to demonstrate the status of shoulder replacement. If nothing else, it allows the surgeon an opportunity to be aware of this situation should he or she elect to refer a patient for consideration of joint replacement. Overall, the shoulder is a very active area of growth in orthopedics, and hopefully this is reflected in the literature that has been reviewed in this section.

Bernard F. Morrey, MD

A retrospective analysis of 509 consecutive interscalene catheter insertions for ambulatory surgery
Marhofer P, Anderl W, Heuberer P, et al (Med Univ of Vienna, Austria; St. Vincent Hosp, Vienna, Austria)
Anaesthesia 70:41-46, 2015

Effective pain therapy after shoulder surgery is the main prerequisite for safe management in an ambulatory setting. We evaluated adverse events and hospital re-admission using a database of 509 interscalene catheters inserted during ambulatory shoulder surgery. Adverse events were recorded for 34 (6.7%) patients (9 (1.8%) catheter dislocations diagnosed in the recovery room, 9 (1.8%) catheter dislocations at home with pain, 2 (0.4%) pain without catheter dislocation, 1 (0.2%) 'secondary' pneumothorax without intervention and 13 (2.6%) other). Twelve (2.4%) patients were re-admitted to hospital (8 (1.6%) for pain, 2 (0.4%) for dyspnoea and 2 (0.4%) for nausea and vomiting), 9 of whom had rotator cuff repair. A well-organised infrastructure, optimally trained medical professionals and appropriate patient selection are the main prerequisites for the safe, effective implementation of ambulatory interscalene catheters in routine clinical practice.

▶ With the growing tendency for outpatient surgery, an essential element in the process includes home-going pain control. A complication rate of about 6% after more than 500 shoulder procedures is impressive. A readmission rate of only about 2% supports the authors' conclusion that an indwelling scalene catheter is a safe and effective means of pain control. That this study originates from Austria underscores the reality of cost-effective outpatient surgery as desirable globally.

B. F. Morrey, MD

Cytotoxic Effects of Ropivacaine, Bupivacaine, and Lidocaine on Rotator Cuff Tenofibroblasts

Sung C-M, Hah Y-S, Kim J-S, et al (Gyeongsang Natl Univ, Jinju, Korea; Gyeongsang Natl Univ Hosp, Jinju, Korea; Eulji Univ, Seoul, Korea; et al)
Am J Sports Med 42:2888-2896, 2014

Background.—Concern has recently arisen over the safety of local anesthetics used on human tissues.

Hypothesis.—Aminoamide local anesthetics have cytotoxic effects on human rotator cuff tenofibroblasts.

Study Design.—Controlled laboratory study.

Methods.—Cultured human rotator cuff tenofibroblasts were divided into control, phosphate buffered saline (PBS), and local anesthetic study groups; the PBS study group was further subdivided by pH level (pH 7.4, 6.0, and 4.4). The 6 local anesthetic subgroups (0.2% and 0.75% ropivacaine, 0.25% and 0.5% bupivacaine, and 1% and 2% lidocaine) were also studied at 10% dilutions of their original concentrations. Exposure times were 5, 10, 20, 40, or 60 minutes for the higher concentrations and 2, 6, 12, 24, 48, or 72 hours for the lower concentrations. Cell viability was evaluated through live, apoptotic, and necrotic cell rates using the annexin V–propidium iodide double-staining method. Intracellular reactive oxygen species (ROS) and the activity of mitogen-activated protein kinases (MAPKs) and caspase-3/7 were investigated.

Results.—The control and PBS groups showed no significant differences in cell viability ($P > .999$). In the local anesthetic study groups, cell viability decreased significantly with increases in anesthetic concentrations ($P < .001$) and exposure times ($P < .001$), with the exception of the lidocaine subgroups, where this effect was masked by the very high cytotoxicity of even low concentrations. Among the studied local anesthetic subgroups, 0.2% ropivacaine was the least toxic. The levels of intracellular ROS of

Higher concentration study

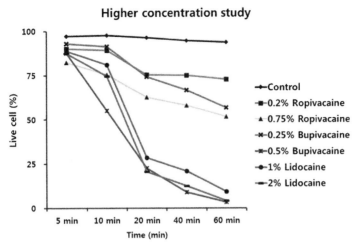

FIGURE 1.—Cytotoxicity of various aminoamide local anesthetics. (A) The higher concentration study demonstrated significant differences between the rate of live cells in the control group and the rate in each of the local anesthetic subgroups ($P < .001$). The live cell rates decreased significantly in an exposure time−dependent manner in all the local anesthetic subgroups ($P < .001$) in both the higher concentration and lower concentration studies. (Reprinted from Sung C-M, Hah Y-S, Kim J-S, et al. Cytotoxic effects of ropivacaine, bupivacaine, and lidocaine on rotator cuff tenofibroblasts. *Am J Sports Med.* 2014;42:2888-2896, with permission from The Author(s).)

each local anesthetic subgroup also increased significantly ($P < .05$). The studied local anesthetics showed increases in the phosphorylation of extracellular signal−regulated kinase 1/2 (ERK1/2), c-Jun N-terminal kinase (JNK), and p38 as well as in levels of caspase-3/7 activity ($P < .001$).

Conclusion.—The cytotoxicity of the anesthetics studied to tenofibroblasts is dependent on exposure time and concentration. Of the evaluated anesthetics, ropivacaine is the least toxic in the clinically used concentration. The studied anesthetics induce tenofibroblast cell death, mediated by the increased production of ROS, by the increased activation of ERK1/2, JNK, and p38 and by the activation of caspase-3/7.

Clinical Relevance.—This study identified the cytotoxic mechanisms of aminoamide local anesthetics acting on rotator cuff tenofibroblasts. The greatest margin of safety was found in lower anesthetic concentrations in general and more specifically in the use of ropivacaine (Fig 1).

▶ The adverse effects of local anesthetic on normal cartilage have been recognized in recent years, especially when administered to the shoulder joint. This study furthers our understanding of the potential adverse effects of various local anesthetic agents on the potential healing of the rotator cuff tenofibroblasts. The precise mechanism of the cytotoxicity was clearly elucidated. Of relevance to the surgeon is that there is wide variation among the 3 agents studied, with ropivacaine being less toxic than lidocaine or bupivacaine (Fig 1A). As demonstrated in the figure, there is wide variation according to agent, concentration, and duration of exposure.

B. F. Morrey, MD

Are Serum Lipids Involved in Primary Frozen Shoulder? A Case-Control Study

Sung C-M, Jung TS, Park HB (Gyeongsang Natl Univ, Jinju, Republic of Korea)
J Bone Joint Surg Am 96:1828-1833, 2014

Background.—Hyperlipidemia is a proposed, but unproven, risk factor for primary frozen shoulder. The purpose of this study was to evaluate the association between serum lipid profiles and primary frozen shoulder.

Methods.—This was a case-control study. The case group comprised 300 patients diagnosed with frozen shoulder from October 2009 to April 2013. Patients with diabetes, thyroid disease, or previous shoulder surgery or trauma were excluded. The control group comprised 900 age and sex-matched persons with normal shoulder function who visited our health promotion center for general check-ups during the same period. We calculated the odds ratios and 95% confidence intervals to identify any association between serum lipid level and primary frozen shoulder, using conditional logistic regression analysis. We evaluated continuous data on the serum levels of total cholesterol, calculated low-density lipoprotein, measured low-density lipoprotein, high-density lipoprotein, triglyceride, and non-high-density lipoprotein cholesterol. We also evaluated categorical data on hyper-cholesterolemia, hyper-low-density lipoproteinemia (calculated and measured), hyper-high-density lipoproteinemia, hyper-triglyceridemia, and hyper-non-high-density lipoprotein cholesterolemia.

Results.—Univariate analysis of the continuous data showed total cholesterol (odds ratio, 1.010 [95% confidence interval, 1.006 to 1.013]; $p < 0.001$), calculated low-density lipoprotein (odds ratio, 1.008 [95% confidence interval, 1.004 to 1.012]; $p < 0.001$), measured low-density lipoprotein (odds ratio, 1.007 [95% confidence interval, 1.003 to 1.011]; $p = 0.001$), high-density lipoprotein (odds ratio, 1.015 [95% confidence interval, 1.006 to 1.024]; $p = 0.001$), and non-high-density lipoprotein cholesterol (odds ratio, 1.007 [95% confidence interval, 1.004 to 1.011]; $p < 0.001$) to be significantly associated with primary frozen shoulder. Univariate analysis of categorical values showed hyper-cholesterolemia (odds ratio, 1.789 [95% confidence interval, 1.366 to 2.343]; $p < 0.001$), calculated hyper-low-density lipoproteinemia (odds ratio, 1.609 [95% confidence interval, 1.210 to 2.138]; $p = 0.001$), measured hyper-low-density lipoproteinemia (odds ratio, 1.643 [95% confidence interval, 1.190 to 2.269]; $p = 0.003$), hyper-high-density lipoproteinemia (odds ratio, 1.440 [95% confidence interval, 1.062 to 1.953]; $p = 0.019$), and hyper-non-high-density lipoprotein cholesterolemia (odds ratio, 1.645 [95%

TABLE 2.—Univariate Conditional Logistic Regression Analyses for Various Serum Lipids

	Odds Ratio*	P Value
Total cholesterol	1.010 (1.006 to 1.013)	<0.001
Calculated low-density lipoprotein	1.008 (1.004 to 1.012)	<0.001
Measured low-density lipoprotein	1.007 (1.003 to 1.011)	0.001
High-density lipoprotein	1.015 (1.006 to 1.024)	0.001
Triglyceride	1.001 (0.999 to 1.002)	0.451
Non-high-density lipoprotein cholesterol	1.007 (1.004 to 1.011)	<0.001

*The values are given as the odds ratio, with the 95% CI in parentheses.
Sung C-M, Jung TS, Park HB. Are Serum Lipids Involved in Primary Frozen Shoulder? A Case-Control Study. *J Bone Joint Surg Am.* 2014;96:1828-1833. http://jbjs.org/.

confidence interval, 1.259 to 2.151]; $p < 0.001$) to be significantly associated with primary frozen shoulder.

Conclusions.—We conclude that hypercholesterolemia and inflammatory lipoproteinemias, particularly hyper-low-density lipoproteinemia and hyper-non-high-density lipoprotein cholesterolemia, have a significant association with primary frozen shoulder. Further research is needed to evaluate whether a non-optimal serum lipid level is a cause, a related co-factor, or a result of primary frozen shoulder (Table 2).

▶ Frozen shoulder is not only a common condition, but the etiology is still poorly understood. This current study is well controlled with sufficient power ($n = 300$) to allow the hypothesis to be validly addressed. Simply stated, this analysis reveals a statistical correlation between hyperlipidemia and the presence of frozen shoulder. All elements of the lipid panel are elevated, with the exception of triglycerides (Table 2). Although this is an important finding, it does not define whether this association has a true cause-and-effect influence or is associated with a third variable. Regardless, it is interesting to speculate and to consider assessing and treating hyperlipidemia in this patient population.

B. F. Morrey, MD

Hill-Sachs Lesions in Shoulders With Traumatic Anterior Instability: Evaluation Using Computed Tomography With 3-Dimensional Reconstruction

Ozaki R, Nakagawa S, Mizuno N, et al (Toyonaka Municipal Hosp, Osaka, Japan; Yukioka Hosp, Osaka, Japan; et al)
Am J Sports Med 42:2597-2605, 2014

Background.—In patients with traumatic anterior shoulder instability, a large Hill-Sachs lesion is a risk factor for postoperative recurrence. However, there is no consensus regarding the occurrence and enlargement of Hill-Sachs lesions.

Purpose.—To investigate the influence of the number of dislocations and subluxations on the prevalence and size of Hill-Sachs lesions evaluated by computed tomography (CT) with 3-dimensional reconstruction.

Study Design.—Cohort study (diagnosis); Level of evidence, 2.

Methods.—The prevalence and size of Hill-Sachs lesions were evaluated preoperatively by CT in 142 shoulders (30 with primary instability and 112 with recurrent instability) before arthroscopic Bankart repair. First, the prevalence of Hill-Sachs lesions was compared with the arthroscopic findings. Then, the size of Hill-Sachs lesions confirmed by arthroscopy was remeasured using the previous CT data. In addition, the relationship of Hill-Sachs lesions with the number of dislocations and subluxations was investigated.

Results.—Hill-Sachs lesions were detected in 90 shoulders by initial CT evaluation and were found in 118 shoulders at arthroscopy. The Hill-Sachs lesions missed by initial CT were 15 chondral lesions and 13 osseous lesions. However, all 103 osseous Hill-Sachs lesions were detected by reviewing the CT data. In patients with primary subluxation, the prevalence of Hill-Sachs lesions was 26.7%, and the mean length, width, and depth of the lesions (calculated as a percentage of the diameter of the humeral head) were 9.0%, 5.3%, and 2.1%, respectively, while the corresponding numbers for primary dislocation were 73.3%, 27.7%, 14.8%, and 7.0%, all showing statistically significant differences. Among all 142 shoulders, the corresponding numbers were, respectively, 56.3%,

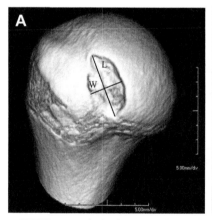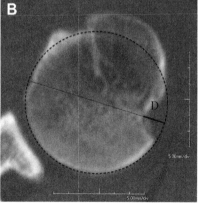

FIGURE 1.—Methods of measuring the size of the Hill-Sachs lesions. (A) Measurement of the length and width of the Hill-Sachs lesion was performed with the Aquarius Net Station with en face 3-dimensional reconstructed computed tomography images showing the lesion. The length of the major axis was measured as the length of the Hill-Sachs lesion, L, and the length of the minor axis was measured as the width, W. (B) On the axial images obtained perpendicular to the longitudinal axis of the humeral shaft, a virtual circle that included the articular surface of the humeral head was drawn, and the longest length between the base of the Hill-Sachs lesion and the corresponding arc was measured as the depth, D. In the axial slice with the largest circle, the diameter of the circle was defined as that of the humeral head. Each measurement was divided by the diameter of the humeral head and calculated as a percentage. (Reprinted from Ozaki R, Nakagawa S, Mizuno N, et al. Hill-sachs lesions in shoulders with traumatic anterior instability: Evaluation using computed tomography with 3-dimensional reconstruction. *Am J Sports Med.* 2014;42:2597-2605, with permission from The Author(s).)

TABLE 1.—Prevalence of Hill-Sachs Lesions: Comparison Between CT (Initial Evaluation) and Arthroscopic Findings[a]

Hill-Sachs Lesion by CT, n	Hill-Sachs Lesion at Arthroscopy, n	
	Positive	Negative
Positive	90	0
Negative	28	24

[a]CT, computed tomography.

Reprinted from Ozaki R, Nakagawa S, Mizuno N, et al. Hill-sachs lesions in shoulders with traumatic anterior instability: Evaluation using computed tomography with 3-dimensional reconstruction. *Am J Sports Med.* 2014;42:2597—2605, with permission from The Author(s).

TABLE 4.—Correlation Between Prevalence and Size of Hill-Sachs Lesions and Number of Dislocations: All Shoulders (in Percentages)

	No. of Dislocations			
	0 (n = 64)	1 (n = 30)	≥2 (n = 48)	P Value
Prevalence	56.3	83.3	87.5	<.001
Size, mean ± SD[a]				
Length	20.7 ± 22.1	33.4 ± 20.2	46.8 ± 21.9	<.001
Width	11.2 ± 11.5	19.1 6 10.9	22.2 ± 10.2	<.001
Depth	4.8 ± 4.8	7.6 ± 4.5	10.2 ± 5.4	<.001

[a]Calculated as a percentage of the diameter of the humeral head.

Reprinted from Ozaki R, Nakagawa S, Mizuno N, et al. Hill-sachs lesions in shoulders with traumatic anterior instability: Evaluation using computed tomography with 3-dimensional reconstruction. *Am J Sports Med.* 2014;42:2597—2605, with permission from The Author(s).

20.7%, 11.2%, and 4.8% in patients who had subluxations but never a dislocation; 83.3%, 33.4%, 19.1%, and 7.6% in patients with 1 episode of dislocation; and 87.5%, 46.8%, 22.2%, and 10.2% in patients with ≥2 episodes, all showing statistically significant differences. There were no differences in lesion measurements in relation to the number of subluxations.

Conclusion.—Computed tomography is a useful imaging modality for evaluating Hill-Sachs lesions except for purely cartilaginous lesions. Hill-Sachs lesions were more frequent and larger when the primary episode was dislocation than when it was subluxation. Among patients with recurrent episodes of complete dislocation, the prevalence of Hill-Sachs lesions is increased, and the lesions are larger (Fig 1, Tables 1 and 4).

▶ Shoulder dislocation is the most common traumatic event of the shoulder requiring physician attention. The role of the Hill-Sachs lesion in recurrence and the implication for proper management is continuing to be elucidated. Emphasis is placed on the inability of a 2-dimensional image to properly characterize the size of the lesion. The computed tomography (CT) scan has been widely adopted to better estimate the size and significance of this osseous defect (Fig 1). The data from this study clearly show the high degree of sensitivity and specificity of the CT scan (Table 1). Finally, the significance of understanding the presence and size of the lesion is demonstrated with a direct correlation between the presence and size of the lesion and subsequent instability (Table 4).

B. F. Morrey, MD

Evidence in managing traumatic anterior shoulder instability: a scoping review

Monk AP, Roberts PG, Logishetty K, et al (Rheumatology and Musculoskeletal Sciences, Oxford, UK; Nuffield Orthopaedic Centre, Oxford, UK; et al)
Br J Sports Med 49:307-311, 2015

Background.—Traumatic anterior shoulder instability (TASI) accounts for 95% of glenohumeral dislocations and is associated with soft tissue and bony pathoanatomies. Non-operative treatments include slings, bracing and physiotherapy. Operative treatment is common, including bony and soft-tissue reconstructions performed through open or arthroscopic approaches. There is management variation in patient pathways for TASI including when to refer and when to operate.

Methods.—A scoping review of systematic reviews, randomised controlled trials, comparing operative with non-operative treatments and different operative treatments were the methods followed. Search was conducted for online bibliographic databases and reference lists of relevant articles from 2002 to 2012. Systematic reviews were appraised using AMSTAR (assessment of multiple systematic reviews) criteria. Controlled trials were appraised using the CONSORT (consolidation of standards of reporting trials) tool.

Results.—Analysis of the reviews did not offer strong evidence for a best treatment option for TASI. No studies directly compare open, arthroscopic and structured rehabilitation programmes. Evaluation of arthroscopic studies and comparison to open procedures was difficult, as many of the arthroscopic techniques included are no longer used. Recurrence rate was generally considered the best measure of operative success, but was poorly documented throughout all studies. There was conflicting evidence on the optimal timing of intervention and no consensus on any scoring system or outcome measure.

Conclusions.—There is no agreement about which validated outcome tool should be used for assessing shoulder instability in patients. There is limited evidence regarding the comparative effectiveness of surgical and non-surgical treatment of TASI, including a lack of evidence regarding the optimal timing of such treatments. There is a need for a well-structured randomised control trial to assess the efficacy of surgical and non-surgical interventions for this common type of shoulder instability.

▶ I accepted this report based on its topic, then rejected it because I thought it did not say much, then decided to include it if for no other reason than to introduce the concept of a "scoping review." This is defined as "critical appraisal of the quality and content of published evidence." Hence, it includes assessing pooled meta-analyses or literature reviews. In fact, 12 such articles were included in the 63 reviewed in the report. The topic is important because there is no evidence-based consensus on the management of traumatic anterior shoulder instability. What is important to understand is that even though the literature does not support nonoperative, arthroscopic, or open stabilization, this does not mean there is no difference. It does mean we need better-constructed studies.

B. F. Morrey, MD

External Rotation Immobilization for Primary Shoulder Dislocation: A Randomized Controlled Trial

Whelan DB, Conjunction with the Joint Orthopaedic Initiative for National Trials of the Shoulder (JOINTS) (Univ of Toronto, Toronto, Ontario, Canada; et al)
Clin Orthop Relat Res 472:2380-2386, 2014

Background.—The traditional treatment for primary anterior shoulder dislocations has been immobilization in a sling with the arm in a position of adduction and internal rotation. However, recent basic science and clinical data have suggested recurrent instability may be reduced with immobilization in external rotation after primary shoulder dislocation.

Questions/Purposes.—We performed a randomized controlled trial to compare the (1) frequency of recurrent instability and (2) disease-specific quality-of-life scores after treatment of first-time shoulder dislocation using either immobilization in external rotation or immobilization in internal rotation in a group of young patients.

Methods.—Sixty patients younger than 35 years of age with primary, traumatic, anterior shoulder dislocations were randomized (concealed, computer-generated) to immobilization with either an internal rotation sling (n = 29) or an external rotation brace (n = 31) at a mean of 4 days after closed reduction (range, 1–7 days). Patients with large bony lesions or polytrauma were excluded. The two groups were similar at baseline. Both groups were immobilized for 4 weeks with identical therapy protocols thereafter. Blinded assessments were completed by independent observers for a minimum of 12 months (mean, 25 months; range, 12–43 months). Recurrent instability was defined as a second documented anterior dislocation or multiple episodes of shoulder subluxation severe enough for the patient to request surgical stabilization. Validated disease-specific quality-of-life data (Western Ontario Shoulder Instability index [WOSI], American Shoulder and Elbow Surgeons evaluation [ASES]) were also collected. Ten patients (17%, five from each group) were lost to followup. Reported compliance with immobilization in both groups was excellent (80%).

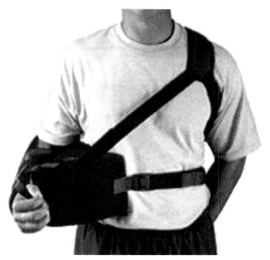

FIGURE 1.—The external rotation immobilization brace is shown. A certified orthopaedic technologist will adjust the brace. Reprinted with permission from DJI, LLC. (With kind permission from Springer Science+Business Media: Whelan DB, Conjunction with the Joint Orthopaedic Initiative for National Trials of the Shoulder (JOINTS). External rotation immobilization for primary shoulder dislocation: a randomized controlled trial. *Clin Orthop Relat Res.* 2014;472:2380-2386, with permission from The Association of Bone and Joint Surgeons.)

TABLE 2.—Results at Minimum 12 Months' Followup

Outcome	External Rotation Brace Group, n = 27 (Number, %)	Internal Rotation Sling Group, n = 25 (Number, %)	P Value
Recurrent dislocation	6 (22)	8 (32)	0.42
Recurrent instability*	10 (37)	10 (40)	0.82
Recurrent instability requiring surgical stabilization	6 (22)	7 (28)	0.63
WOSI score (%)†	87 (14)	84 (21)	0.74
ASES score (points)†	95 (5)	89 (14)	0.05
Mean ROM (°) (index versus opposite)	70 versus 76	76 versus 78	0.15 versus 0.67

*Includes frank recurrent dislocations and subluxations.
†Values are expressed as mean with SD in parentheses.
WOSI = Western Ontario Shoulder Instability index; ASES = American Shoulder and Elbow Surgeons evaluation.
With kind permission from Springer Science+Business Media: Whelan DB, Conjunction with the Joint Orthopaedic Initiative for National Trials of the Shoulder (JOINTS). External rotation immobilization for primary shoulder dislocation: a randomized controlled trial. *Clin Orthop Relat Res.* 2014;472:2380–2386, with permission from The Association of Bone and Joint Surgeons.

Results.—With the numbers available, there was no difference in the rate of recurrent instability between groups: 10 of 27 patients (37%) with the external rotation brace versus 10 of 25 patients (40%) with the sling redislocated or developed symptomatic recurrent instability

($p = 0.41$). WOSI scores were not different between groups ($p = 0.74$) and, although the difference in ASES scores approached statistical significance ($p = 0.05$), the magnitude of this difference was small and of uncertain clinical importance.

Conclusions.—Despite previous published findings, our results show immobilization in external rotation did not confer a significant benefit versus sling immobilization in the prevention of recurrent instability after primary anterior shoulder dislocation. Further studies with larger numbers may elucidate whether functional outcomes, compliance, or comfort with immobilization can be improved with this device.

Level of Evidence.—Level I, therapeutic study. See Instructions for Authors for a complete description of levels of evidence (Fig 1, Table 2).

▶ Despite its inconclusive results, I selected this contribution because it employed acceptable rigor to address an important clinical question. The selection and exclusion criteria avoid many confounding variables. The use of the external rotation position has been accepted by some (Fig 1), based on clinical and basic investigations of its superiority over the conventional sling with the arm internally rotated. The bottom line of this study is that no difference could be demonstrated with the sample size entered into the study (Table 2). The major criticism is the study was underpowered. Even if this is the case, and it probably is, the difference between the 2 positions appears not to be too clinically relevant.

B. F. Morrey, MD

Latarjet, Bristow, and Eden-Hybinette Procedures for Anterior Shoulder Dislocation: Systematic Review and Quantitative Synthesis of the Literature
Longo UG, Loppini M, Rizzello G, et al (Campus Bio-Medico Univ, Rome, Italy)
Arthroscopy 30:1184-1211, 2014

Purpose.—The aim of this study was to evaluate clinical outcome, rate of recurrence, complications, and rate of postoperative osteoarthritis in patients with anterior shoulder instability managed with Latarjet, Bristow, or Eden-Hybinette procedures.

Methods.—A systematic review of the literature on management of anterior dislocation of the shoulder with glenoid bony procedures was performed. A comprehensive search of PubMed, MEDLINE, CINAHL, Cochrane, EMBASE, and Google Scholar databases using various combinations of the keywords "shoulder," "dislocation," "treatment," "Latarjet," "Bristow," "bone loss," "Eden-Hybinette," "iliac," "bone," "block," "clinical," "outcome," and "Bankart." The following data

Study or Subgroup	Bone block procedures Events	Total	Bankart repair Events	Total	Weight	Odds Ratio M-H, Fixed, 95% CI	Odds Ratio M-H, Fixed, 95% CI
Bonnevialle et al., 2013	1	6	0	5	6.6%	3.00 [0.10-90.96]	
Hovelius et al., 2001	2	30	3	26	47.1%	0.55 [0.08-3.56]	
Hovelius et al., 2011	0	97	1	88	24.5%	0.30 [0.01-7.44]	
Weaver et al., 1994	2	61	1	24	21.8%	0.78 [0.07-9.02]	
Total (95% CI)		**194**		**143**	**100.0%**	**0.70 [0.21-2.31]**	
Total events	5		5				

Heterogeneity: $\chi^2 = 1.04$, df = 3 ($P = .79$); $I^2 = 0\%$
Test for overall effect: $z = 0.59$ ($P = .56$)

0.01 0.1 1 10 100
Bone block procedures   Bankart repair

FIGURE 2.—Forest plot of osteoarthritis after bone block procedures and Bankart repair. (CI, confidence interval; M-H, Mantel-Haenszel). *Editor's Note:* Please refer to original journal article for full references. (Reprinted from Arthroscopy: The Journal of Arthroscopic and Related Surgery. Longo UG, Loppini M, Rizzello G, et al. Latarjet, bristow, and eden-hybinette procedures for anterior shoulder dislocation: systematic review and quantitative synthesis of the literature. *Arthroscopy.* 2014;30:1184-1211, Copyright 2014, with permission the Arthroscopy Association of North America.)

were extracted: demographics, bone defects and other lesions, type of surgery, outcome measurement, range of motion (ROM), recurrence of instability, complications, and osteoarthritis. A quantitative synthesis of all comparative studies was performed to compare bone block procedures and Bankart repair in terms of postoperative recurrence of instability and osteoarthritis.

Results.—Forty-six studies were included and 3,211 shoulders were evaluated. The mean value of the Coleman Methodology Score (CMS) was 65 points. Preoperatively, the injuries detected most were glenoid bone loss and Bankart lesions. The Eden-Hybinette procedure had the highest rate of postoperative osteoarthritis and recurrence. Pooled results from comparative studies showed that the bone block procedures were associated with a lower rate of recurrence when compared with Bankart repair (odds ratio [OR], 0.45; 95% confidence interval [CI], 0.28 to 0.74; $P = .002$), whereas there was no significant difference between the 2 groups in terms of postoperative osteoarthritis ($P = .79$).

Conclusions.—The open Bristow-Latarjet procedure continues to be a valid surgical option to treat patients with anterior shoulder instability. Bone block procedures were associated with a lower rate of recurrence when compared with the Bankart repair. The Eden-Hybinette procedure has clinical outcomes very similar to the Bristow-Latarjet technique but has a higher rate of postoperative osteoarthritis and recurrence. An arthroscopic Bristow-Latarjet procedure seems to be better in terms of prevention of recurrence and rehabilitation, but randomized studies are needed to reach definitive conclusions.

Level of Evidence.—Level IV, systematic review of Level II, III, and IV studies (Fig 2).

▶ This systematic review of the literature provides some clarity to one of the topics of debate in the world of shoulder surgery. The authors sanctioned almost

3000 papers while retaining 46 for review. The assessment stratified the clinical features into those with and without osseous deficiency. The conclusions are not only likely to be valid, they are clinically relevant. If there is an osseous deficiency, the Bankart procedure is inadequate (Fig 2). Furthermore, the Bristow-Latarjet is superior to the Eden-Hybinette procedure from the perspectives of both fewer recurrences and less likelihood of late degenerative changes. The conclusion is obvious.

B. F. Morrey, MD

A Survey of Expert Opinion Regarding Rotator Cuff Repair
Acevedo DC, Paxton ES, Williams GR, et al (Thomas Jefferson Univ, Philadelphia, PA)
J Bone Joint Surg Am 96:e123(1-7), 2014

Many patients with rotator cuff tears have questions for their surgeons regarding the surgical procedure, perioperative management, restrictions, therapy, and ability to work after a rotator cuff repair. The purpose of our study was to determine common clinical practices among experts regarding rotator cuff repair and to assist them in counseling patients. We surveyed 372 members of the American Shoulder and Elbow Surgeons (ASES) and the Association of Clinical Elbow and Shoulder Surgeons (ACESS); 111 members (29.8%) completed all or part of the survey, and 92.8% of the respondents answered every question. A consensus response (>50% agreement) was achieved on 49% (24 of 49) of the questions. Variability in responses likely reflects the fact that clinical practices have evolved over time based on clinical experience (Table 1).

▶ I thought the general orthopedic surgeon might find this survey of interest. The survey is of the members of the American Shoulder and Elbow Surgeons' management of a patient with a moderate-sized rotator cuff tear undergoing surgery. Table 1 summarizes those questions for which there was agreement in the response that exceeded 50%. The lack of routine imaging to determine healing was of interest to me, as was the lack of routine deep vein thrombosis prophylaxis. The period of sling usage averaged about 5 to 6 weeks, and most surgeons told workers' compensation patients that they would be off work for

TABLE 1.—Important Clinical Questions with Majority Agreement (>50%)

	Response (%)
In general, will you operate on a smoker?	
Yes	91.3
Do you use DVT prophylaxis (Lovenox, ASA*, Coumadin) routinely after rotator cuff surgery for a majority of your patients?	
No	86.4
Do you routinely use an imaging modality to assess for healing in your postoperative rotator cuffs? And if so, what is your preferred imaging modality?	
No	87.4
Do you give the patient a VIDEO of their arthroscopic cuff repair?	
No	76.7
Do you tell your patients to sleep in an inclined position after surgery for their comfort?	
Yes	73.8
Do you have a lifting guideline you recommend patients to follow at 6 months?	
Let pain be your guide	62.7
Do you have a lifting guideline you recommend patients to follow at 1 year?	
Let pain be your guide	72.8
After a rotator cuff repair, when do you tell patients that they should expect to be "as good as it gets"?	
1 year	69.9
Do you give the patient a copy of their surgical arthroscopy pictures?	
Yes	68.6
When do you tell a Workers' Compensation patient that they will be able to return to work (assuming a laborer) after repair of a LARGE tear (2-4 cm)?	
6 months	68.
In the setting of a full-thickness rotator cuff tear with a significantly degenerated biceps, what is your preferred method of treatment (sex and age not being a factor)?	
Tenodesis	66
Do you allow your patients to take off their slings while sitting down or while sleeping in the immediate postoperative period?	
No	66
On average, how long do you have your patients wear a sling after rotator cuff repair for a LARGE tear (2-4 cm)?	
5-6 weeks	65
How often do you admit patients to the hospital the night of surgery (for pain control, patient requests, etc.)?	
Almost never	62.1
On average how long do you have your patients wear a sling after rotator cuff repair for a MASSIVE tear (>5 cm)?	
5-6 weeks	58.3
When do you tell Workers' Compensation patients that they will be able to return to work (assuming a laborer) after repair of a SMALL tear (<2 cm)?	
6 months	56.6
In general, when do you allow patients to drive a car after a rotator cuff repair?	
When the patient is out of the sling full time	55.3
What type of sling do you place your patient in after a standard rotator cuff repair (supraspinatus)?	
Sling with a pillow (i.e., UltraSling)	54.5
What pain medications do you prescribe for your patients for postoperative pain control? (May choose more than one)	
Percocet	54.5
In general, how do you treat full-thickness subscapularis tendon tears?	
Arthroscopic	54.4
In general, do you allow your patients to take NSAIDs after surgery (within the first 4 weeks)?	
Yes	51
In what setting do you perform the majority of your rotator cuff repairs?	
Hospital	51
In general, how long do you follow your postoperative cuff repairs?	
6 months to 1 yr	50.5
What percent healing rates do you quote your patients if any for SMALL tears (<2 cm)?	
80-90%	50

*ASA = acetylsalicylic acid.
Reprinted from Acevedo DC, Paxton ES, Williams GR, et al. A Survey of Expert Opinion Regarding Rotator Cuff Repair. J Bone Joint Surg Am. 2014;96:e123(1-7). http://jbjs.org/.

6 months. I recommend reading the full survey to better appreciate how these data might be useful in your practice.

B. F. Morrey, MD

A Prospective Evaluation of Survivorship of Asymptomatic Degenerative Rotator Cuff Tears

Keener JD, Galatz LM, Teefey SA, et al (Washington Univ, St Louis, MO; et al)
J Bone Joint Surg Am 97:89-98, 2015

Background.—The purpose of this prospective study was to report the long-term risks of rotator cuff tear enlargement and symptom progression associated with degenerative asymptomatic tears.

Methods.—Subjects with an asymptomatic rotator cuff tear in one shoulder and pain due to rotator cuff disease in the contralateral shoulder enrolled as part of a prospective longitudinal study. Two hundred and twenty-four subjects (118 initial full-thickness tears, fifty-six initial partial-thickness tears, and fifty controls) were followed for a median of 5.1 years. Validated functional shoulder scores were calculated (visual analog pain scale, American Shoulder and Elbow Surgeons [ASES], and simple shoulder test [SST] scores). Subjects were followed annually with shoulder ultrasonography and clinical evaluations.

Results.—Tear enlargement was seen in 49% of the shoulders, and the median time to enlargement was 2.8 years. The occurrence of tear-enlargement events was influenced by the severity of the final tear type, with enlargement of 61% of the full-thickness tears, 44% of the partial-thickness tears, and 14% of the controls ($p < 0.05$). Subject age and sex were not related to tear enlargement. One hundred subjects (46%) developed new pain. The final tear type was associated with a greater risk of pain development, with the new pain developing in 28% of the controls, 46% of the shoulders with a partial thickness tear, and 50% of those with a full-thickness tear ($p < 0.05$). The presence of tear enlargement was associated with the onset of new pain ($p < 0.05$). Progressive degenerative changes of the supraspinatus muscle were associated with tear enlargement, with supraspinatus muscle degeneration increasing in 4% of the shoulders with a stable tear compared with 30% of the shoulders with tear enlargement ($p < 0.05$). Nine percent of the shoulders with a stable tear showed increased infraspinatus muscle degeneration compared with 28% of those in which the tear had enlarged ($p = 0.07$).

Conclusions.—This study demonstrates the progressive nature of degenerative rotator cuff disease. The risk of tear enlargement and progression of muscle degeneration is greater for shoulders with a full-thickness tear, and tear enlargement is associated with a greater risk of pain development across all tear types.

Level of Evidence.—Prognostic Level II. See Instructions for Authors for a complete description of levels of evidence.

▶ I think this will become a classic. Rotator cuff tear is the condition most commonly requiring shoulder surgery. For this reason, there is controversy as to whether all cuff tears should be fixed, and if so, when? If they do not all need to be fixed, then which ones do, and which ones do not, need intervention? One reason this is such an important question is that a smaller tear that progresses to a larger tear is associated with poorer outcome from repair. So, the central finding is important: Full thickness tears, even if they are without pain initially, do progress and become symptomatic. In my opinion, this well done study with adequate power does justify fixing the full thickness tear, especially when symptoms are present or have developed over time.

B. F. Morrey, MD

Arthroscopic Versus Mini-Open Rotator Cuff Repair: An Up-to-Date Meta-analysis of Randomized Controlled Trials

Ji X, Bi C, Wang F, et al (Shanghai Jiao Tong Univ, China)
Arthroscopy 31:118-124, 2015

Purpose.—The aim of this meta-analysis was to compare the clinical outcomes of arthroscopic and mini-open rotator cuff repairs based on recently published Level I randomized controlled trials (RCTs).

Methods.—We systematically searched electronic databases to identify RCTs that compared arthroscopic and mini-open rotator cuff repairs from 1980 to October 2013. The clinical outcome scores, including the University of California, Los Angeles score and the Constant-Murley score, were converted to a common 100-point outcome score for further analysis. The results of the pooled studies were analyzed in terms of surgery time, weighted 100-point score, pain on a visual analog scale (VAS), and range of motion. Study quality was assessed and relevant data were extracted independently by 2 reviewers.

Results.—Five RCTs, including 166 patients in the arthroscopic repair group and 163 patients in the mini-open repair group, were included in this meta-analysis. The results of the meta-analysis showed that there were no significant differences in surgery time ($P = .11$), weighted 100-point score ($P = .65$), VAS pain score ($P = 87$), or range of motion ($P = .29$ for forward flexion and $P = .82$ for external rotation).

Conclusions.—On the basis of current literature, no differences in surgery time, functional outcome score, VAS pain score, and range of motion were found at the end of follow-up between the arthroscopic and mini-open rotator cuff repair techniques. In addition, there was no significant difference in VAS pain score in the early phase between the 2 repairs.

Level of Evidence.—Level I, meta-analysis of Level I studies.

▶ I found this to be an interesting study for several reasons. First, the conclusion: No difference between the 2 techniques in any measured parameter, including recovery, is straightforward and easy to remember. This is the kind of study we have been selecting more and more because it is a debatable topic, without a clear answer. The answer is clear, based on what has been published. This is the interesting point: The conclusions were drawn from only 5 studies that qualified, according to the selection parameters. The reviews covered 23 years, but the only ones that qualified were from 2009 to 2014 literature. Finally, it is worthy of note that of the 5 articles, 3 are from Asia and 2 are from Europe.

B. F. Morrey, MD

Knot Impingement After Rotator Cuff Repair: Is It Real?

Park YE, Shon MS, Lim TK, et al (Sungkyunkwan Univ, Seoul, Korea; Natl Med Ctr, Seoul, Korea; Wonkwang Univ Sanbon Hosp, Gyeonggi-do, Korea; et al)
Arthroscopy 30:1055-1060, 2014

Purpose.—The purpose of this study was to compare morphologic features of the acromion after 2 different repair methods (single-row [SR] repair with a minimum of 4 knots and suture-bridge [SB] repair with minimal knots) in medium to large rotator cuff tears.

Methods.—From May 2005 to July 2012, 1,693 rotator cuff repairs were performed, among them medium to large tears requiring more than 2 anchors for repair; those who had 6-month postoperative magnetic resonance imaging (MRI) scans were included (221 shoulders). They were divided into 2 groups; group A (SR repair) and group B (SB repair). Acromial morphologic characteristics were evaluated using MRI 6 months postoperatively. An acromial defect was defined as an irregular defect or erosion on the flat acromion. Clinical measurements were performed using the American Shoulder and Elbow Surgeons (ASES) score, Constant score, visual analogue scale (VAS) pain score, and range of motion (ROM).

Results.—Erosion in the acromion was observed in 2 of 118 patients (1.7%) in group A and in 1 of 103 (1%) patients in group B. There was no statistically significant difference between the 2 groups ($P = .796$). A statistically significant improvement was observed in the clinical scores measured ($P = .0043$). ROM was not fully recovered to the preoperative level at 6 months postoperatively. Acromioplasty was performed in 2 of 3 patients with acromial erosion. There was acromial erosion in one patient in group A without performing subacromial decompression.

Conclusions.—Our study showed that there was no difference in acromial erosion in high-profile knots made by an SR compared with double-row (DR) SB low-profile repairs.

Level of Evidence.—Level III, retrospective comparative study.

▶ These investigators have addressed a question I have long asked myself, often in reference to different procedures. Nonetheless, the question is not only valid, it is one that occurs regularly when dealing with rotator cuff repair. That these investigators found a low incidence, < 2%, of problems attributed to the knot is noteworthy. It is also important to observe that there was no difference from a standard and a low-profile knot. This was a difficult study to complete, and the information is clinically useful.

B. F. Morrey, MD

Is Arthroscopic Distal Clavicle Resection Necessary for Patients With Radiological Acromioclavicular Joint Arthritis and Rotator Cuff Tears? A Prospective Randomized Comparative Study

Oh JH, Kim JY, Choi JH, et al (Chung-Ang Univ, Seoul, Korea)
Am J Sports Med 42:2567-2573, 2014

Background.—The failure of subacromial decompression may be attributed to persistent symptoms of acromioclavicular joint (ACJ) arthritis, while inferior clavicular spurs of the ACJ may be associated with failed healing of repaired rotator cuffs.

Purpose.—To evaluate the clinical effectiveness of arthroscopic distal clavicle resection (DCR) in patients with rotator cuff tears and concomitant asymptomatic radiological ACJ arthritis.

Study Design.—Randomized controlled trial; Level of evidence, 1.

Methods.—A total of 78 patients with rotator cuff tears in addition to radiological and asymptomatic ACJ arthritis who were scheduled for arthroscopic rotator cuff repair were prospectively randomized into 2 groups. Patients underwent arthroscopic rotator cuff repair with acromioplasty. Patients in group 1 (39 patients) underwent additional arthroscopic DCR, while patients in group 2 (39 patients) did not. Clinical outcomes of the 2 groups were compared using the visual analog scale (VAS) for pain, range of motion, Constant score, and American Shoulder and Elbow Surgeons (ASES) score up to at least 24 months. The structural integrity of repaired rotator cuffs was assessed using ultrasonography, computed tomography arthrography, or MRI at least 6 months after surgery. To evaluate ACJ instability, weighted stress radiography of the ACJ was studied at 6 and 12 months postoperatively.

Results.—Patients in both groups showed significant improvement in the VAS score and all functional scores at final follow-up (mean, 29.2 months; range, 24-46 months) without significant differences between the 2 groups ($P > .05$). Results (mean ± SD) for preoperative group 1/group 2 and postoperative group 1/group 2 were as follows, respectively: $7.2 \pm 1.8/6.1 \pm 1.9$ ($P = .02$) and $0.6 \pm 1.8/0.6 \pm 0.9$ ($P = .97$) for the VAS score, $74.1 \pm 5.7/73.8 \pm 8.0$ ($P = .87$) and

96.3 ± 5.7/95.7 ± 4.6 (*P* =.77) for the Constant score, and 47.0 ± 10.3/ 50.8 ± 14.1 (*P* =.22) and 91.5 ± 15.5/94.5 ± 11.8 (*P* =.55) for the ASES score. Failed cuff healing occurred in 9 patients (23%) in group 1 and 10 patients (26%) in group 2, with no significant difference (*P* =.95). In group 1, there were 2 patients (5.0%) with ACJ subluxation on weighted stress radiography at 6 months postoperatively. These patients complained of gross protrusion and ACJ tenderness.

Conclusion.—Preventive arthroscopic DCR in patients with rotator cuff tears and concomitant asymptomatic radiological ACJ arthritis did not result in better clinical or structural outcomes, and it did lead to symptomatic ACJ instability in some patients. Preventive arthroscopic DCR is not recommended in patients with radiological but asymptomatic ACJ arthritis. Further long-term follow-up is needed to confirm the development of symptoms in ACJ arthritis.

▶ This is an excellent prospective randomized study that should have consequences for clinical decision making. The study is clean with valid and measurable end points. The fact is, there is no merit to an arthroscopic distal clavicle resection for asymptomatic arthritis of the acromioclavicular joint. Note that such a practice results in asymptomatic distal clavicle instability. Also note that this conclusion is for the asymptomatic acromioclavicular arthritic condition.

B. F. Morrey, MD

Arthroscopic Repair of Full-Thickness Rotator Cuff Tears With and Without Acromioplasty: Randomized Prospective Trial With 2-Year Follow-up

Abrams GD, Gupta AK, Hussey KE, et al (Stanford Univ, CA; Florida Orthopedic Inst, Tampa; Rush Univ Med Ctr, Chicago, IL; et al)
Am J Sports Med 42:1296-1303, 2014

Background.—Acromioplasty is commonly performed during arthroscopic rotator cuff repair, but its effect on short-term outcomes is debated.

Purpose.—To report the short-term clinical outcomes of patients undergoing arthroscopic repair of full-thickness rotator cuff tears with and without acromioplasty.

Study Design.—Randomized controlled trial; Level of evidence, 2.

Methods.—Patients undergoing arthroscopic repair of full-thickness rotator cuff tears were randomized into acromioplasty or nonacromioplasty groups. The Simple Shoulder Test (SST), American Shoulder and Elbow Surgeons (ASES) score, Constant score, University of California—Los Angeles (UCLA) score, and Short Form-12 (SF-12) health assessment were collected along with physical examination including range of motion and dynamometer strength testing. Intraoperative data including tear size, repair configuration, and concomitant procedures were recorded. Follow-up examination was performed at regular intervals up to 2 years.

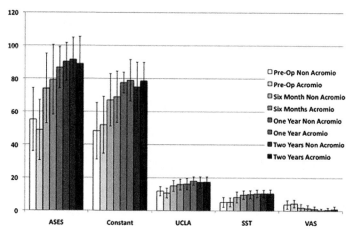

FIGURE 4.—Preoperative functional scores versus those at 6-month, 1-year, and minimum 2-year follow-up for the nonacromioplasty (Non Acromio) and acromioplasty (Acromio) groups. There were no significant differences between groups at any time point during the study period. ASES, American Shoulder and Elbow Surgeons score; Constant, Constant score; SST, Simple Shoulder Test score; UCLA, University of California—Los Angeles score; VAS, visual analog scale score. (Reprinted from Abrams GD, Gupta AK, Hussey KE, et al. Arthroscopic repair of full-thickness rotator cuff tears with and without acromioplasty: randomized prospective trial with 2-year follow-up. *Am J Sports Med.* 42:1296-1303, 2014, with permission from The Author(s).)

Preoperative imaging was reviewed to classify the acromial morphologic type, acromial angle, and lateral acromial angulation.

Results.—A total of 114 patients were initially enrolled in the study, and 95 (83%; 43 nonacromioplasty, 52 acromioplasty) were available for a minimum 2-year follow-up. There were no significant differences in baseline characteristics, including number of tendons torn, repair configuration, concomitant procedures, and acromion type and angles. Within groups, there was a significant ($P < .001$) improvement in all functional outcome scores from preoperatively to all follow-up time points, including 2 years, for the nonacromioplasty and acromioplasty groups (ASES score: 55.1-91.5, 48.8-89.0; Constant score: 48.3-75.0, 51.9-78.7, respectively). There were no significant differences in functional outcomes between nonacromioplasty and acromioplasty groups or between subjects with different acromial features at any time point.

Conclusion.—The results of this study demonstrate no difference in clinical outcomes after rotator cuff repair with or without acromioplasty at 2 years postoperatively (Fig 4).

▶ We must commend the authors for designing and conducting this prospective randomized study that investigates a controversial issue regarding rotator cuff surgery. Does an acromioplasty improve the outcome of a rotator cuff repair? The study is sufficiently powered with a sample size of 114 procedures. The surveillance of 2 years would seem adequate to discriminate any differences, should they exist. They do not (Fig 4). It is too bad the distinctions among the various assessment parameters and the 2 groups is not more evident in this figure. Regardless, one can tell at a glance, these data are the same. No difference. This is an important finding, but like so many worthwhile studies, I have reservations that it will change clinical practice. It will be rationalized that it is a flawed study. In reality, the criticism of the study is, I fear, motivated by something else.

B. F. Morrey, MD

Early Passive Motion Versus Immobilization After Arthroscopic Rotator Cuff Repair

Riboh JC, Garrigues GE (Duke Univ, Durham, NC)
Arthroscopy 30:997-1005, 2014

Purpose.—To provide a synthesis of the highest-quality literature available comparing early passive motion (EPM) with strict sling immobilization during the first 4 to 6 weeks after surgery.

Methods.—The Medline, Cochrane, and Embase databases were searched for eligible studies. We reviewed 886 citations, and 5 randomized clinical trials (RCTs) (Level II) met the inclusion criteria for meta-analysis. Four RCTs contributed to the analysis of range of motion, and 5 contributed to the analysis of retear rates. A single Level IV study was available for qualitative review. Random-effects models were used for meta-analysis, computing mean differences for continuous variables and risk ratios for dichotomous variables.

Results.—EPM resulted in improved shoulder forward flexion at 3 months (mean difference, 14.70°; 95% confidence interval [CI], 5.52° to 23.87°; $P=.002$), 6 months (mean difference, 4.31°; 95% CI, 0.17° to 8.45°; $P=.04$), and 12 months (mean difference, 4.18°; 95% CI, 0.36° to 8.00°; $P=.03$). External rotation at the side was only superior with EPM at 3 months (mean difference, 10.43°; 95% CI, 4.51° to 16.34°; $P=.0006$). Rotator cuff retear rates (16.3% for immobilization v 21.1% for EPM; risk ratio, 0.82; 95% CI, 0.57 to 1.20; $P=.31$) were not significantly different between EPM and immobilization at a minimum of 1 year of follow-up.

Conclusions.—A small number of RCTs with low to moderate risks of bias are currently available. Meta-analysis suggests that after primary arthroscopic rotator cuff repair of small to medium tears, EPM results in 15° of improved forward flexion at 3 months and approximately 5° at 6 and 12 months. External rotation is improved by 10° with EPM at 3 months only. The clinical importance of these differences has yet to be determined. Retear rates at a minimum of 1 year of follow-up are not clearly affected by type of rehabilitation.

Level of Evidence.—Level II, meta-analysis of Level II studies and qualitative review of Level IV study (Figs 3 and 4).

▶ This is an interesting article from several perspectives. As is so often the case, the question is valid, the answer is unknown, and the clinical relevance is high.

A

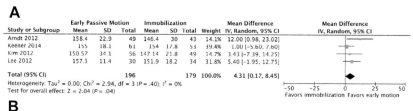

B

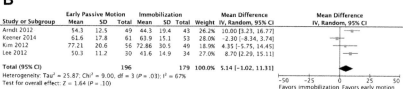

FIGURE 3.—Range of motion (in degrees) at 6 months after surgery. (A) EPM results in improved forward flexion. (B) EPM and immobilization result in statistically equivalent external rotation at the side. Meta-analysis results are shown for the 4 included studies. Data are reported as mean differences between the EPM and immobilization groups with 95% CIs. A positive mean difference indicates superiority of the EPM group. The size of each box is proportional to the study weight in the meta-analysis. The bars on either side of the boxes represent the 95% CI. (IV, inverse variance; Random, random-effects model.) (Reprinted from Arthroscopy: The Journal of Arthroscopic and Related Surgery. Riboh JC, Garrigues GE. Early passive motion versus immobilization after arthroscopic rotator cuff repair. *Arthroscopy.* 2014;30:997-1005, Copyright 2014, with permission from the Arthroscopy Association of North America.)

A

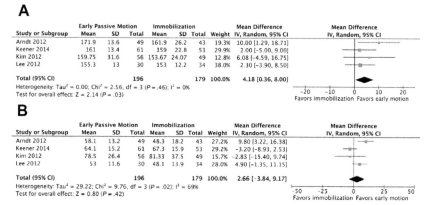

B

FIGURE 4.—Range of motion (in degrees) at 12 months after surgery. (A) EPM results in improved forward flexion. (B) External rotation at the side is no different between the EPM and immobilization groups. Meta-analysis results are shown for the 4 included studies. Data are reported as mean differences between the EPM and immobilization groups with 95% CIs. A positive mean difference indicates superiority of the EPM group. The size of each box is proportional to the study weight in the metaanalysis. The bars on either side of the boxes represent the 95% CI. (IV, inverse variance; Random, random-effects model.) (Reprinted from Arthroscopy: The Journal of Arthroscopic and Related Surgery. Riboh JC, Garrigues GE. Early passive motion versus immobilization after arthroscopic rotator cuff repair. *Arthroscopy.* 2014;30:997-1005, Copyright 2014, with permission from the Arthroscopy Association of North America.)

Only 5 usable studies from more than 880 citations were worthy of assessment. These few studies show improved motion at 3 months but not at 6 or 12 months (Fig 3). Furthermore, the retear rate of 16% in the immobilized and 22% in the early motion group is not statistically significant.

Frankly, however, I question whether this is not in fact clinically relevant (Fig 4). To me, this study, although technically accurate, is actually helpful to the clinician in forming treatment plans. In a word, early motion resulting in less than 5 degrees of improved motion is not worth a 25% increased risk of retear of the cuff repair. This is a different conclusion than is drawn by the investigators.

B. F. Morrey, MD

How often do surgeons intervene on shoulder labral lesions detected at MR examination? A retrospective review of MR examinations correlated with arthroscopy

Magee T (Univ of Central Florida School of Medicine, Orlando)
Br J Radiol 87:20130736, 2014

Objective.—We report the prevalence of surgical intervention on shoulder labral lesions detected at MR examinations and how surgeons describe labral tears seen at MR examinations in their arthroscopy reports.

Methods.—A retrospective review of 100 consecutive patients aged 50 years or younger who had shoulder labral tears on MR and went on to have surgery performed. It was determined whether surgical intervention was performed on the MR lesions.

Results.—Of these 100 patients, 72 had superior labral anterior to posterior (SLAP) tears, 38 had posterior labral tears and 28 had anterior labral tears on MR examination. All 100 patients went on to arthroscopy. All lesions described on MRI were described on arthroscopy. Of the 72 SLAP tears, 64 were described as fraying on arthroscopy with 51 debrided. The remaining eight SLAP tears were tacked surgically. Of the 38 posterior labral tears, 36 were described as fraying on arthroscopy with 29 debrided and 2 had surgical tacking performed. Of the 28 anterior labral tears described on MR examination, 26 had surgical tacking performed and 2 were debrided. There were four SLAP tears, two anterior labral tears and three posterior labral tears seen on arthroscopy but not seen on MR examination.

Conclusion.—In this series, a high percentage of SLAP tears and posterior labral tears described on MR examination did not have surgical tacking. Most anterior labral tears had surgical tacking. Based on the above, our surgeons request we describe superior and posterior labral lesions as fraying and/or tearing, unless we can see a displaced tear. Most anterior labral lesions are treated with surgical tacking.

Advances in Knowledge.—MRI allows for sensitive detection of labral tears. The tears often are not clinically significant.

▶ This topic was interesting to me. Labral tears are sometimes difficult to diagnose clinically, and the surgeon often relies heavily on the MRI report. It is therefore of interest that the vast majority of interventions of posterior, anterior, and superior lesions were only fraying and were debrided. Few, if any, anatomic sector were repaired (Table 1 in the original article). One can legitimately ask whether a debridement is indicated. Often I think it is not. Unfortunately, to me this study confirms my concern and suspicion that we are tending to operate on the image rather than the patient. I hope not.

B. F. Morrey, MD

Hospital Readmissions After Surgical Treatment of Proximal Humerus Fractures: Is Arthroplasty Safer Than Open Reduction Internal Fixation?
Zhang AL, Schairer WW, Feeley BT (Univ of California San Francisco)
Clin Orthop Relat Res 472:2317-2324, 2014

Background.—With technologic advances such as locked periarticular plating, hemiarthroplasty of the humeral head, and more recently reverse total shoulder replacement, surgical treatment of proximal humerus fractures has become more commonplace. However, there is insufficient information regarding patient outcomes after surgery, such as the frequency of unplanned hospital readmissions and factors contributing to readmission.

Questions/Purposes.—We measured (1) the frequency of unplanned hospital readmissions after surgical treatment of proximal humerus fractures, (2) the medical and surgical causes of readmission, and (3) the risk factors associated with unplanned readmissions.

Methods.—The State Inpatient Database from seven different states was used to identify patients who underwent treatment for a proximal humerus fracture with open reduction and internal fixation (ORIF), hemiarthroplasty of the humeral head, or reverse total shoulder arthroplasty from 2005 through 2010. The database was used to measure the 30-day and 90-day readmission rates and identify causes and risk factors for readmission. Multivariate modeling and a Cox proportional hazards model were used for statistical analysis.

Results.—A total of 27,017 patients were included with an overall 90-day readmission rate of 14% (15% for treatment with ORIF, 15% for reverse total shoulder arthroplasty, and 13% for hemiarthroplasty). The majority of readmissions were associated with medical diagnoses (75%), but treatment with ORIF was associated with the most readmissions from surgical complications, (29%) followed by reverse total shoulder arthroplasty (20%) and hemiarthroplasty (16%) ($p < 0.001$). Risk of readmission was greater for patients who were female, African American, discharged to a nursing facility, or had Medicaid insurance.

Conclusions.—As the majority of unplanned hospital readmissions were associated with medical diagnoses, it is important to consider patient medical comorbidities before surgical treatment of proximal humerus fractures and during the postoperative care phase.

Level of Evidence.—Level III, therapeutic study. See the Instructions for Authors for a complete description of levels of evidence.

▶ I think this is a useful study for providing basic information. Most of the readmissions (70%) after proximal humeral fractures are for medical reasons. The frequency of readmission is rather high at 14%. This is consistent with the fact that most fractures occur in the older patient with associated medical comorbidities. It is also of value to note that when the hospital readmission is correlated with the type of fracture treatment, open reduction and internal fixation is most commonly associated with readmission, reverse in the middle, and the hemi-replacement the least common ($P < .001$). Such information does not reflect the clinical outcome or the selection factors favoring 1 treatment selection over another.

B. F. Morrey, MD

High Incidence of Hemiarthroplasty for Shoulder Osteoarthritis Among Recently Graduated Orthopaedic Surgeons

Mann T, Baumhauer JF, O'Keefe RJ, et al (Univ of Rochester, NY; et al)
Clin Orthop Relat Res 472:3510-3516, 2014

Background.—Primary glenohumeral osteoarthritis is a common indication for shoulder arthroplasty. Historically, both total shoulder arthroplasty (TSA) and hemi-shoulder arthroplasty (HSA) have been used to treat primary glenohumeral osteoarthritis. The choice between procedures is a topic of debate, with HSA proponents arguing that it is less invasive, faster, less expensive, and technically less demanding, with quality of life outcomes equivalent to those of TSA. More recent evidence suggests TSA is superior in terms of pain relief, function, ROM, strength, and patient satisfaction. We therefore investigated the practice of recently graduated orthopaedic surgeons pertaining to the surgical treatment of this disease.

Questions/Purposes.—We hypothesized that (1) recently graduated, board eligible, orthopaedic surgeons with fellowship training in shoulder surgery are more likely to perform TSA than surgeons without this training (2) younger patients are more likely to receive HSA than TSA (3) patient sex affects the choice of surgery (4) US geographic region affects practice patterns and (5) complication rates for HSA and TSA are not different.

Methods.—We queried the American Board of Orthopaedic Surgery's database to identify practice patterns of orthopaedic surgeons taking their board examination. We identified 771 patients with primary glenohumeral osteoarthritis treated with TSA or HSA from 2006 to 2011. The rates of TSA and HSA were compared based on the treating surgeon's fellowship training, patient age and sex, US geographic region, and reported surgical complications.

Results.—Surgeons with fellowship training in shoulder surgery were more likely (86% versus 72% OR 2.32 95% CI, 1.56–3.45, $p < 0.001$) than surgeons without this training to perform TSA rather than HSA. The mean age for patients receiving HSA was not different from that for patients receiving TSA (66 versus 68, years, $p = 0.057$). Men were more likely to receive HSA than TSA when compared to women (RR 1.54 95% CI, 1.19–2.00, $p = 0.0012$). The proportions of TSA and HSA were similar regardless of US geographic region (Midwest HSA 21%, TSA 79% Northeast HSA 25%, TSA 75% Northwest HSA 16%, TSA 84% South HSA 27%, TSA 73% Southeast HSA 24%, TSA 76% Southwest HSA 23%, TSA 77% overall $p = 0.708$). The overall complication rates were not different with the numbers available: 8.4% (15/179) for HSA and 8.1% (48/592) for TSA ($p = 0.7555$).

Conclusions.—The findings of this study are at odds with the recommendations in the current clinical practice guidelines for the treatment of glenohumeral osteoarthritis published by the American Academy of Orthopaedic Surgeons. These guidelines favor using TSA over HSA in the treatment of shoulder arthritis. Further investigation is needed to clarify if these practice patterns are isolated to recently graduated board eligible orthopaedic surgeons or if the use of HSA continues with orthopaedic surgeons applying for recertification.

Level of Evidence.—Level III, therapeutic study. See Instructions for Authors for a complete description of levels of evidence.

▶ As the authors point out, over the years, the long-term superiority of total shoulder arthroplasty compared with hemireplacement is clear. This reality is well recognized by those who subspecialize in shoulder surgery. This interesting survey confirms what one might suspect: Eighty-five percent of those with specific training in shoulder surgery perform total replacement compared with 70% of recent graduates but without shoulder surgery fellowship training ($P < .001$). The study demonstrates that our practice does not follow the data. This, of course, may be explained on the basis of lack of awareness of the data, lack of experience doing the complete replacement, or both. Either way, it demonstrates, once again, that as a specialty we sometimes (often?) do not allow ourselves to be evidence driven.

B. F. Morrey, MD

Arthroscopic Tissue Culture for the Evaluation of Periprosthetic Shoulder Infection

Dilisio MF, Miller LR, Warner JJP, et al (Brigham and Women's Hosp/Harvard Med School, Boston, MA; Massachusetts General Hosp, Boston)
J Bone Joint Surg Am 96:1952-1958, 2014

Background.—Periprosthetic shoulder infections can be difficult to diagnose. The purpose of this study was to investigate the utility of arthroscopic tissue culture for the diagnosis of infection following shoulder arthroplasty. Our hypothesis was that culture of arthroscopic biopsy tissue is a more reliable method than fluoroscopically guided shoulder aspiration for diagnosing such infection.

Methods.—A retrospective review identified patients who had undergone culture of arthroscopic biopsy tissue during the evaluation of a possible chronic periprosthetic shoulder infection. The culture results of the arthroscopic biopsies were compared with those of fluoroscopically guided glenohumeral aspiration and open tissue biopsy samples obtained at the time of revision surgery.

Results.—Nineteen patients had undergone arthroscopic biopsy to evaluate a painful shoulder arthroplasty for infection. All subsequently underwent revision surgery, and 41% of those with culture results at that time had a positive result, which included *Propionibacterium* acnes in each case. All arthroscopic biopsy culture results were consistent with the culture results obtained during the revision surgery, yielding 100% sensitivity, specificity, positive predictive value, and negative predictive value. In contrast, fluoroscopically guided glenohumeral aspiration yielded a sensitivity of 16.7%, specificity of 100%, positive predictive value of 100%, and negative predictive value of 58.3%.

Conclusions.—Arthroscopic tissue biopsy is a reliable method for diagnosing periprosthetic shoulder infection and identifying the causative organism.

Level of Evidence.—Diagnostic Level I. See Instructions for Authors for a complete description of levels of evidence.

▶ The authors assess an important and emerging problem, especially with shoulder and elbow prosthetic infections. A painful shoulder replacement today is considered infected unless another cause is obvious. The problem is that erythrocyte sedimentation rate and C-reactive protein markers are often normal. Further, as demonstrated here, joint fluid aspiration is unreliable if the culture is negative. In this experience, tissue culture obtained arthroscopically was specific and sensitive. We have adopted this approach in selected cases, but not routinely. If the treatment is planned to be a staged procedure, this information is a little less necessary. The study is straightforward and valuable.

B. F. Morrey, MD

6 Spine

Introduction

The articles chosen for the Spine chapter of the YEAR BOOK OF ORTHOPEDICS 2015 are a wonderful reflection of the current dynamic spine practice environment and are representative of the challenges musculoskeletal surgical specialists face in their work today. We have reviewed almost 900 different articles representing the depth and breadth of the published peer-reviewed literature in the English-speaking world and have selected 20 articles relevant to both the general orthopedic care provider and the spine specialist.

Selections discussing the diagnostic accuracy of history-taking to assess lumbosacral nerve root compression, cost savings analysis of intrawound vancomycin powder in posterior spinal surgery, nasal MRSA colonization and its impact on surgical site infection following spine surgery, and complications related to the growing burden of osteoporotic fractures should assist the practitioner and student with common real-world challenges that increasingly stress the busy practice today.

Perhaps more controversially, several articles concerning case volume variation, training, and outcomes between orthopedic and neurologic surgery spine graduates testing for board certification are presented. A number of reviews include queries about trends in variations of bone morphogenic protein utilization. Medicare payments for spinal procedures and the longitudinal cost associated with non–value-added presurgical testing with MRI should provoke discussion and controversy. Keeping in mind the growing epidemic of obesity and its associated complications challenging the care professional, I have included reviews regarding patient outcomes related to BMI during elective spinal surgery, as well as cost variations related to different common techniques of lumbar fusion with or without the diagnosis of diabetes mellitus. The very frustrating outcome of reoperation is addressed with a discussion on variations in recurrent lumbar disk herniation, and the increasing confidence on the sports-field sidelines, in regards to screening of pediatric neck trauma, is examined. Finally, we look at costs and outcomes of incidental durotomy, as the utility of epidural steroid injections, non-operative treatment of thoracolumbar burst fractures, nasal MRSA preoperative screening benefits, and detailed cost analysis of minimally invasive versus open transforaminal interbody fusion are critiqued.

As healthcare design focuses on systems and populations of care, the articles selected have a bias toward some of the newer large database repositories spanning multiple healthcare systems, states, and regions. I hope that this concentrated review not only provides the reader with the most relevant and interesting content of the year and helps with practical common surgical challenges but is also forward-looking enough to help with understanding of the coming healthcare changes.

Paul M. Huddleston, MD

Comparison of complications, costs, and length of stay of three different lumbar interbody fusion techniques: an analysis of the Nationwide Inpatient Sample database
Goz V, Weinreb JH, Schwab F, et al (NYU Hosp for Joint Diseases, NY)
Spine J 14:2019-2027, 2014

Background Context.—Lumbar interbody fusion (LIF) techniques have been used for years to treat a number of pathologies of the lower back. These procedures may use an anterior, posterior, or combined surgical approach. Each approach is associated with a unique set of complications, but the exact prevalence of complications associated with each approach remains unclear.

Purpose.—To investigate the rates of perioperative complications of anterior lumbar interbody fusion (ALIF), posterior/transforaminal lumbar interbody fusion (P/TLIF), and LIF with a combined anterior-posterior interbody fusion (APF).

Study Design/Setting.—Retrospective review of national data from a large administrative database.

Patient Sample.—Patients undergoing ALIF, P/TLIF, or APF.

Outcome Measures.—Perioperative complications, length of stay (LOS), total costs, and mortality.

Methods.—The Nationwide Inpatient Sample database was queried for patients undergoing ALIF, P/TLIF, or APF between 2001 and 2010 as identified via International Classification of Diseases, ninth revision codes. Univariate analyses were carried out comparing the three cohorts in terms of the outcomes of interest. Multivariate analysis for primary outcomes was carried out adjusting for overall comorbidity burden, race, gender, age, and length of fusion. National estimates of annual total number of procedures were calculated based on the provided discharge weights. Geographic distribution of the three cohorts was also investigated.

Results.—An estimated total of 923,038 LIFs were performed between 2001 and 2010 in the United States. Posterior/transforaminal lumbar interbody fusions accounted for 79% to 86% of total LIFs between 2001 and 2010, ALIFs for 10% to 15%, and APF decreased from 10% in 2002 to less than 1% in 2010. On average, P/TLIF patients were oldest (54.55 years), followed by combined approach (47.23 years) and ALIF (46.94 years) patients ($p < .0001$). Anterior lumbar interbody fusion, P/TLIF, and combined surgical costs were $75,872, $65,894, and $92,249, respectively ($p < .0001$). Patients in the P/TLIF cohort had the greatest number of comorbidities, having the highest prevalence for 10 of 17 comorbidities investigated. Anterior-posterior interbody fusion group was associated with the greatest number of complications, having the highest incidence of 12 of the 16 complications investigated.

Conclusions.—These data help to define the perioperative risks for several LIF approaches. Comparison of outcomes showed that a combined approach is more expensive and associated with greater LOS, whereas ALIF is associated with the highest postoperative mortality. These trends should be taken into consideration during surgical planning to improve clinical outcomes (Fig 1).

▶ Lumbar interbody fusions (LIFs) remain a versatile technique for spinal arthrodesis, allowing surgeons the ability to correct deformity, increase healing rates, and indirectly decompress neural elements. With a series of anterior lumbar interbody fusions being reported for salvage of failed arthrodesis in the early 1970s,[1] by the time the mid-1990s rolled around, the interbody "cage rage" was in full swing. With increased visualization and exposure of the anterior spine came increased complications previously uncommon to spine surgeons, such as injury to the great vessels, ureters, or neurologic structures in proximity to the anterior lumbar spine. Although anterior lumbar spine exposure revolutionized fusion of the lumbar spine, some surgeons did not perform the technique or did not practice in proximity to general or vascular surgeons that could perform the exposure. This limitation, combined with the desire to minimize the often-horrific complications associated with the anterior approach, led to the development of hybrid techniques, such as anterior/posterior or 360-degree techniques. This allowed the placement of posterior spinal instrumentation away from the anterior structures and provided posterior exposure for decompression and autologous bone grafting. With the development of posterior minimally invasive techniques and the Infuse implant, surgeons felt empowered to perform circumferential or "360" approaches from a posterior alone technique. These posterior LIFs (or PLIFs) and their newer technical cousins, the transformational interbody fusion (TLIFs), finally allowed surgeons to approach the anterior/posterior fusion rate techniques with fewer complications and no need to find an anterior spinal exposure surgeon.

This publication uses the Medicare National Inpatient sample database to describe trends in LIF prevalence over the first decade of the 21st century. Although the authors are limited in their ability to suggest causation as to the different techniques and the resultant complications, the power of the large data set still provides some interesting statistics. The best part of the article is probably the sole figure (Fig 1), which provides an illustration of the geographic distribution of LIFs over the study period. The anterior lumbar fusions were performed predominantly in the large urban areas where one would expect to find a nucleus of academic spine surgeons with access to general surgeons familiar with the exposure. The techniques of PLIF and TLIF, which do not require a 2-surgeon team were more widely dispersed. Another interesting fact is that anterior and anterior/posterior fusion rates fell precipitously from 10% to 1% over the time period.

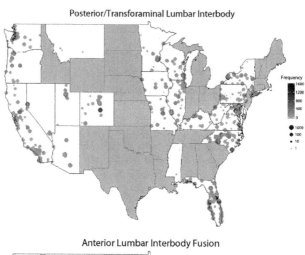

Posterior/Transforaminal Lumbar Interbody

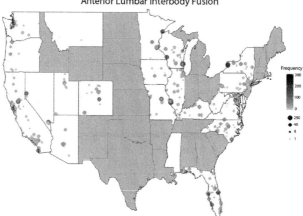

Anterior Lumbar Interbody Fusion

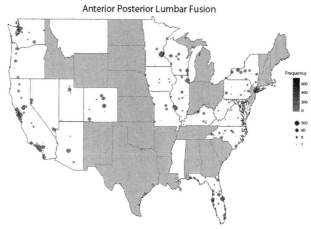

Anterior Posterior Lumbar Fusion

FIGURE 1.—Geographic distribution of posterior/transforaminal lumbar interbody fusion (Top), anterior lumbar interbody fusion (Middle), and combined anterior-posterior interbody fusions (Bottom) based on the data from 2001 to 2010. Size and color of points are proportional to the number of procedures. States in gray did not report hospital-identifying information for a minimum of 3 years. (Reprinted from The Spine Journal. Goz V, Weinreb JH, Schwab F, et al. Comparison of complications, costs, and length of stay of three different lumbar interbody fusion techniques: an analysis of the nationwide inpatient sample database. *Spine J.* 2014;14:2019-2027, Copyright 2014, with permission from Elsevier.)

With the development of improved anterior lumbar fixation, it is possible there might be a rebound in the future for anterior alone surgeries, but I believe this is unlikely. With the increasing emphasis on demonstrating medical value in health care, the increased costs and complications of the anterior and anterior/ posterior approaches set a high enough bar that it might not be possible to sufficiently increase the outcomes, safety, and satisfaction of the patients and payers to overcome posterior techniques. Laterally based interspinal fusion techniques are unlikely to overcome the convenience of posterior-based approaches because the extreme LIFs (or XLIFs) have their own complication profile related to lumbar plexus and viscera injury.

P. Huddleston, MD

Reference

1. Stauffer RN, Coventry MB. Anterior interbody lumbar spine fusion. Analysis of Mayo clinic series. *J Bone Joint Surg Am.* 1972;54:756-768.

Outcomes and Complications of Diabetes Mellitus on Patients Undergoing Degenerative Lumbar Spine Surgery

Guzman JZ, Iatridis JC, Skovrlj B, et al (Icahn School of Medicine at Mount Sinai, NY)
Spine 39:1596-1604, 2014

Study Design.—Retrospective database analysis.

Objective.—To assess the effect glycemic control has on perioperative morbidity and mortality in patients undergoing elective degenerative lumbar spine surgery.

Summary of Background Data.—Diabetes mellitus (DM) is a prevalent disease of glucose dysregulation that has been demonstrated to increase morbidity and mortality after spine surgery. However, there is limited understanding of whether glycemic control influences surgical outcomes in patients with DM undergoing lumbar spine procedures for degenerative conditions.

Methods.—The Nationwide Inpatient Sample was analyzed from 2002 to 2011. Hospitalizations were isolated on the basis of *International Classification of Diseases, Ninth Revision, Clinical Modification,* procedural codes for lumbar spine surgery and diagnoses codes for degenerative conditions of the lumbar spine. Patients were then classified into 3 cohorts: controlled diabetic, uncontrolled diabetic, and nondiabetic. Patient de ographic data, acute complications, and hospitalization outcomes were determined for each cohort.

Results.—A total of 403,629 (15.7%) controlled diabetic patients and 19,421 (0.75%) uncontrolled diabetic patients underwent degenerative lumbar spine surgery from 2002 to 2011. Relative to nondiabetic patients, uncontrolled diabetic patients had significantly increased odds of cardiac complications, deep venous thrombosis, and postoperative shock; in addition, uncontrolled diabetic patients also had an increased mean length of stay (approximately, 2.5 d), greater costs (1.3-fold), and a greater risk of inpatient mortality (odds ratio = 2.6, 95% confidence interval = 1.5–4.8, $P < 0.0009$). Controlled diabetic patients also had increased risk of acute complications and inpatient mortality when compared with nondiabetic patients, but not nearly to the same magnitude as uncontrolled diabetic patients.

Conclusion.—Suboptimal glycemic control in diabetic patients undergoing degenerative lumbar spine surgery leads to increased risk of acute complications and poor outcomes. Patients with uncontrolled DM, or poor glucose control, may benefit from improving glycemic control prior to surgery.

Level of Evidence.—3.

▶ Because diabetes mellitus (DM) is a common associated medical morbidity in obese patients, this research publication can rightly serve as a companion article on another of the YEAR BOOK selections on the relationship of obesity to spine surgery outcomes. Obesity has been described by the Centers for Disease Control and Prevention (CDC) as an "epidemic" and costs the country more than $150 billion a year, or almost 10% of the nation's medical costs.[1] Strongly associated with this epidemic has been the astronomical increase in type 2 DM, or adult onset diabetes. Whether caused by eating too much, exercising too little, or both, the diagnosis bodes poorly for the patient, and the consequences after spine surgery can be significant and life threatening. The authors leverage the enormous power of the National Inpatient Sample to examine a large cohort of more than 2 500 000 million patients who underwent degenerative lumbar spinal surgery between 2002 and 2011, focusing on controlled (> 400 000 patients) and uncontrolled (> 19 000 patients) diabetics.

Postoperative spine surgery patients with DM, either controlled or uncontrolled, all had more medical morbidities that those without DM. What is impressive is that congestive heart failure and renal disease increased 3-fold and 5-fold, respectively. Additionally, the uncontrolled DM patients were significantly more obese than controlled diabetics and had increased costs and length of stay.

The moral and professional questions remain unanswered with this investigation. Should spine surgeons be performing elective spine surgery on degenerative lumbar conditions in this population when resources are limited and the subsequent outcomes are so significantly poor? If so, how would a policy in this context be implemented? What associated DM control pathway or disease management program should be implemented, and is this the surgeon's responsibility? Or should patients be barred from even visiting with the surgeon until the DM is under control? Similarly, if a surgeon is consistently getting poor outcomes after elective degenerative lumbar surgery in the context of DM and fails to implement interventions preoperatively to normalize glucose control, is it unprofessional and/or unethical? I believe the rapid implementation of value-based purchasing and reimbursement of medical procedures in the Medicare population will provide the strong change that current peer pressure, professionalism, and ethics have not brought into effect.

P. Huddleston, MD

Reference

1. Centers for Disease Control and Prevention, Division of Nutrition, Physical Activity, and Obesity. www.cdc.gov. http://www.cdc.gov/nccdphp/dnpao/index.html. Accessed April 7, 2015.

A Review of Osteoporotic Vertebral Fracture Nonunion Management

Yang H, Pan J, Wang G (First Affiliated Hosp of Soochow Univ, Suzhou, China)
Spine 39:S142-S144, 2014

Osteoporotic vertebral fractures are a frequently encountered clinical problem, and like other fractures, they may develop nonunion that can often go unrecognized. The aim of this study is to review the related articles reporting the osteoporotic vertebral fracture nonunion and discuss the radiological characteristics, diagnosis, and treatment of osteoporotic vertebral fractures.

▶ In 2009, the oldest orthopedic society in the world, the American Orthopedic Association (AOA), promoted the "Own the Bone" campaign. This educational program was seen as a valuable tool for hospitals and providers to positively affect fragility care. Although some surgeons may see themselves as specialists or "proceduralists," the AOA vision for fragility fractures visualized the orthopedist as a key figure both in the diagnosis and treatment of osteoporotic compression fractures and as a valuable coordinator for the patient with various medical specialties involved in ideal care. The changing demographics of Western civilization will ensure that all practicing musculoskeletal specialists will encounter an increasingly aged but active population that is simultaneously more informed and demanding of a high level of functioning and quality of life. Providers must have a passing familiarity with the proper diagnosis of osteoporosis and the various classes of bone-sparing agents, as well as a rudimentary knowledge of the anabolic agents available for treatment.

This review focuses on an unfortunate but common complication of osteoporotic fracture, nonunion, also known by its eponym Kummell disease, a painful, progressive kyphosis, marked by a vertebral vacuum sign. For practitioners of invasive procedural, but not surgical, treatment of vertebral osteoporotic compressions fractures, the article contains several valuable skills and "tricks" for improving patient outcomes with vertebroplasty and kyphoplasty. Vertebroplasty has been found to be less effective because of its challenges in controlling the injected "cement," polymethyl methacrylate (PMMA). In contrast, vertebroplasty treatment of the nonunion "cleft" of Kummell disease involves the creation of a cavity within the vertebral body that allowed for a viscous injection of PMMA. This reduces the predilection of the cement to flow radially out of the vertebral body and endanger the host, either by injury to the adjacent neural structures or by embolism through adjacent veins.

It is still hotly disputed as to the proper role of vertebroplasty and kyphoplasty in acute vertebral body fractures. Musculoskeletal providers should not shy away from osteoporosis care and might consider these procedures as a way to "own the bone" and prevent the chronic pain, deformity, and dysfunction inherent in unrecognized Kummell disease.

P. Huddleston, MD

The Cascade of Medical Services and Associated Longitudinal Costs Due to Nonadherent Magnetic Resonance Imaging for Low Back Pain

Webster BS, Choi Y, Bauer AZ, et al (Liberty Mutual Res Inst for Safety, Hopkinton, MA; Univ of Massachusetts-Lowell)
Spine 39:1433-1440, 2014

Study Design.—Retrospective cohort study.

Objective.—To compare type, timing, and longitudinal medical costs incurred after adherent *versus* nonadherent magnetic resonance imaging (MRI) for work-related low back pain.

Summary of Background Data.—Guidelines advise against MRI for acute uncomplicated low back pain, but is an option for persistent radicular pain after a trial of conservative care. Yet, MRI has become frequent and often nonadherent. Few studies have documented the nature and impact of medical services (including type and timing) initiated by nonadherent MRI.

Methods.—A longitudinal, workers' compensation administrative data source was accessed to select low back pain claims filed between January 1, 2006 and December 31, 2006. Cases were grouped by MRI timing (early, timely, no MRI) and subgrouped by severity ("less severe," "more severe") (final cohort = 3022). Health care utilization for each subgroup was evaluated at 3, 6, 9, and 12 months post-MRI. Multivariate logistic regression models examined risk of receiving subsequent diagnostic studies and/or treatments, adjusting for pain indicators and demographic covariates.

Results.—The adjusted relative risks for MRI group cases to receive electromyography, nerve conduction testing, advanced imaging, injections, and surgery within 6 months post-MRI risks in the range from 6.5 (95% CI: 2.20−19.09) to 54.9 (95% CI: 22.12−136.21) times the rate for the referent group (no MRI less severe). The timely and early MRI less severe subgroups had similar adjusted relative risks to receive most services. The early MRI more severe subgroup cases had generally higher adjusted relative risks than timely MRI more severe subgroup cases. Medical costs for both early MRI subgroups were highest and increased the most over time.

Conclusion.—The impact of nonadherent MRI includes a wide variety of expensive and potentially unnecessary services, and occurs relatively soon post-MRI. Study results provide evidence to promote provider and patient conversations to help patients choose care that is based on evidence, free from harm, less costly, and truly necessary.

Level of Evidence.—N/A.

▶ In discussions about resource utilization and cost containment, no procedure will generate as much spirited discussion as MRI. Patients with spine conditions can be very expensive, not only in the sense of lost wages and degree of suffering, but also as in the cost of medical investigations. Radiographs, imaging, injections, and the proliferation of nonsurgical but procedural treatments for disc joints, facet joints, and nerves have proliferated like weapons in an arms race. Many of these interventions burgeon from the interpretation of the index MRI after an injury, insult, or incident. It has been well detailed that the incidental findings seen on these scans and those of the injured often frighten patients or excite providers to perpetuate a "cascade of medical services."

This institutional review board-approved research project was the product of Liberty Mutual Research Institute for Safety and included resource utilization and cost-based data on workers' compensation patients reporting low back injuries in 2006. The final cohort of 3022 patients were studied to determine a correlation between the severity of reported injury and the timing of the first MRI after injury. Workers suffering from low back pain after injury were 17 and 54 times more likely to undergo subsequent diagnostic services and invasive treatments within 6 months after injury than those who received no MRI. Cases with "red-flag" diagnoses of severe trauma, infection, cancer, or caudal equine syndrome were excluded.

The findings from this study are distressing to those who would advocate for an evidence-based evaluation of work-related low back pain as most of the subsequent resource utilization and cost seemed to emanate from the original MRI. Although it is common knowledge that the asymptotic population will manifest radiographic findings that are asymptomatic if screenings are performed, the discovery of these "injuries" on MRI (eg, bone spurs, osteophytes, and disc joint bulges) in the context of a recent injury will allot the asymptomatic finding an unwarranted association with the temporally related injury. Waiting for a period of approximately 6 weeks postinjury was associated with much lower imaging and procedural use, suggesting patients were healing, adapting, or accommodating their injury by that time and not interested in or suggested to pursue further treatment. Incentivization is another matter entirely. The MRI facility is often owned by the treating medical groups for these patients and can be a large source of income. Providers and health care organizations may consciously or unconsciously be influenced to obtain MRIs at the behest of the patient, employer, or qualified rehabilitation consultant to diagnose the worker. I have often heard, "Let's get the MRI so that we can see what's wrong so you can 'fix' me" in my practice. The challenge as the provider is to have the discipline and integrity to advocate for only the care that is supported by evidence, free from harm, and truly necessary.

P. Huddleston, MD

Impact of Increased Body Mass Index on Outcomes of Elective Spinal Surgery

Seicean A, Alan N, Seicean S, et al (Case Western Reserve Univ School of Medicine, Cleveland, OH; Univ Hosps, Cleveland, OH; et al)
Spine 39:1520-1530, 2014

Study Design.—Observational retrospective cohort study of prospectively collected database.

Objective.—To determine whether overweight body mass index (BMI) influences 30-day outcomes of elective spine surgery.

Summary of Background Data.—Obesity is prevalent in the United States, but its impact on the outcome of elective spine surgery remains controversial.

Methods.—We used National Surgical Quality Improvement Program, a prospective clinical database with proven validity and reproducibility consisting of 256 perioperative standardized variables from surgical patients at nearly 400 academic and nonacademic hospitals nationwide. We identified 49,314 patients who underwent elective fusion, laminectomy or both between 2006 and 2012. We divided patients according to BMI (kg/m^2) as normal (18.5−24.9), preobese (25.0−29.9), obese I (30.0−34.9), obese II (35.0−39.9), and obese III ($\geq$40). Relationship between increased BMI and outcome of surgery measured as prolonged hospitalization, complications, return to the operating room, discharged with continued care requirement, readmission, and death was determined using logistic regression before and after propensity score matching.

Results.—All overweight patients (BMI $\geq$25 kg/m^2) showed increased odds of an adverse outcome compared with normal patients in unmatched analyses, with maximal effect seen in obese III group. In the propensity-matched sample, obese III patients continued to show increased odds for complications (odds ratio, 1.6; 95% confidence interval, 1.1−2.3), readmission (odds ratio, 2.3; 95% confidence interval, 1.1−4.9), and return to the operating room (odds ratio, 1.8; 95% confidence interval, 1.1−3.1).

Conclusion.—Impact of obesity on elective spine surgery outcome is mediated, at least in part, by comorbidities in patients with BMI between 25.0 and 39.9 kg/m^2. However, BMI itself is an independent risk factor for adverse outcomes in morbidly obese patients.

Level of Evidence.—3.

▶ It has been surprising to see the many studies showing minimal differences in spinal outcome after spinal surgery in obese patients, even in the Spine Patient Outcomes Research Trial.[1] How could this be? A contrarian result has been selected for this spine review, and I believe it is more consistent with my professional experience. This interesting research from investigators using the National Surgical Quality Improvement Program (NSQIP) database uses a large cohort (50 000 patients) and some interesting statistics to suggest otherwise. The investigators from Case Western, the Ohio State University, and the Cleveland Clinic in fact prove what most surgeons have suspected all along, that obese patients have more complications within 30 days of surgery. It is interesting to consider how much of the angst in caring for this patient population is related to latent discomfort and anxiety related to the surgical technique. Decreased visibility, difficulty getting exposure, and performing closure all leave lasting imprints on an experienced surgeon's memory. This is separate and distinct from the challenges related to comorbidities that are often associated with the obese patient, such as diabetes, wound-healing issues, malnutrition, and mobility.

Limitations of the study include its short end point (30 days) and the fact that it does not incorporate patient-reported outcome measures. Further, although the database is enormous, it is retrospective in nature and does not represent patients who were denied surgery because of their body mass index (BMI) due to surgeon preference. However, NSQIP data do represent patients cared for in more than 400 academic and community hospitals and are collected in a standardized, deidentified, and randomized manner.

In factoring in mortality, the researchers did not notice any increase across the various increasing categories of BMI but did note that in the morbidly obese (BMI greater than 40), high BMI itself was predictive of complications, increased length of stay, and requiring skilled nursing postdischarge. This result should suggest strongly to even the most prepared and medically supported surgeon that surgical case selection can minimize postsurgical spine complications independent of the provider's ability to mitigate the risk of concomitant morbidities.

P. Huddleston, MD

Reference

1. Rihn JA, Radcliff K, Hilibrand AS, et al. Does obesity affect outcomes of treatment for lumbar stenosis and degenerative spondylolisthesis? analysis of the spine patient outcomes research trial (SPORT). *Spine*. 2012;37:1933-1946.

Variations in Medicare payments for episodes of spine surgery
Schoenfeld AJ, Harris MB, Liu H, et al (Univ of Michigan, Ann Arbor; Brigham and Women's Hosp, Boston, MA)
Spine J 14:2793-2798, 2014

Background Context.—Although the high cost of spine surgery is generally recognized, there is little information on the extent to which payments vary across hospitals.

Purpose.—To examine the variation in episode payments for spine surgery in the national Medicare population. We also sought to determine the root causes for observed variations in payment at high cost hospitals.

Study Design.—All patients in the national fee for service Medicare population undergoing surgery for three conditions (spinal stenosis, spondylolisthesis, and lumbar disc herniation) between 2005 and 2007 were included.

Patient Sample.—Included 185,954 episodes of spine surgery performed between 2005 and 2007.

Outcome Measures.—Payments per episode of spine surgery.

Methods.—All patients in the national fee for service Medicare population undergoing surgery for three conditions (spinal stenosis, spondylolisthesis, and lumbar disc herniation) between 2005 and 2007 were identified (n = 185,954 episodes of spine surgery). Hospitals were ranked on least to most expensive and grouped into quintiles. Results were risk- and price-adjusted using the empirical Bayes method. We then assessed the contributions of index hospitalization, physician services, readmissions, and postacute care to the overall variations in payment.

Results.—Episode payments for hospitals in the highest quintile were more than twice as high as those made to hospitals in the lowest quintile ($34,171 vs. $15,997). After risk- and price-adjustment, total episode payments to hospitals in the highest quintile remained $9,210 (47%) higher. Procedure choice, including the use of fusion, was a major determinant of the total episode payment. After adjusting for procedure choice, however, hospitals in the highest quintile continued to be 28% more expensive than those in the lowest. Differences in the use of postacute care accounted for most of this residual variation in payments across hospitals. Hospital episode payments varied to a similar degree after subgroup analyses for disc herniation, spinal stenosis, and spondylolisthesis. Hospitals expensive for one condition were also found to be expensive for services provided for other spinal diagnoses.

Conclusions.—Medicare payments for episodes of spine surgery vary widely across hospitals. As they respond to the new financial incentives inherent in health care reform, high cost hospitals should focus on the use of spinal fusion and postacute care.

▶ Although the title of this research article references the seemingly colorless topic of Medicare payments, the substance touches on a truly provocative point about human behavior. The authors, from the University of Michigan and Harvard University, describe the tremendous variation in the cost of providing spine care for Medicare beneficiaries for 3 standard conditions: spinal stenosis, spondylolisthesis, and lumbar disc herniation. At first glance, there is a variation of more than 100% in the cost of care from the least to most expensive. Even after adjusting for risk and procedure of choice, the variation approached 50%. How is this possible, you might ask? Follow the money! In the 1976 movie *All The President's Men*, screenwriter William Goldman attributed this phrase to Deep Throat, the Watergate informant eventually outed to be FBI Deputy Director W. Mark Felt. Felt's suggestion that the key to understanding the investigations into the Watergate controversy at the time were to understand the path and influence of campaign money. In the spinal care world, our parallel would be "follow the fusion!" Introduction of a spinal arthrodesis into the care of these 3 diseases, although warranted in many cases, also interjects great cost with inconsistent benefit. Even if there were universally agreement on the indication for arthrodesis, there still exist many technique options for even a straightforward diagnosis of L4-L5 degenerative spondylolisthesis. Some surgeons might insist on an uninstrumented posterior lateral technique, whereas others might still use a 360 or even transforaminal interbody procedure, and each with different risk profiles and reimbursement rates. This dramatic and persistent cost in care variation, in the face of widespread and easily obtainable medical evidence, suggests that individual health care providers are being effectively motivated, consciously or unconsciously, not by medical evidence but by economic incentives. As the variation in care and cost destroys the efficient delivery of value to all participants in health care delivery, it becomes clear that current incentives need to be realigned to effect any meaningful and durable change in health delivery variation and its downstream influence on cost of care. The current trend toward outcomes-based reimbursement is currently the most likely alternative. As Mitt Romney noted, "The answer for health care is market incentives, not a Godzilla-sized government bureaucracy."

P. Huddleston, MD

The use of bone morphogenetic protein in thoracolumbar spine procedures: analysis of the MarketScan longitudinal database
Veeravagu A, Cole TS, Jiang B, et al (Stanford Univ School of Medicine, Palo Alto, CA; et al)
Spine J 14:2929-2937, 2014

Background Context.—The use of recombinant human bone morphogenetic protein (BMP) in the thoracolumbar spine remains controversial, with many questioning the risks and benefits of this new biologic.

Purpose.—To describe national trends, incidence of complications, and revision rates associated with BMP use in thoracolumbar spine procedures.

Study Design/Setting.—Administrative database study.

Patient Sample.—A matched cohort of 52,259 patients undergoing thoracolumbar fusion surgery from 2006 to 2010 were identified in the MarketScan database. Patients without BMP treatment were matched 2:1 to patients receiving intraoperative BMP.

Outcome Measures.—Revision rates and postoperative complications.

Methods.—The MarketScan database was used to select patients undergoing thoracolumbar fusion procedures, with and without intraoperative BMP. We ascertained outcome measures using either *International Classification of Disease, ninth revision*, or Current Procedural Terminology coding, and matched groups were evaluated using a bivariate and multivariate analyses. Kaplan-Meier estimates of fusions failure rates were also calculated.

Results.—Patients receiving intraoperative BMP underwent fewer refusions, decompressions, posterior and anterior revisions, or any revision procedure (single level 4.53% vs. 5.85%, $p < .0001$; multilevel 5.02% vs. 6.83%, $p < .0001$; overall cohort 4.73% vs. 6.09%, $p < .0001$). After adjusting for comorbidities, demographics, and levels of procedure, BMP was not associated with the postoperative development of cancer (odds ratio 0.92). Bone morphogenetic protein use was associated with an increase in any complication at 30 days (15.8% vs. 14.9%, $p = .0065$), which is only statistically significant among multilevel procedures (19.74% vs. 18.02%, $p = .0013$). Thirty-day complications in multilevel procedures associated with BMP use included new dysrhythmia (4.68% vs. 4.01%, $p = .0161$) and delirium (1.08% vs. 0.69%, $p = .0024$). A new diagnosis of chronic pain was associated with BMP use in both single-level (2.74% vs. 2.15%, $p = 0019$) and multilevel (3.7% vs. 2.52%, $p < .0001$) procedures. Bone morphogenetic protein was negatively associated with infection in single-level procedures (2.12% vs. 2.64%, $p = .0067$) and wound dehiscence in multilevel procedures (0.84% vs. 1.18%, $p = .0167$).

Conclusions.—In national data analysis of thoracolumbar procedures, we found that BMP was associated with decreased incidence of revision spinal surgery and with a slight increased risk of overall complications at 30 days. Although no BMP-associated increased risk of malignancy was found, lack of long-term follow-up precludes detection of between-group differences in malignancies and other rare events that may not appear until later.

▶ The product Infuse or bone morphogenic protein-2 (BMP) continues to be a controversial and important adjunct to spine surgery. With the intense media focus on the product, it is important to remember the staff and consumer enthusiasm for the drug/implant in its early years. Some casual anecdotes I remember hearing in meetings, clinics, and the surgical halls were, "it's a 'bone bomb'," it would "eliminate the need for autograft," it "guaranteed fusion," and that it was going to eliminate anterior spine surgery and enable minimally invasive surgery in the spine, just like the knee. As large data sets become available to better reflect on and understand the effect of BMP on spine surgery in the United States, a better profile of its impact and the needed requirement for studies ahead is clear.

The authors published data from Thomson Reuters Market Scan Commercial Claims and Encounters database combined with data from Medicare. This enabled an analysis of more than 100 payers and inpatient, outpatient, and pharmacy services from a wide range of large employers, health plans, and organizations. The final data set had information on a cohort of more than 52 000 patients who underwent thoracolumbar surgery from 2006 to 2010. They studied readmission and reparation rates as well as the relationship between BMP use and malignant neoplasm. Mean follow-up was about a year and a half for both groups. Members of the BMP groups were seen to have a higher risk of postoperative complications, but they used less pain medicine as a group up to 180 days postoperation. This cohort did not show an increase in malignancy, contrary to the previously reported Food and Drug Administration AMPLIFY data on posterior lateral fusions.

One of the interesting insights into this study is the possibility that there may be something fundamentally different in the surgeons who use BMP and those that do not. If the conclusions of this study and others are consciously or unconsciously known to the surgeons and caregivers that perform spine surgery, what does it say about the differences in the providers. Is one group "comfortable" or accepting of a higher complication rate at 30 days? Do they "like" taking the phone calls to console the patients for their leg pain or retrograde ejaculation that has been noted with Infuse use? Are surgeons who do not use BMP indifferent to the fact that their reapportion is higher? Do the Infuse users not have access or training in anterior procedures and have lower reported use of this procedure to increase fusion rate? Are the patients, surgeons, and hospitals aware that the utilization of BMP has added $900 million in hospital charges without failing to reduce the frequency of autograft bone harvest, and does this influence their behavior? These are rhetorical questions, but they attempt to pose the following question for dialogue: What are the surgeon differences, if any, between cohorts that received BMP vs those that did not? Only a double-blind prospective randomized trial will be able to provide the information to help answer and provide insight into these questions and many others.

P. Huddleston, MD

Surgeon Specialty and Outcomes After Elective Spine Surgery

Seicean A, Alan N, Seicean S, et al (Case Western Reserve Univ School of Medicine, Cleveland, OH; Univ Hosps, Cleveland, OH; et al)
Spine 39:1605-1613, 2014

Study Design.—Retrospective cohort analysis of prospectively collected clinical data.

Objective.—To compare outcomes of elective spine fusion and laminectomy when performed by neurological and orthopedic surgeons.

Summary of Background Data.—The relationship between primary specialty training and outcome of spinal surgery is unknown.

Methods.—We analyzed the 2006 to 2012 American College of Surgeons National Surgical Quality Improvement Project database of 50,361 patients, 33,235 (66%) of which were operated on by a neurosurgeon. We eliminated all differences in preoperative and intraoperative risk factors between surgical specialties by matching 17,126 patients who underwent orthopedic surgery (OS) to 17,126 patients who underwent neurosurgery (NS) on propensity scores. Regular and conditional logistic regressions were used to predict adverse postoperative outcomes in the full sample and matched sample, respectively. The effect of perioperative transfusion on outcomes was further assessed in the matched sample.

Results.—Diagnosis and procedure were the only factors that were found to be significantly different between surgical subspecialties in the full sample. We found that compared with patients who underwent NS, patients who underwent OS were more than twice as likely to experience prolonged length of stay (LOS) (odds ratio: 2.6, 95% confidence interval: 2.4-2.8), and significantly more likely to receive a transfusion perioperatively, have complications, and to require discharge with continued care.

After matching, patients who underwent OS continued to have slightly higher odds for prolonged LOS, and twice the odds for receiving perioperative transfusion compared with patients who underwent NS. Taking into account perioperative transfusion did not eliminate the difference in LOS between patients who underwent OS and those who underwent NS.

Conclusion.—Patients operated on by OS have twice the odds for undergoing perioperative transfusion and slightly increased odds for prolonged LOS. Other differences between surgical specialties in 30-day postoperative outcomes were minimal. Analysis of a large, multi-institutional sample of prospectively collected clinical data suggests that surgeon specialty has limited influence on short-term outcomes after elective spine surgery.

Level of Evidence.—3.

▶ Common in military jargon, a "BLUF," or "bottom line up front," places the conclusion or recommendation at the beginning to facilitate rapid decision making. In this YEAR BOOK selection, patients who undergo spine surgery have a significantly higher risk of requiring transfusion and more than twice the odds of prolonged length of stay (LOS). This provocative conclusion once again represents the research power of researchers using large, standardized patient health databases such as the Medicare National Inpatient Sample (NIS) or, in the case of this article, the American College of Surgeons National Surgical Quality improvement Project (NSQIP). As a companion article to another selection for this YEAR BOOK,[1] this work might lull readers into concluding that the increased spine caseload of neurologic surgeons is leading to improved outcomes. Au contraire, mon frère! This conclusion by researchers should not serve as a call to arms for all orthopedist in a struggle for market share and influence but serve as another excellent example of the strengths and weaknesses of the NSQIP database.

In this study, more than 50 000 patients were analyzed with 66% of them being operated on by neurosurgeons (NS). Although initial comparisons revealed even larger differences between the operated groups when analyzed by specialty type, a 1-to-1 match between NS and orthopedic surgeons (OS) showed very little difference. OS were more likely to operate on older patients and perform fusion with laminectomy. NS were more commonly performing surgeries on patients with spondylosis (ie, arthritis) presumably for spinal stenosis and resultant nerve compression and for patients with the diagnosis of disc displacement or herniation. This mirrors what I have observed in my training and practice experience. Thinking about the risk of transfusion and increased LOS, it seems reasonable that there might be an increased transfusion rate in arthrodesis patients, and on further scrutiny, the risk of increased LOS was for "prolonged LOS," defined as more than 4 days. Average LOS between the groups was not significant.

Still, practitioners should take this information as support for further development of common pathways to protocols and define standard care for fusion and nonfusion spinal procedures. As the science of spine surgery is further refined, both OS and NS spine specialists should strive to blur the differences in care to achieve similar, best outcomes for the benefit of patients; providers and payers should not be able to tell the difference between the 2 disciplines with regard to spine care. I think we will know when our work is done when we no longer hear the question I have heard from patients dozens of times over my career: "Are you a NS or OS spine specialist, and what's the difference?"

P. Huddleston, MD

Reference

1. Daniels AH, Ames CP, Smith JS, Hart RA. Variability in spine surgery procedures performed during orthopaedic and neurological surgery residency training: an analysis of ACGME case log data. *J Bone Joint Surg Am.* 2014;96:e196.

Variability in Spine Surgery Procedures Performed During Orthopaedic and Neurological Surgery Residency Training: An Analysis of ACGME Case Log Data

Daniels AH, Ames CP, Smith JS, et al (Brown Univ, Providence, RI; Univ of California San Francisco; Univ of Virginia, Charlottesville; et al)

J Bone Joint Surg Am 96:e196(1-7), 2014

Background.—Current spine surgeon training in the United States consists of either an orthopaedic or neurological surgery residency, followed by an optional spine surgery fellowship. Resident spine surgery procedure volume may vary between and within specialties.

Methods.—The Accreditation Council for Graduate Medical Education surgical case logs for graduating orthopaedic surgery and neurosurgery residents from 2009 to 2012 were examined and were compared for spine surgery resident experience.

Results.—The average number of reported spine surgery procedures performed during residency was 160.2 spine surgery procedures performed by orthopaedic surgery residents and 375.0 procedures performed by neurosurgery residents; the mean difference of 214.8 procedures (95% confidence interval, 196.3 to 231.7 procedures) was significant ($p = 0.002$). From 2009 to 2012, the average total spinal surgery procedures logged by orthopaedic surgery residents increased 24.3% from 141.1 to 175.4 procedures, and those logged by neurosurgery residents increased 6.5% from 367.9 to 391.8 procedures. There was a significant difference ($p < 0.002$) in the average number of spinal deformity procedures between graduating orthopaedic surgery residents (9.5 procedures) and graduating neurosurgery residents (2.0 procedures). There was substantial variability in spine surgery exposure within both specialties; when comparing the top 10% and bottom 10% of 2012 graduates for spinal instrumentation or arthrodesis procedures, there was a 13.1-fold difference for orthopaedic surgery residents and an 8.3-fold difference for neurosurgery residents.

Conclusions.—Spine surgery procedure volumes in orthopaedic and neurosurgery residency training programs vary greatly both within and between specialties. Although orthopaedic surgery residents had an increase in the number of spine procedures that they performed from 2009 to 2012, they averaged less than half of the number of spine procedures performed by neurological surgery residents. However, orthopaedic surgery residents appear to have greater exposure to spinal deformity than neurosurgery residents. Furthermore, orthopaedic spine fellowship training provides additional spine surgery case exposure of approximately 300 to 500 procedures; thus, before entering independent practice, when compared with neurosurgery residents, most orthopaedic spine surgeons complete as many spinal procedures or more. Although case volume is not the sole determinant of surgical skills or clinical decision making, variability in spine surgery procedure volume does exist among residency programs in the United States.

▶ The specialty of spine surgery lies within 2 disciplines of procedural care, much as radiology and vascular medicine straddled the interventional vascular specialties in the early to late 1990s. Over the past 20 years, innovations in medical technology have driven many of the improvements in that discipline, with the development of arterial and venous stents leading the way. It seems that both disciplines have maintained a healthy presence in this common anatomic space within institutions with which I am familiar, with vascular surgeons continuing to place stents and perform open surgeries while radiologists have continued to provide services in diagnostic angiography imaging and inferior vena cava filter placement. As the content of the fellowship training has converged, the groups have moved closer together; I believe this will serve as a template for the spine specialties within orthopedics and neurologic sciences going forward.

The authors nicely review data from Accreditation Council for Graduate Medical Education (ACGME) credited programs to describe the information available from 2009 through 2012 on 148 orthopedic and 85 neurological surgery programs. As professionals in this space might suppose, the neurologic surgery residents are exposed to almost twice as many spine cases on their residency than that of orthopedics surgery residents. The orthopedics residents had more than 4 times as many deformity cases as their neurologic surgery colleagues even as the neurosurgery residents documented more spinal instrumentation cases and fusion cases. Factoring in the variability between the 90th and 10th percentile within the 2 groups, they revealed a high degree of variability in both. When considering the finished product of completing an additional spine fellowship for an orthopedic trainee, this would add another 300 to 500 cases to their case logs because most spine fellowship trained orthopedists will have logged more spine cases than their neurologic surgeon equivalents.

Weaknesses in this report included the fact that it encompasses the ACGME accredited programs and assumes all trainees accurately log their cases and that these representative cases actually represent a true exposure to spine surgery. This report additionally did not capture or make any conclusions regarding work-hour restrictions and their possible effects on case numbers and quality.

What seems obvious to me is that the current arguments about competency and proficiency in the spine field should focus more on the commonalities of the training and attempt to minimize the differences going forward. Much as the vascular and radiologic specialists have found, the patient does not really care about the degree of the result. Both orthopedic surgery and neurologic surgery should work toward a shared or combined curriculum in the area to assist in the training and education to standardize the specialty. The patients and general public, as well as the shared science, will benefit only in the long term.

P. Huddleston, MD

Diagnostic accuracy of history taking to assess lumbosacral nerve root compression

Verwoerd AJH, Peul WC, Willemsen SP, et al (Erasmus MC Univ Med Ctr, Rotterdam, The Netherlands; Leiden Univ Med Ctr, The Netherlands)
Spine J 14:2028-2037, 2014

Background Context.—The diagnosis of sciatica is primarily based on history and physical examination. Most physical tests used in isolation show poor diagnostic accuracy. Little is known about the diagnostic accuracy of history items.

Purpose.—To assess the diagnostic accuracy of history taking for the presence of lumbosacral nerve root compression or disc herniation on magnetic resonance imaging in patients with sciatica.

Study Design.—Cross-sectional diagnostic study.

Patient Sample.—A total of 395 adult patients with severe disabling radicular leg pain of 6 to 12 weeks duration were included.

Outcome Measures.—Lumbosacral nerve root compression and disc herniation on magnetic resonance imaging were independently assessed by two neuroradiologists and one neurosurgeon blinded to any clinical information.

Methods.—Data were prospectively collected in nine hospitals. History was taken according to a standardized protocol. There were no study-specific conflicts of interest.

Results.—Exploring the diagnostic odds ratio of 20 history items revealed a significant contribution in diagnosing nerve root compression for "male sex," "pain worse in leg than in back," and "a non-sudden onset." A significant contribution to the diagnosis of a herniated disc was found for "body mass index <30," "a non-sudden onset," and "sensory loss." Multivariate logistic regression analysis of six history items preselected from the literature (age, gender, pain worse in leg than in back, sensory loss, muscle weakness, and more pain on coughing/sneezing/straining) revealed an area under the receiver operating characteristic curve of 0.65 (95% confidence interval, 0.58−0.71) for the model diagnosing nerve root compression and an area under the receiver operating characteristic curve of 0.66 (95% confidence interval, 0.58−0.74) for the model diagnosing disc herniation.

Conclusions.—A few history items used in isolation had significant diagnostic value and the diagnostic accuracy of a model with six pre-selected items was poor.

▶ In a companion article in this YEAR BOOK OF ORTHOPEDICS SPINE collection, "The Cascade of Medical Services and Associated Longitudinal Costs Due to Nonadherent magnetic Resonance Imaging for Low Back Pain" by Webster et al, the authors point out the fascinating and detailed financial associations between obtaining an magnetic resonance (MR) early in the time line of acute back pain and sciatica with its high costs and association with subsequent interventions. In our health care environment, the influence of cost controls and a push for value has placed greater emphasis on history, physical examination, and clinical pathways.[1] Because value in health care can be described as Value = Quality divided by Cost, large increases in health care delivery cost will always lower delivered value in the absence of an increase in quality. As medical imaging continues to be a prime determinant of surgical intervention, any attempt to decrease cost in spine care must address MR indications.

The authors of this report performed a prospective study of the predictive value of a small battery of questions to predict herniated disc and nerve compression, as validated by an actual MR of the affected lumber spine. Significant findings included identifying variables such as male sex, pain worse in the leg than in the back, and a non-sudden onset as having a significant positive value in diagnosing lumbosacral nerve root compression on MRI. Variable body mass index < 30, non-sudden onset, and having a sensory loss were associated with predicting lumbar disc herniation on MRI. Unfortunately, predictions based on 6 published questions from the literature performed poorly.

If readers find frustrating the conclusion that a standard collection of familiar low back pain questions published in the literature is of mediocre usefulness but a couple of specific questions in the right patient might be helpful, this editor would agree. It suggests that there is more to the effectiveness of the spine history than just the questions. I would always advocate for the simultaneous alignment of the patient's symptoms, the physical findings, and the imaging to best predict the diagnosis and predict a positive outcome after appropriate intervention. The pressure to avoid advanced imaging will increasingly stress the musculoskeletal specialist to do more with less. The evidence-based practice is still insufficient regarding spine care; successful outcomes will continue to involve the wise distillation of patient and disease variables, which is difficult to quantify and value (ie, experience). The ability to appreciate this gestalt represents the art of medicine and the key to positive outcomes in spine care.

P. Huddleston, MD

Reference

1. Vroomen PC, de Krom MC, Wilmink JT, Kester AD, Knottnerus JA. Diagnostic value of history and physical examination in patients suspected of lumbosacral nerve root compression. *J Neurol Neurosurg Psychiatry.* 2002;72:630-634.

Cost savings analysis of intrawound vancomycin powder in posterior spinal surgery

Emohare O, Ledonio CG, Hill BW, et al (Regions Hosp, Saint Paul, MN; Univ of Minnesota, Minneapolis; Saint Louis Univ, MO)
Spine J 14:2710-2715, 2014

Background Context.—Recent studies have shown that prophylactic use of intrawound vancomycin in posterior instrumented spine surgery substantially decreases the incidence of wound infections requiring repeat surgery. Significant cost savings are thought to be associated with the use of vancomycin in this setting.

Purpose.—To elucidate cost savings associated with the use of intrawound vancomycin in posterior spinal surgeries using a budget-impact model.

Study Design.—Retrospective cohort study.

Patient Sample.—Data from a cohort of 303 patients who underwent spinal surgery (instrumented and noninstrumented) over 2 years were analyzed; 96 of these patients received prophylactic intrawound vancomycin powder in addition to normal intravenous (IV) antibiotic prophylaxis, and 207 received just routine IV antibiotic prophylaxis. Patients requiring repeat surgical procedures for infection were identified, and the costs of these additional procedures were elucidated.

Outcome Measure.—Cost associated with the additional procedure to remediate infection in the absence of vancomycin prophylaxis.

Methods.—We retrospectively reviewed the cost of return procedures for treatment of surgical site infection (SSI). The total reimbursement received by the health care facility was used to model the costs associated with repeat surgery, and this cost was compared with the cost of a single local application of vancomycin costing about $12.

Results.—Of the 96 patients in the treatment group, the return-to-surgery rate for SSI was 0. In the group without vancomycin, seven patients required a total of 14 procedures. The mean cost per episode of surgery, based on the reimbursement, the health care facility received was $40,992 (range, $14,459–$114,763). A total of $573,897 was spent on 3% of the 207-patient cohort that did not receive intrawound vancomycin, whereas a total of $1,152 ($12×96 patients) was spent on the cohort treated with vancomycin.

Conclusions.—This study shows a reduction in SSIs requiring a return-to-surgery—with large cost savings—with use of intrawound vancomycin powder. In our study population, the cost savings totaled more than half a million dollars.

▶ With the terrible price in patient suffering, hospital expense, and the cost to society and how it's related to surgical site infection (SSI), surgeons have aggressively moved toward the prophylactic use of powdered vancomycin applied directly to the surgical wounds. Previously reported results from other studies have suggested a reduction in SSIs with this technique in spine trauma patients.[1] There is some concern that the more prevalent use of antibiotics will provide selection pressure on the organisms endemic to local SSIs and either encourage antibiotic resistance or shift the representative spectrum or organisms.

The authors from the University of Minnesota and Regions Hospital in St Paul, Minnesota have suggested with this retrospective review a decrease in deep wound infection when comparing a group of 96 patients who received prophylactic vancomycin to the wound and 206 patients who did not. There were 5 superficial infections reported in each group and 7 deep infections in the control group. Cost data were generated that suggested more than $1.2 million were billed in the 7 infected patients with just over $500 00 in reimbursement. Three of the 7 infected accounted for 10 of the 14 readmissions.

The differences in the 2 populations, which were not case matched, are too different to draw any conclusions. Previous publications examining the association between vancomycin use and SSI have noted a much higher reported complication rate in the wound powdered antibiotic groups. Additionally, at our institution, we have seen an increase in reported Gram-negative organisms infecting the vancomycin use groups. This editor cautions readers to maintain a healthy skepticism with this technique but supports the future prospective randomized study of its use.

P. Huddleston, MD

Reference

1. Godil SS, Parker SL, O'Neill KR, Devin CJ, McGirt MJ. Comparative effectiveness and cost-benefit analysis of local application of vancomycin powder in posterior spinal fusion for spine trauma: clinical article. *J Neurosurg Spine.* 2013;19: 331-335.

A retrospective study of iliac crest bone grafting techniques with allograft reconstruction: do patients even know which iliac crest was harvested?
Pirris SM, Nottmeier EW, Kimes S, et al (Mayo Clinic, Rochester, MN; Mayo Clinic College of Medicine in Florida, Jacksonville; et al)
J Neurosurg Spine 21:595-600, 2014

Object.—Considerable biological research has been performed to aid bone healing in conjunction with lumbar fusion surgery. Iliac crest autograft is often considered the gold standard because it has the vital properties of being osteoconductive, osteoinductive, and osteogenic. However, graft site pain has been widely reported as the most common donor site morbidity. Autograft site pain has led many companies to develop an abundance of bone graft extenders, which have limited proof of efficacy. During the surgical consent process, many patients ask surgeons to avoid harvesting autograft because of the reported pain complications. The authors sought to study postoperative graft site pain by simply asking patients whether they knew which iliac crest was grafted when a single skin incision was made for the fusion operation.

Methods.—Twenty-five patients underwent iliac crest autografting with allograft reconstruction during instrumented lumbar fusion surgery. In all patients the autograft was harvested through the same skin incision but with a separate fascial incision. At various points postoperatively, the patients were asked if they could tell which iliac crest had been harvested, and if so, how much pain did it cause (10-point Numeric Rating Scale).

Results.—Most patients (64%) could not correctly determine which iliac crest had been harvested. Of the 9 patients who correctly identified the side of the autograft, 7 were only able to guess. The 2 patients who confidently identified the side of grafting had no pain at rest and mild pain with activity. One patient who incorrectly guessed the side of autografting did have significant sacroiliac joint degenerative pain bilaterally.

Conclusions.—Results of this study indicate the inability of patients to clearly define their graft site after iliac crest autograft harvest with allograft reconstruction of the bony defect unless they have a separate skin incision. This simple, easily reproducible pilot study can be expanded into a larger, multiinstitutional investigation to provide more definitive answers regarding the ideal, safe, and cost-effective bone graft material to be used in spinal fusions.

▶ It has been the teaching in spine surgery that iliac crest donor-site pain is often worse than spine surgical-site pain for so long that it has become mantra. But is it, and can patients really tell the difference? The authors from Jacksonville, Florida, asked this very question and found that patients were less likely to be able to predict the side of their iliac crest bone grafting than the chance of a coin flip. In fact, only 36% of patients guessed correctly, and most of those admitted freely they had guessed! Although the very real potential complications of iliac crest autographing cannot be denied, the concern of pain at the door site may not actually be consistent or clinically relevant. Ten years ago in spine practice, it was common for iliac crest grafting to be performed through a posterior vertical incision from the posterior superior iliac spine (PSIS) to the posterior inferior iliac spine (PIIS) or a diagonal incision originating over the skin superficial to the posterior inferior iliac spine, continuing cranial and superiorly toward the iliac crest. That particular approach, although easy to create and providing good visibility, often strayed close to the path of the clonal nerves. These nerves are vulnerable to injury; whether during the approach and cut or burned with an electric knife or caught up in the closure and sutured together in the repair, such events can cause chronic and severe paresthesias and dysesthesias in the area of the incision. In an effort to minimize such complications, I began taking iliac crest graft from supra fascial incision but using the same skin incision. This minimizes the potential to traumatize the nerve bundles of the mid to lateral iliac crest and, when accompanied with a vertical incision rom the PSIS to the PIIS, places the incision directly over the largest portion of cancellous bone available using a posterior approach.

The authors freely and correctly acknowledge the limitation of the study but do encourage others to challenge their own beliefs and patients' perceptions before summarily dismissing the role of iliac crest autograft, the gold standard, from the surgical armamentarium in the future.

P. Huddleston, MD

Epidural Steroid Injections, Conservative Treatment, or Combination Treatment for Cervical Radicular Pain: A Multicenter, Randomized, Comparative-effectiveness Study
Cohen SP, Hayek S, Semenov Y, et al (Johns Hopkins School of Medicine, Baltimore, MD; Case Western Reserve School of Medicine, Cleveland, OH; Massachusetts General Hosp, Boston; et al)
Anesthesiology 121:1045-1055, 2014

Background.—Cervical radicular pain is a major cause of disability. No studies have been published comparing different types of nonsurgical therapy.

Methods.—A comparative-effectiveness study was performed in 169 patients with cervical radicular pain less than 4 yr in duration. Participants received nortriptyline and/or gabapentin plus physical therapies, up to three cervical epidural steroid injections (ESI) or combination treatment over 6 months. The primary outcome measure was average arm pain on a 0 to 10 scale at 1 month.

Results.—One-month arm pain scores were 3.5 (95% CI, 2.8 to 4.2) in the combination group, 4.2 (CI, 2.8 to 4.2) in ESI patients, and 4.3 (CI, 2.8 to 4.2) in individuals treated conservatively ($P = 0.26$). Combination group patients experienced a mean reduction of -3.1 (95% CI, -3.8 to -2.3) in average arm pain at 1 month *versus* -1.8 (CI, -2.5 to -1.2) in the conservative group and -2.0 (CI, -2.7 to -1.3) in ESI patients ($P = 0.035$). For neck pain, a mean reduction of -2.2 (95% CI, -3.0 to -1.5) was noted in combination patients *versus* -1.2 (CI, -1.9 to -0.5) in conservative group patients and -1.1 (CI, -1.8 to -0.4) in those who received ESI; ($P = 0.064$). Three-month posttreatment, 56.9% of patients treated with combination therapy experienced a positive outcome *versus* 26.8% in the conservative group and 36.7% in ESI patients ($P = 0.006$).

Conclusions.—For the primary outcome measure, no significant differences were found between treatments, although combination therapy provided better improvement than stand-alone treatment on some measures. Whereas these results suggest an interdisciplinary approach to neck pain may improve outcomes, confirmatory studies are needed.

▶ Better patient outcomes and pain relief were found in this prospective study randomizing patients with cervical radiculopathy to conservative pharmacotherapy with physical therapy (PT), epidural steroid injection, or combination treatment with PT and at least 1 injection and oral medication. Surprising? Not really, but it reinforces the potential value of a multidisciplinary method to address this condition and the patients who suffer. These studies are a tremendous effort to run and complete, and the authors in this largely military intervention deserve a lot of credit for bringing the effort to completion and reporting their findings. Just over one-third of the patients who were eligible enrolled and completed the investigation. Patients were followed over a 6-month timeframe.

If you have suffered from a bad cervical radiculopathy, you will understand and remember the often terrible and relentless nature of the discomfort. Although many well-done studies will appropriately report the long-term (1- and 2-year) outcomes to make decisions about durability, it is important to appreciate that 1-month pain scores for both the neck and the arm were lower in the combination treatment group. Although it may be difficult to demonstrate value in such a short time period, the humane aspect of an early effect is always an added bonus whether you are the patient or the physician. In their analysis, the authors found at both the 3- and 6-month follow-ups, providers had more comfortable patients with combination therapy. I believe that even if these results were not strongly statistically significant, the trend would suggest that, for certain populations of patients, the outcomes will be improved if the solo orthopedist incorporates a team of therapists of physiatrists, anesthesiologist, or interventional radiologists to participate in a multimodal and multidisciplinary interventions. From the provider's standpoint, the burden of care can be shared among providers, and a consistent treatment algorithm can decrease variation within a practice and increase value delivered to the patient. Additionally, the opportunity to standardize the care for this diagnosis and condition allows for the implementation and intervention at the entry into the medical system. In a properly organized clinic, the surgical specialist would then see only the patients who had failed such an organized and evidenced-based intervention; improving efficiency. Weaknesses of the study include the lack of standardization of both the PT and the pharmacotherapeutic arms. Again, these authors present a wonderful opportunity to standardize the creation of a integrated intervention that should improve satisfaction for both providers and patients.

P. Huddleston, MD

Differences in the surgical treatment of recurrent lumbar disc herniation among spine surgeons in the United States

Mroz TE, Lubelski D, Williams SK, et al (Cleveland Clinic Foundation, OH; Univ of Miami Miller School of Medicine, FL; et al)
Spine J 14:2334-2343, 2014

Background Context.—There are often multiple surgical treatment options for a spinal pathology. In addition, there is a lack of data that define differences in surgical treatment among surgeons in the United States.

Purpose.—To assess the surgical treatment patterns among neurologic and orthopedic spine surgeons in the United States for the treatment of one- and two-time recurrent lumbar disc herniation.

Study Design.—Electronic survey.

Patient Sample.—An electronic survey was delivered to 2,560 orthopedic and neurologic surgeons in the United States.

Outcome Measures.—The response data were analyzed to assess the differences among respondents over various demographic variables. The probability of disagreement is reported for various surgeon subgroups.

Methods.—A survey of clinical and radiographic case scenarios that included a one- and two-time lumbar disc herniation was electronically delivered to 2,560 orthopedic and neurologic surgeons in the United States. The surgical treatment options were revision microdiscectomy, revision microdiscectomy with in situ fusion, revision microdiscectomy with posterolateral fusion using pedicle screws, revision microdiscectomy with posterior lumbar interbody fusion/transforaminal lumbar interbody fusion (PLIF/TLIF), anterior lumbar interbody fusion (ALIF) with percutaneous screws, ALIF with open posterior instrumentation, or none of these. Significance of $p = .01$ was used to account for multiple comparisons.

Results.—Four hundred forty-five surgeons (18%) completed the survey. Surgeons in practice for 15+ years were more likely to select revision microdiscectomy compared with surgeons with fewer years in practice who were more likely to select revision microdiscectomy with PLIF/TLIF ($p < .001$). Similarly, those surgeons performing 200+ surgeries per year were more likely to select revision microdiscectomy with PLIF/TLIF than those performing fewer surgeries ($p = .003$). No significant differences were identified for region, specialty, fellowship training, or practice type. Overall, there was a 69% and 22% probability that two randomly selected spine surgeons would disagree on the surgical treatment of two- and one-time recurrent disc herniations, respectively. This probability of disagreement was consistent over multiple variables including geographic, practice type, fellowship training, and annual case volume.

Conclusions.—Significant differences exist among US spine surgeons in the surgical treatment of recurrent lumbar disc herniations. It will become increasingly important to understand the underlying reasons for these differences and to define the most cost-effective surgical strategies for these common lumbar pathologies as the United States moves closer to a value-based health-care system.

▶ The scenario put forth by the authors deals with 1 common and then 1 not so common complication of a standard lumbar discectomy: recurrent herniation and twice recurrent lumbar disc herniation, respectively. Although there may be little variation in treatment recommendation with a first-time herniation, after a second herniation, things get interesting. In real life, this is often a difficult situation. Patients are in pain and suffering, and even if they were adequately informed as to the risk of recurrent herniation, they still feel a complicated morass of emotions ranging from anger and regret to anxiety of another procedure to distrust of their provider. From the surgeon's perspective, as I am considering the merits of discectomy vs fusion for the twice herniated, I can sometimes hear the old saying in my mind, "the definition of insanity is doing the same thing over and over again and expecting a different result." How many times am I, as a surgeon, willing to risk going back to do the same thing (ie, discectomy) again and expect a different result? If you perform a surgical fusion after the second herniation, hopefully the patient will be improved with resolution of their radicular pain. If successful with the arthrodesis, you would have also eliminated the patient's chances of suffering a recurrent disc herniation at that level ever again. In contrast, by taking the chance of a second disc fragment incision, you will have engineered a success with the smallest amount of surgery available, ensuring a grateful patient and a speedier recovery. That does not exclude the possibility of postdiscectomy back pain, which may lead to a fusion anyway at a *fourth* surgery. Sisyphus could relate!

My professional concern is that in the evolution of value-based care, the surgeon will come to see the fusion option as having unreasonably high cost and low value, even though it may produce a high satisfaction and outcome in the right patient. The issue becomes the surgeon's inability to see the future. But I guess if we could do that, we would be buying lottery tickets!

It is interesting to see that, although the study had a lot of responses (> 400), this represented only a small (< 15%) response rate from the initial cohort. I like the Research Electronic Data Capture software and have used it with success for both surveys; it demonstrates robust ability to coordinate questions within a branching logic and relations database. It is notable that unlike research studies using the National Surgical Quality Improvement Program and Nationwide Inpatient Sample databases, orthopedists outnumber the neurosurgeons 3 to 1 in their responses. Also, the busier surgeons (> 200 cases per year) were more likely to perform revision discectomy with fusion, as were the least experienced surgeons (< 15 years in practice). Perhaps most interestingly, there was no significant difference in technique selection based on geography, specialty, practice type, or fellowship training.

This study, although limited by low response rate, suggests that differences in training and geography can become less with experience and caseload. Leaders should consider these facts and incentives attempt to shape and steer physicians in the upcoming value-based health care world.

P. Huddleston, MD

Imaging, Clearance, and Controversies in Pediatric Cervical Spine Trauma
Tat ST, Mejia MJ, Freishtat RJ (Children's Natl Med Ctr, Washington, DC; Georgetown Univ School of Medicine, Washington, DC)
Pediatr Emerg Care 30:911-918, 2014

Diagnosing cervical spine injury in children can be difficult because the clinical examination can be unreliable, and evidence-based consensus guidelines for cervical spine injury evaluation in children have not been established. However, the consequences of cervical spine injuries are significant. Therefore, practitioners should understand common patterns of cervical spine injury in children, the evidence and indications for cervical spine imaging, and which imaging modalities to use. Herein, we review the epidemiology and unique anatomical features of pediatric cervical spine injury. In addition, we will summarize current practice for clearance and imaging of the pediatric cervical spine in trauma.

▶ Taking care of trauma patients with suspected cervical spine injuries is a common task of any practitioner in an emergency department setting, rink-side at the hockey game, or on the sidelines at the neighborhood soccer tournament. What is an often rite of passage for young orthopedic physicians covering the local Friday night game has changed over the past decade. Players seem to have gotten bigger, the games faster, and the injuries complicated with return to play and the specter of closed head and traumatic brain injuries. Although many of these games involve young adults or skeletally mature young men and women, many athletes will be skeletally immature and some younger than 10 years of age. Certain general rules of trauma apply to the young and the old, but the skeletally immature have their own risks and injury patterns, and it is worth reviewing the differences and helpful strategies to assist the musculoskeletal provider in imaging clearance and pitfalls of pediatric cervical spine trauma.

This review article by pediatrics and emergency department providers from the Washington, DC, area highlights the stresses and uncertainty often associated with pediatric spinal injuries. Pediatric cervical spine injury is reported to occur at a frequency of about 1% to 1.5% with an average age of injury around 9 to 11 years. Whereas sports injuries are the cause of most cervical injuries in children older than 8 years old, falls are the most common in those younger than 8 years. Abuse is an uncommon course. Although mortality can vary from 13% to 28%, those injured are more likely than adults to regain some useful function after an injury. The different proportions of the head and neck and flexible nature of tissues and unclassified bones make the child susceptible to different patterns of injury because young children are more susceptible to injury at the C2-C3 level rather than the C5-C6 as adults. As for the routine immobilization of the patient with a suspected injury, there is variable evidence with data suggesting that prolonged extraction and immobilization times in polytrauma patients can lead to increased neurologic disability. Several studies have found use of both the NEXUS criteria and the Canadian C-Spine Rule to assist the provider in clearing the spine and considering advanced imaging. Because many children cannot maintain still during these evaluations, magnetic resonance use usually requires sedation and has not been of great additional value over routine lateral radiographs, which are seen to be helpful; however, the risk of radiation exposure must be measured with greater weight than in adults and has not been seen to be of great value other than in obtunded patients.

Although limited as a review article, this work does synthesize the authors' message into several important points. Do not hesitate to clear the pediatric cervical spine without radiographs if the child suffered a low-risk injury or does not raise any red flags on the NEXUS criteria. Odontoid and routine flexion and extension radiographs are difficult to obtain and are unlikely to provide improved sensitivity detecting ligamentous injury compared with nondynamic views. There is currently no evidence to suggest the routine CT scanning of children is useful or standard of care, but the authors do recommend CT scanning for children with persistent pain and limited range of motion after initial evaluations.

Although all of our fears over missing an injury in any patient are warranted, this review and its relevant points should go a long way in helping musculoskeletal providers improve their confidence and quality of care when evaluating the after effects of falls and injuries.

P. Huddleston, MD

Nasal MRSA colonization: Impact on surgical site infection following spine surgery

Thakkar V, Ghobrial GM, Maulucci CM, et al (Thomas Jefferson Univ, Philadelphia, PA)
Clin Neurol Neurosurg 125:94-97, 2014

Background.—Prior studies published in the cardiothoracic, orthopedic and gastrointestinal surgery have identified the importance of nasal (methicillin-resistant *Staphylococcus aureus*) MRSA screening and subsequent decolonization to reduce MRSA surgical site infection (SSI). This is the first study to date correlating nasal MRSA colonization with postoperative spinal MRSA SSI.

Objective.—To assess the significance of nasal MRSA colonization in the setting of MRSA SSI.

Methods.—A retrospective electronic chart review of patients from year 2011 to June 2013 was conducted for patients with both nasal MRSA colonization within 30 days prior to spinal surgery. Patients who tested positive for MRSA were put on contact isolation protocol. None of these patients received topical antibiotics for decolonization of nasal MRSA.

Results.—A total of 519 patients were identified; 384 negative (74%), 110 MSSA-positive (21.2%), and 25 (4.8%) MRSA-positive. Culture positive surgical site infection (SSI) was identified in 27 (5.2%) cases and was higher in MRSA-positive group than in MRSA-negative and MSSA-positive groups (12% vs. 5.73% vs. 1.82%; $p = 0.01$). The MRSA SSI rate was 0.96% ($n = 5$). MRSA SSI developed in 8% of the MRSA-positive group as compared to only in 0.61% of MRSA-negative group, with a calculated odds ratio of 14.23 ($p = 0.02$). In the presence of SSI, nasal MRSA colonization was associated with MRSA-positive wound culture (66.67 vs. 12.5%; $p < 0.0001$).

Conclusion.—Preoperative nasal MRSA colonization is associated with postoperative spinal MRSA SSI. Preoperative screening and subsequent decolonization using topical antibiotics may help in decreasing the incidence of MRSA SSI after spine surgery. Nasal MRSA+ patients undergoing spinal surgery should be informed regarding their increased risk of developing surgical site infection.

▶ Researchers from the Departments of Neurological and Orthopedic Surgery of Thomas Jefferson University make a strong argument for routinely screening spine surgery patients in the 30 days before surgery. In their report, patients undergoing elective surgery in their Philadelphia facility developed culture-positive surgical site infection (SSI) in 5.2% cases; this was higher in the methicillin-resistant *Staphylococcus aureus* (MRSA)-positive group than in MRSA-negative and methicillin-sensitive *S aureus* (MSSA)-positive groups (12% vs 5.73% vs 1.82%; $P = .01$). These results mirror findings from the literature in gastrointestinal, cardiac, and orthopedic surgeries where patients with documented colonization show a higher rate of infections peri- and postoperatively. Significant limitations of the study are its retrospective nature and the irregular use of topical vancomycin in selected patients. Nevertheless, I believe the biggest weapon in this population is awareness. It may be best to use nasal MSSA and MRSA screening to stratify various interventions according to the risk, and knowing the patients colonization before surgery may enable a more tailored application of topical antibiotics and overall patient risk assessment. Further studies should examine the cost-effectiveness of widespread screening.

P. Huddleston, MD

A perioperative cost analysis comparing single-level minimally invasive and open transforaminal lumbar interbody fusion

Singh K, Nandyala SV, Marquez-Lara A, et al (Rush Univ Med Ctr, Chicago, IL; et al)
Spine J 14:1694-1701, 2014

Background Context.—Emerging literature suggests superior clinical short- and long-term outcomes of MIS (minimally invasive surgery) TLIFs (transforaminal lumbar interbody fusion) versus open fusions. Few studies to date have analyzed the cost differences between the two techniques and their relationship to acute clinical outcomes.

Purpose.—The purpose of the study was to determine the differences in hospitalization costs and payments for patients treated with primary single-level MIS versus open TLIF. The impact of clinical outcomes and their contribution to financial differences was explored as well.

Study Design/Setting.—This study was a nonrandomized, nonblinded prospective review.

Patient Sample.—Sixty-six consecutive patients undergoing a single-level TLIF (open/MIS) were analyzed (33 open, 33 MIS). Patients in either cohort (MIS/open) were matched based on race, sex, age, smoking status, medical comorbidities (Charlson Comorbidity index), payer, and diagnosis. Every patient in the study had a diagnosis of either degenerative disc disease or spondylolisthesis and stenosis.

Outcome Measures.—Operative time (minutes), length of stay (LOS, days), estimated blood loss (EBL, mL), anesthesia time (minutes), Visual Analog Scale (VAS) scores, and hospital cost/payment amount were assessed.

Methods.—The MIS and open TLIF groups were compared based on clinical outcomes measures and hospital cost/payment data using SPSS version 20.0 for statistical analysis. The two groups were compared using bivariate chi-squared analysis. Mann-Whitney tests were used for non-normal distributed data. Effect size estimate was calculated with the Cohen *d* statistic and the *r* statistic with a 95% confidence interval.

Results.—Average surgical time was shorter for the MIS than the open TLIF group (115.8 minutes vs. 186.0 minutes respectively; $p = .001$). Length of stay was also reduced for the MIS versus the open group (2.3 days vs. 2.9 days, respectively; $p = .018$). Average anesthesia time and EBL were also lower in the MIS group ($p < .001$). VAS scores decreased for both groups, although these scores were significantly lower for the MIS group ($p < .001$). Financial analysis demonstrated lower total hospital direct costs (blood, imaging, implant, laboratory, pharmacy, physical therapy/occupational therapy/speech, room and board) in the MIS versus the open group ($19,512 vs. $23,550, $p < .001$). Implant costs were similar ($p = .686$) in both groups, although these accounted for about two-thirds of the hospital direct costs in the MIS cohort ($13,764) and half of these costs ($13,778) in the open group. Hospital payments were $6,248 higher for open TLIF patients compared with the MIS group ($p = .267$).

Conclusions.—MIS TLIF technique demonstrated significant reductions of operative time, LOS, anesthesia time, VAS scores, and EBL compared with the open technique. This reduction in perioperative parameters translated into lower total hospital costs over a 60-day perioperative period. Although hospital reimbursements appear higher in the open group over the MIS group, shorter surgical times and LOS days in the MIS technique provide opportunities for hospitals to reduce utilization of resources and to increase surgical case volume.

▶ The authors from Rush University in Chicago have attempted to describe the value of single-level transformational lumbar interbody fusions using a unilateral minimally invasive technique compared with a unilaterally instrumented open technique. They compared preoperative costs related to implants used and length of stay in an attempt to measure differences in value. With the continued, relentless changes in health care finance related to Patient Protection and Affordable Care Act, health care providers will no longer be paid solely on production and will be increasingly compensated on patient outcomes, satisfaction, safety, and costs over time. In a comparison of procedures, equivalent outcomes will be measured differently if 1 method is different in how much it costs the health insurer, hospital, or patient. For example, 2 identical patient-care episodes providing the same services for the same condition for the same patient type will differ in value delivered if the costs vary over time. This study attempts to describe lower costs and is an interesting example of the use of unilateral instrumentation for single-level degenerative lumbar spine issues. It is limited in its final analysis by not standardizing the indications, order sets, and biologics.

In my practice, I would try to hold the same standard for preparing the lumbar interbody disc space for a standard open vs a minimally invasive surgery (MIS) case, and it is not clear that this was done as these cases were collected. Without the use of an operating microscope leveraging better light and magnification, the visualization could not definitely be stated to be improved with an MIS technique over open. If the standard open operation would require 25-minute time window to allow for maximal removal of the intervertebral disc joint and preparation of the bony end plates, why would a shorter time be acceptable in an MIS case for the same amount of work? This has not been proven to be so in previously reported studies, and I believe it is fair to describe the discectomy accomplished by a transforaminal lumbar interbody fusion using any technique as "subtotal" compared with the gold-standard anterior lumbar approach. The general premise in MIS cases was first described as "less is more." I believe this has morphed into "less is equivalent" and now "less is cheaper." My concern for making too much of this study's conclusions is that the study design is not truly patient-centric in that it fails to answer our original question of which procedure delivers the highest value. The authors and all orthopedists have a wonderful opportunity to build on this study and standardize the indications, hospital order sets, and perioperative clinical pathways over a 2-year timeframe and report value in that construct. Particular focus should be on revision and admission rates, fusion rates as defined by CT scans, and costs over the follow-up period including readmission, revision, and failure rates defined by visual analog scores and an Oswestry Disability Index.

P. Huddleston, MD

Orthosis versus no orthosis for the treatment of thoracolumbar burst fractures without neurologic injury: a multicenter prospective randomized equivalence trial
Bailey CS, Urquhart JC, Dvorak MF, et al (Univ of Western Ontario, London, Canada; Univ of British Columbia, Vancouver, Canada; et al)
Spine J 14:2557-2564, 2014

Background Context.—Thoracolumbar burst fractures have good outcomes when treated with early ambulation and orthosis (TLSO). If equally good outcomes could be achieved with early ambulation and no brace, resource utilization would be decreased, especially in developing countries where prolonged bed rest is the default option because bracing is not available or affordable.

Purpose.—To determine whether TLSO is equivalent to no orthosis (NO) in the treatment of acute AO Type A3 thoracolumbar burst fractures with respect to their functional outcome at 3 months.

Study Design.—A multicentre, randomized, nonblinded equivalence trial involving three Canadian tertiary spine centers. Enrollment began in 2002 and 2-year follow-up was completed in 2011.

Patient Sample.—Inclusion criteria included AO-A3 burst fractures between T11 and L3, skeletally mature and older than 60 years, 72 hours from their injury, kyphotic deformity lower than 35°, no neurologic deficit. One hundred ten patients were assessed for eligibility for the study; 14 patients were not recruited because they resided outside the country (3), refused participation (8), or were not consented before independent ambulation (3).

Outcome Measures.—Roland Morris Disability Questionnaire score (RMDQ) assessed at 3 months postinjury. The equivalence margin was set at $\delta = 5$ points.

Methods.—The NO group was encouraged to ambulate immediately with bending restrictions for 8 weeks. The TLSO group ambulated when the brace was available and weaned from the brace after 8 to 10 weeks. The following competitive grants supported this work: VHHSC Interdisciplinary Research Grant, Zimmer/University of British Columbia Research Fund, and Hip Hip Hooray Research Grant. Aspen Medical provided the TLSOs used in this study. The authors have no financial or personal relationships that could inappropriately influence this work.

Results.—Forty-seven patients were enrolled into the TLSO group and 49 patients into the NO group. Forty-six participants per group were available for the primary outcome. The RMDQ score at 3 months postinjury was 6.8 ± 5.4 (standard deviation [SD]) for the TLSO group and 7.7 ± 6.0 (SD) in the NO group. The 95% confidence interval (-1.5 to 3.2) was within the predetermined margin of equivalence. Six patients required surgical stabilization, five of them before initial discharge.

Conclusions.—Treating these fractures using early ambulation without a brace avoids the cost and patient deconditioning associated with a brace and complications and costs associated with long-term bed rest if a TLSO or body cast is not available.

▶ In the classic study by Wood et al,[1] the researchers reported the stunning finding that patients treated with cast or bracing for the treatment of thoracolumbar fractures without neurologic deficit performed as well as, or better, than controls who were treated operatively. Body-casted patients had a shorter hospital stay and no difference at follow-up in posttraumatic kyphosis. These were truly impressive results and highly persuasive in supporting a simple but effective nonoperative treatment for a difficult problem.

But as one of my spine fellowship mentors once told me, "Spine body casting is low tech and high art." So what options does the community, rural, or nonacademic provider have to treat neurologically intact thoracolumbar fractures if he or she was never exposed to the "high art of casting" or has experienced a loss of the knowledge due to the passage of time? This is the thrust of the selected article on the use of orthosis vs no orthosis for the treatment of thoracolumbar fractures, an investigation that took place in the western provinces of Canada by researchers in Alberta, British Columbia, and Ontario. The vast distances between cities and often rugged geography of the area challenge hospitals and providers to deliver and fit available casts and orthoses used to treat patients suffering from neurologically intact thoracolumbar spine injuries. Nonoperative management has evolved from bed rest to casting to newer off-the-shelf thoracolumbar orthoses with an associated decrease in morbidity and increase in mobility. The authors constructed the study to further test the logic of rapid mobilization of thoracolumbar fractures in a protocol comparing brace wear to no brace wear and early mobilization.

One of the limitations of the study is that it did not factor any differences in immediate pain levels in patients as they mobilized into the results; scores were recorded at 3 months' postintervention. Initial and follow-up posttraumatic kyphosis measurements were similar between the groups, and there were no follow-up differences in pain, disability as measured by the Roland-Morris tool, and length of stay.

This study should give orthopedists and other musculoskeletal specialists who participate in the care of patients with stable thoracolumbar burst fractures without neurologic deficit confidence that they can mobilize their patients quickly and avoid prolonged bed rest waiting for a brace, without fretting about compromising patient length of stay or outcome at 3 months. The challenge for orthopedists and other specialists will be getting patients, families, and some of their colleagues to believe them!

P. Huddleston, MD

Reference

1. Wood K, Buttermann G, Mehbod A, Garvey T, Jhanjee R, Sechriest V. Operative compared with nonoperative treatment of a thoracolumbar burst fracture without neurological deficit: a prospective, randomized study. *J Bone Joint Surg Am*. 2003; 85:773-781.

Cost Analysis of Incidental Durotomy in Spine Surgery
Nandyala SV, Elboghdady IM, Marquez-Lara A, et al (Rush Univ Med Ctr, Chicago, IL)
Spine 39:E1042-E1051, 2014

Study Design.—Retrospective database analysis.

Objective.—To characterize the consequences of an incidental durotomy with regard to perioperative complications and total hospital costs

Summary of Background Data.—There is a paucity of data regarding how an incidental durotomy and its associated complications may relate to total hospital costs.

Methods.—The Nationwide Inpatient Sample database was queried from 2008 to 2011. Patients who underwent cervical or lumbar decompression and/or fusion procedures were identified, stratified by approach, and separated into cohorts based on a documented intraoperative incidental durotomy. Patient demographics, comorbidities (Charlson Comorbidity Index), length of hospital stay, perioperative outcomes, and costs were assessed. Analysis of covariance and multivariate linear regression were used to assess the adjusted mean costs of hospitalization as a function of durotomy.

Results.—The incidental durotomy rate in cervical and lumbar spine surgery is 0.4% and 2.9%, respectively. Patients with an incidental durotomy incurred a longer hospitalization and a greater incidence of perioperative complications including hematoma and neurological injury ($P < 0.001$). Regression analysis demonstrated that a cervical durotomy and its postoperative sequelae contributed an additional adjusted \$7638 (95% confidence interval, 6489–8787; $P < 0.001$) to the total hospital costs. Similarly, lumbar durotomy contributed an additional adjusted \$2412 (95% confidence interval, 1920-2902; $P < 0.001$) to the total hospital costs. The approach-specific procedural groups demonstrated similar discrepancies in the mean total hospital costs as a function of durotomy.

Conclusion.—This analysis of the Nationwide Inpatient Sample database demonstrates that incidental durotomies increase hospital resource utilization and costs. In addition, it seems that a cervical durotomy and its associated complications carry a greater financial burden than a lumbar durotomy. Further studies are warranted to investigate the long-term financial implications of incidental durotomies in spine surgery and to reduce the costs associated with this complication.

Level of Evidence.—3.

▶ This article is a nice contrast to the companion article on durotomies selected for this Year Book. The most significant difference is the data source, and for readers this will make all the difference. This study leverages the National Inpatient Sample database, which is a representative sample of all Medicare patients hospitalized in the United States. Researchers can access the data set,[1] which is the largest publicly available all-payer inpatient health care database in the United States, yielding national estimates of hospital inpatient stays. It differs from some of the specialty registries by documenting a 20% sample of all discharges from community hospitals participating nationwide. It represents the common and the relevant if you are a practicing community spine surgeon, not a sample biased by potential academic bias.

In this report, the authors from Rush University in Chicago found a statistically significant ($P < .001$) difference across the variables of complications, length of stay, and total hospital costs compared with patients without durotomy. As we have seen with other analyses, increasing the denominator of the value equation decreases value if other variables in the nominator (quality = outcomes, safety, and satisfaction) are held constant. Data such as those from this report appropriately emphasize the effect on the patient and the system and do not attempt to justify the status quo regarding durotomy rates whether using minimally invasive surgical techniques or not.

P. Huddleston, MD

Reference

1. Overview of the National (Nationwide) Inpatient Sample (NIS). https://www.hcup-us.ahrq.gov/nisoverview.jsp. Accessed April 7, 2015.

No difference in postoperative complications, pain, and functional outcomes up to 2 years after incidental durotomy in lumbar spinal fusion: a prospective, multi-institutional, propensity-matched analysis of 1,741 patients
Adogwa O, Huang MI, Thompson PM, et al (Duke Univ Med Ctr, Durham, NC; et al)
Spine J 14:1828-1834, 2014

Background.—Incidental durotomies occur in up to 17% of spinal operations. Controversy exists regarding the short- and long-term consequences of durotomies.

Purpose.—The primary aim of this study was to assess the effect of incidental durotomies on the immediate postoperative complications and patient-reported outcome measures.

Study Design.—Prospective study.

Patient Sample.—A total of 1,741 patients undergoing index lumbar spine fusion were selected from a multi-institutional prospective data registry.

Outcome Measures.—Patient-reported outcome measures used in this study included back pain (BP-Visual Analog Scale), leg pain (LP-Visual Analog Scale), and Oswestry Disability Index.

Methods.—A total of 1,741 patients were selected from a multi-institutional prospective data registry, who underwent primary lumbar fusion for low back pain and/or radiculopathy between January 2003 and December 2010. We collected and analyzed data on patient demographics, postoperative complications, back pain, leg pain, and functional disability over 2 years, with risk-adjusted propensity score modeling.

Results.—Incidental durotomies occurred in 70 patients (4%). Compared with the control group (n = 1,671), there was no significant difference in postoperative infection ($p = .32$), need for reoperation ($p = .85$), or symptomatic neurologic damage ($p = .66$). At 1- and 2-year follow-up, there was no difference in patient-reported outcomes of back pain (BP-Visual Analog Scale), leg pain (LP-Visual Analog Scale), or functional disability (Oswestry Disability Index) ($p > .3$), with results remaining consistent in the propensity-matched cohort analysis ($p > .4$).

Conclusion.—Within the context of an on-going debate on the consequences of incidental durotomy, we found no difference in neurologic symptoms, infection, reoperation, back pain, leg pain, or functional disability over a 2-year follow-up period.

▶ Anyone who has cared for a patient with a symptomatic durotomy after spine surgery knows that the patient, nursing staff, and medical providers all wish the complication had not happened. It is of small consolation to the vomiting, headache, or bed rest-inflicted patient to know that at 2 years, their "outcome" will be equivalent to those without a durotomy at 2 years. But alas, the measurement of such surgical interventions has become more driven by outcomes, and these are defined by the propelling of value; quality divided by cost. In today's health care payment system, quality is defined as outcomes, patient safety, and satisfaction considered over cost over time. Durotomy certainly leads to longer surgery times and may complicate subsequent revision surgery because there might be a bigger laminectomy defect or scarring of the neural elements from the repair or exposure necessary for the repair. Another limitation of this study is the lack of measurement or acknowledgment of headache or length of stay. It would have been helpful to have known additionally what proportion of the cases were done with a minimally invasive approach. From the patient's standpoint, anything affecting the variables on the "Top" of the value equation will decrease the value. This study is attempting to look at this often preventable complication from an administrative viewpoint and will due disservice to the only real measure; the best interests of the patient are the only interest to be considered.

P. Huddleston, MD

7 Total Hip Arthroplasty

Introduction

As everyone knows, the controversies surrounding hip replacement over the past several years have involved bearing surfaces. This is no less true this year, though the frequency of articles discussing this topic has decreased. We have tried to include relevant contributions that continue to explore this very important issue; however, we have identified questions that have been addressed with a large series of procedures being studied by way of the national registries. I found these analyses to be extremely helpful in offering insights into questions that cannot be simply addressed by a single person's practice or even a large multicenter practice. This section also addresses the ongoing problems that are associated with hip replacement surgery, although these frankly continue to be lessened as time moves forward. Finally, I have provided examples of studies addressing the cost-effectiveness of this surgery and analyses of the modes of failure. Fortunately, this continues to be one of the most effective interventions to improve the quality of life.

Bernard F. Morrey, MD

Exercise therapy may postpone total hip replacement surgery in patients with hip osteoarthritis: a long-term follow-up of a randomised trial

Svege I, Nordsletten L, Fernandes L, et al (Oslo Univ Hosp, Norway)
Ann Rheum Dis 74:164-169, 2013

Background.—Exercise treatment is recommended for all patients with hip osteoarthritis (OA), but its effect on the long-term need for total hip replacement (THR) is unknown.

Methods.—We conducted a long-term follow-up of a randomised trial investigating the efficacy of exercise therapy and patient education versus patient education only on the 6-year cumulative survival of the native hip to THR in 109 patients with symptomatic and radiographic hip OA.

Results regarding the primary outcome measure of the trial, self-reported pain at 16 months follow-up, have been reported previously.

Results.—There were no group differences at baseline. The response rate at follow-up was 94%. 22 patients in the group receiving both exercise therapy and patient education and 31 patients in the group receiving patient education only underwent THR during the follow-up period, giving a 6-year cumulative survival of the native hip of 41% and 25%, respectively ($p = 0.034$). The HR for survival of the native hip was 0.56 (CI 0.32 to 0.96) for the exercise therapy group compared with the control group. Median time to THR was 5.4 and 3.5 years, respectively. The exercise therapy group had better selfreported hip function prior to THR or end of study, but no significant differences were found for pain and stiffness.

Conclusions.—Our findings in this explanatory study suggest that exercise therapy in addition to patient education can reduce the need for THR by 44% in patients with hip OA. ClinicalTrials.gov number NCT00319423 (original project protocol) and NCT01338532 (additional protocol for long-term follow-up) (Fig 2).

▶ This Norwegian prospective randomized study is important because it provides scientific basis to recommend modest exercise in those with early hip arthritis. It provides appropriate inclusion and exclusion criteria and uses validated outcome measurement tools. Noteworthy inclusion criteria were the

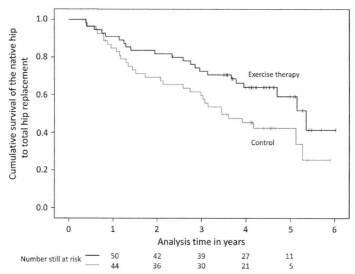

FIGURE 2.—Kaplan—Meier survival estimates over the 6-year follow-up period. The black line represents the exercise therapy group, and the grey line represents the control group. Censored data are marked at each line. The number of patients at risk is given for each year for each group. (Reproduced from Svege I, Nordsletten L, Fernandes L, et al. Exercise therapy may postpone total hip replacement surgery in patients with hip osteoarthritis: a long-term follow-up of a randomised trial. *Ann Rheum Dis.* 2013;74:164-169, with permission from the BMJ Publishing Group Ltd.)

presence of pain for > 3 months and radiographic evidence of minimum narrowing. The wide range of age eligibility, 40 to 80 years, and the lack of defining the degree or amount of pain might be considered deficiencies. Nonetheless, those doing exercises with reasonable compliance did statistically better than the control group at 3 years, and this improvement was maintained for 6 years (Fig 2). Although this is really helpful to know, we cannot say whether exercise avoids the need for hip replacement or simply postpones it.

B. F. Morrey, MD

Age- and health-related quality of life after total hip replacement; Decreasing gains in patients above 70 years of age

Gordon M, Greene M, Frumento P, et al (Swedish Hip Arthroplasty Register, Gothenburg, Sweden; Karolinska Inst, Stockholm, Sweden)
Acta Orthop 85:244-249, 2014

Background.—While age is a common confounder, its impact on health-related quality of life (HRQoL) after total hip replacement is uncertain. This could be due to improper statistical modeling of age in previous studies, such as treating age as a linear variable or by using age categories. We hypothesized that there is a non-linear association between age and HRQoL.

Methods.—We selected a nationwide cohort from the Swedish Hip Arthroplasty Register of patients operated with total hip replacements due to primary osteoarthritis between 2008 and 2010. For estimating HRQoL, we used the generic health outcome questionnaire EQ-5D of the EuroQol group that consists of 2 parts: the EQ-5D index and the EQ VAS estimates.

Using linear regression, we modeled the EQ-5D index and the EQ VAS against age 1 year after surgery. Instead of using a straight line for age, we applied a method called restricted cubic splines that allows the line to bend in a controlled manner. Confounding was controlled by adjusting for preoperative HRQoL, sex, previous contralateral hip surgery, pain, and Charnley classification.

Results.—Complete data on 27,245 patients were available for analysis. Both the EQ-5D index and EQ VAS showed a non-linear relationship with age. They were fairly unaffected by age until the patients were in their late sixties, after which age had a negative effect.

Interpretation.—There is a non-linear relationship between age and HRQoL, with improvement decreasing in the elderly (Table 2).

▶ The question being addressed is of growing importance as society is beginning to recognize and will increasingly have to deal with the aging population expecting a joint replacement. At some point, the quality of life analysis may be factored into whether such a procedure is indicated. Although the analysis is frankly beyond most orthopedic surgeons' background or interest, the results are of interest. In a word, the improvement in life after more than 27 000 hip

TABLE 2.—Raw Comparison of the Median (Interquartile Range) Pre/Postoperative EQ-5D Index and EQ VAS for Various Age Groups

Age, Years	n	EQ-5D (IQR)			EQ VAS (IQR)		
		Preoperative	Postoperative	Change	Preoperative	Postoperative	Change
≤ 50	1,216	0.71 (0.61–0.81)	0.93 (0.87–0.97)	0.19 (0.10–0.27)	50 (32–70)	85 (70–90)	25 (10–45)
51–60	4,726	0.71 (0.61–0.78)	0.93 (0.83–0.97)	0.17 (0.10–0.26)	50 (35–70)	80 (70–91)	25 (8–44)
61–70	12,005	0.74 (0.64–0.81)	0.93 (0.84–0.97)	0.16 (0.07–0.25)	52 (38–71)	80 (70–92)	20 (5–40)
71–80	11,788	0.77 (0.67–0.84)	0.91 (0.81–0.97)	0.12 (0.06–0.20)	54 (40–70)	80 (61–90)	20 (2–38)
81–85	3,356	0.74 (0.64–0.81)	0.87 (0.77–0.97)	0.10 (0.03–0.20)	50 (40–70)	75 (55–89)	15 (0–35)
> 85	1,428	0.71 (0.63–0.80)	0.87 (0.77–0.93)	0.13 (0.03–0.22)	50 (36–70)	70 (50–85)	20 (0–35)

Reprinted from Gordon M, Greene M, Frumento P, et al. Age- and health-related quality of life after total hip replacement; Decreasing gains in patients above 70 years of age. *Acta Orthop.* 2014;85: 244-249, reprinted by permission of Taylor & Francis Ltd, http://www.informaworld.com.

replacements as documented in the Swedish joint registry lessens with age (Table 2). I found it interesting that the abstract concludes less value in those older than 70 years; my interpretation of the authors' data would suggest this occurs after the age of 80 years. Regardless, an awareness of this type of analysis, and its future implications, is important to orthopedic surgeons.

B. F. Morrey, MD

Activity Levels and Functional Outcomes of Young Patients Undergoing Total Hip Arthroplasty
Malcolm TL, Szubski CR, Nowacki AS, et al (Cleveland Clinic, OH)
Orthopedics 37:e983-e992, 2014

The activity demands of young patients undergoing total hip arthro-plasty (THA) have not been clearly defined. University of California Los Angeles (UCLA) activity score, Hip disability and Osteoarthritis Outcome Score (HOOS), Short Form-12 version 2 (SF-12v2), and Functional Comorbidity Index (FCI) questionnaires were administered to 70 young patients who had undergone THA (young THA group; ie, ≤ 30 years old), 158 general patients who had undergone THA (general THA group; ie, ≥ 31 years old), and 106 young, comorbidity-matched patients who had not undergone arthroplasty and had no significant hip disease (nonarthroplasty group). Mean postoperative UCLA activity scores were similar among groups (young THA group, 6.5; general THA group, 6.4; nonarthroplasty group, 6.6) before and after adjustment for comorbidity, sex, and race ($P = .62$ and $P = .47$, respectively). Adjusted analyses also found a negative association between postoperative activity and increases in comorbidity and female sex ($P < .001$). Patients in the young THA group reported higher expectations of postoperative activity (7.7) than those in the general THA group (7.1; $P = .02$). Postoperative HOOS results showed greater hip symptoms ($P = .003$) and poorer hip-related quality of life ($P < .001$) in the young THA group. Patient groups had sim-ilar postoperative SF-12v2 physical health scores ($P = .31$), although men-tal health scores were significantly higher in the general THA group ($P < .001$). The interesting finding of lower postoperative expectations, greater hip-related quality of life, and better mental health scores in the general THA group may indicate a need for better management of expect-ations in young patients undergoing THA, including a discussion of real-istic gains in activity and potential comorbidity-related restrictions.

▶ This article was selected because of the ever-increasing pressure on our spe-cialty by society to restore one to "normalcy." This is especially true of younger patients. The authors assessed an ever more rigorous definition of "young" as being less than 30 years of age. Twenty years ago, "young" was considered less than 50 when considering hip replacement. The measurement tools are appropriate and the sample sizes are adequate to draw the conclusions they describe. In short, the young patient does not do as well subjectively, which the authors correctly speculate to be because of heightened, often unrealistic, expectations. This is important information when discussing risk/benefit with the very young patient.

B. F. Morrey, MD

Associations Between Preoperative Physical Therapy and Post-Acute Care Utilization Patterns and Cost in Total Joint Replacement
Snow R, Granata J, Ruhil AVS, et al (OhioHealth, Columbus; Orthopedic Foot and Ankle Ctr, Westerville; Ohio Univ, Athens; et al)
J Bone Joint Surg Am 96:e165(1)-e165(8), 2014

Background.—Health-care costs following acute hospital care have been identified as a major contributor to regional variation in Medicare spending. This study investigated the associations of preoperative physical therapy and post-acute care resource use and its effect on the total cost of care during primary hip or knee arthroplasty.

Methods.—Historical claims data were analyzed using the Centers for Medicare & Medicaid Services Limited Data Set files for Diagnosis Related Group 470. Analysis included descriptive statistics of patient demographic characteristics, comorbidities, procedures, and post-acute care utilization patterns, which included skilled nursing facility, home health agency, or inpatient rehabilitation facility, during the ninety-day period after a surgical hospitalization. To evaluate the associations, we used bivariate and multivariate techniques focused on post-acute care use and total episode-of-care costs.

Results.—The Limited Data Set provided 4733 index hip or knee replacement cases for analysis within the thirty-nine-county Medicare hospital referral cluster. Post-acute care utilization was a significant variable in the total cost of care for the ninety-day episode. Overall, 77.0% of patients used post-acute care services after surgery. Post-acute care utilization decreased if preoperative physical therapy was used, with only 54.2% of the preoperative physical therapy cohort using post-acute care services. However, 79.7% of the non-preoperative physical therapy cohort used post-acute care services. After adjusting for demographic characteristics and comorbidities, the use of preoperative physical therapy was associated with a significant 29% reduction in post-acute care use, including an $871 reduction of episode payment driven largely by a reduction in payments for skilled nursing facility ($1093), home health agency ($527), and inpatient rehabilitation ($172).

Conclusions.—The use of preoperative physical therapy was associated with a 29% decrease in the use of any post-acute care services. This association was sustained after adjusting for comorbidities, demographic characteristics, and procedural variables.

Clinical Relevance.—Health-care providers can use this methodology to achieve an integrative, cost-effective, patient care pathway using preoperative physical therapy.

▶ We must get used to seeing more of this kind of study. One must question the optimal use of physical therapy in joint replacement surgery. It can, of course, be both over- and underutilized. This interesting study demonstrates that the use of a preoperative therapy program (Table 1 in the original article) can significantly decrease the cost of the episode of care by rescuing the need for costly postoperative rehabilitative services (Table 4 in the original article). This is an important concept and is consistent with the large body of data demonstrating the value of preoperative patient education to reduce the length of hospitalization, the single most important variable to reduce the cost of care.

B. F. Morrey, MD

Effectiveness and safety of different duration of thromboprophylaxis in 16,865 hip replacement patients - A real-word, prospective observational study
Pedersen AB, Sorensen HT, Mehnert F, et al (Aarhus Univ Hosp, Denmark; Univ of Southern Denmark)
Thromb Res 135:322-328, 2015

Introduction.—Clinical trials have provided evidence about efficacy and safety of extended thromboprophylaxis among total hip replacement (THR) patients. There is a lack of evidence on effectiveness and safety of extended treatment in unselected patients from routine clinical practice. We examined the effectiveness and safety of short (1-6 days) and standard (7-27 days) compared with extended ($\geq$28 days) thromboprophylaxis using population-based design.

Material and Methods.—Among all primary THR procedures performed in Denmark from 2010 through 2012 (n = 16,865), we calculated adjusted hazard ratios (aHRs) with 95% confidence intervals (CIs) for risk of symptomatic venous thromboembolism (VTE) and major bleeding, in addition to net clinical benefit, defined as the number of VTE avoided minus the number of excess bleeding events occurring among patients prescribed short-term and standard versus extended treatment.

Results.—The 90-day risks of VTE were 1.1% (short), 1.4% (standard), and 1.0% (extended), yielding aHRs of 0.83 (95% CI: 0.52-1.31) and 0.82 (95% CI: 0.50-1.33) for short and standard versus extended treatment. The risk of major bleeding was 1.1% (short), 1.0% (standard), and 0.7% (extended), resulting in aHRs of 1.64 (95% CI: 0.83-3.21) and 1.24 (95% CI: 0.61-2.51) for short and standard versus extended thromboprophylaxis. Direct comparison between benefits and harms using net clinical benefit analyses did not favor any of the three treatment durations. The same results were found for VTE or death.

TABLE 2.—The Effect of Thromboprophylaxis Treatment Duration on Risk of Venous Thromboembolism (VTE), Other Cardiovascular Events, and Bleeding in Total Hip Replacement Patients Within 90 days of Surgery, with Extended Treatment Duration as the Reference

Outcomes	Short, 0-6 days, N = 4804, n (% of N)	Standard, 7-27 days, N = 6362 n (% of N)	Extended, +28 days, N = 5699 n (% of N)	Hazard ratio (95% CI) Short vs. Extended treatment		Hazard ratio (95% CI) Standard vs. Extended treatment	
				Crude	Adjusted*	Crude	Adjusted*
VTE, including deep venous thrombosis and pulmonary embolism	54 (1.1)	86 (1.4)	57 (1.0)	1.13 (0.78-1.64)	0.83 (0.52-1.31)	1.36 (0.97-1.90)	0.82 (0.50-1.33)
Myocardial infarction	14 (0.3)	35 (0.6)	28 (0.5)	0.59 (0.31-1.13)	0.50 (0.21-1.16)	1.12 (0.68-1.85)	0.71 (0.32-1.57)
Ischemic stroke	21 (0.4)	35 (0.6)	20 (0.4)	1.25 (0.68-2.31)	0.76 (0.42-1.65)	1.53 (0.88-2.66)	0.93 (0.42-2.06)
Any major bleeding	51 (1.1)	66 (1.0)	37 (0.7)	1.79 (1.09-2.94)	1.64 (0.83-3.21)	1.70 (1.05-2.77)	1.24 (0.61-2.51)

*Hazard ratio with 95% CI, adjusted for age; sex; Charlson Comorbidity Index score; anticoagulation drug; and use of acetylsalicylic acid, other platelet inhibitors, and vitamin K antagonists prior to total hip replacement.

Reprinted from Thrombosis Research. Pedersen AB, Sorensen HT, Mehnert F, et al. Effectiveness and safety of different duration of thromboprophylaxis in 16,865 hip replacement patients - A real-word; prospective observational study. *Thromb Res.* 2015;135:322-328, Copyright 2015, with permission from Elsevier.

Conclusions.—In a real-word observational cohort of unselected THR patients, we observed no difference in the risks of symptomatic VTE, VTE/death or bleeding with respect to thromboprophylaxis duration (Table 2).

▶ Another benefit from a national registry. The question of the duration of thromboprophylaxis is huge. It has obvious implications not only regarding protection, but also the potential risk of a bleeding complication must always be considered. In addition, the added cost and inconvenience of prolonged treatment is a concern. Hence, with more than 16 000 cases treated in the recent timeframe over 2 years, there is no real difference neither in the safety provided nor in the complications among any of the 3 time periods of treatment: < 6 days, < 27 days, and > 28 days (Table 2). This really surprised me because there are data to support prolonged treatment. I personally protect, with low-dose warfarin not requiring monitoring, for 21 days. I am not sure I will change my protocol based on this study, but I will continue to follow the literature on this topic.

B. F. Morrey, MD

Factors Affecting Readmission Rates Following Primary Total Hip Arthroplasty
Mednick RE, Alvi HM, Krishnan V, et al (Northwestern Univ, Chicago, IL)
J Bone Joint Surg Am 96:1201-1209, 2014

Background.—Readmissions following total hip arthroplasty are a focus given the forthcoming financial penalties that hospitals in the United States may incur starting in 2015. The purpose of this study was to identify both preoperative comorbidities and postoperative conditions that increase the risk of readmission following total hip arthroplasty.

Methods.—Using the American College of Surgeons—National Surgical Quality Improvement Program data for 2011, a study population was identified using the Current Procedural Terminology code for primary total hip arthroplasty (27130). The sample was stratified into readmitted and non-readmitted cohorts. Demographic variables, preoperative comorbidities, laboratory values, operative characteristics, and surgical outcomes were compared between the groups using univariate and multivariate logistic regression models.

Results.—Of the 9441 patients, there were 345 readmissions (3.65%) within the first thirty days following surgery. Comorbidities that increased the risk for readmission were diabetes ($p < 0.001$), chronic obstructive pulmonary disease ($p < 0.001$), bleeding disorders ($p < 0.001$), preoperative blood transfusion ($p = 0.035$), corticosteroid use ($p < 0.001$), dyspnea ($p = 0.001$), previous cardiac surgery ($p = 0.002$), and hypertension ($p < 0.001$). A multivariate regression model was used to control for potential confounders. Having a body mass index of ≥ 40 kg/m^2 (odds ratio, 1.941 [95% confidence interval, 1.019 to 3.696]; $p = 0.044$) and using corticosteroids preoperatively (odds ratio, 2.928 [95% confidence interval, 1.731 to 4.953]; $p < 0.001$) were independently associated with a higher likelihood of readmission, and a high preoperative serum albumin (odds ratio, 0.688 [95% confidence interval, 0.477 to 0.992]; $p = 0.045$) was independently associated with a lower risk for readmission. Postoperative surgical site infection, pulmonary embolism, deep venous thrombosis, and sepsis ($p < 0.001$) were also independent risk factors for readmission.

Conclusions.—The risk of readmission following total hip arthroplasty increases with growing preoperative comorbidity burden, and is specifically increased in patients with a body mass index of ≥40 kg/m^2, a history of corticosteroid use, and low preoperative serum albumin and in patients with postoperative surgical site infection, a thromboembolic event, and sepsis.

Level of Evidence.—Prognostic Level III. See Instructions for Authors for a complete description of levels of evidence (Table 2).

▶ Using the American College of Surgeon's database allows significant granularity of the data to provide legitimacy to the conclusions of this article. For me, the bottom line is contained in Table 2. Note that approximately 40% of

TABLE 2.—Postoperative Complications

	Not Readmitted*,† (N — 9096)	Readmitted*,† (N = 345)	P Value‡
Overall complications	2152 (23.66%)	212 (61.45%)	<0.001
Surgical complications	95 (1.04%)	109 (31.59%)	<0.001
Superficial surgical site infection	48 (0.53%)	34 (9.86%)	<0.001
Deep or incisional surgical site infection	3 (0.03%)	16 (4.64%)	<0.001
Organ or space surgical site infection	2 (0.02%)	24 (6.96%)	<0.001
Wound dehiscence	5 (0.05%)	13 (3.77%)	<0.001
Pulmonary embolism	13 (0.14%)	14 (4.06%)	<0.001
Peripheral nerve injury	4 (0.04%)	0 (0.00%)	1
Graft or prosthesis failure	0 (0.00%)	1 (0.29%)	0.037
Deep venous thrombosis	22 (0.24%)	19 (5.51%)	<0.001
Medical complications	2101 (23.10%)	136 (39.42%)	<0.001
Pneumonia	23 (0.25%)	11 (3.19%)	<0.001
Unplanned intubation	16 (0.18%)	6 (1.74%)	<0.001
Ventilator for more than forty-eight hours	7 (0.08%)	1 (0.29%)	0.258
Acute renal failure	7 (0.08%)	1 (0.29%)	0.258
Urinary tract infection	93 (1.02%)	19 (5.51%)	<0.001
Stroke or cerebrovascular accident	7 (0.08%)	7 (2.03%)	<0.001
Coma	1 (0.01%)	0 (0.00%)	1
Cardiac arrest	5 (0.05%)	2 (0.58%)	0.025
Myocardial infarction	19 (0.21%)	6 (1.74%)	<0.001
Blood transfusion	1989 (21.87%)	109 (31.59%)	<0.001
Sepsis or septic shock	40 (0.44%)	5 (1.45%)	0.08

*Some patients had more than one postoperative complication, which is reflected in the values for the specific complications; the values for the overall, surgical, and medical complications only reflect the total number of patients who had complications.

†The values are given as the number of patients, with the percentage in parentheses.

‡Significance was set at $p \leq 0.05$.

Reprinted from Mednick RE, Alvi HM, Krishnan V, et al. Factors Affecting Readmission Rates Following Primary Total Hip Arthroplasty. *J Bone Joint Surg Am.* 2014;96:1201-1209. http://jbjs.org/.

the overall rate or about 4% readmissions are for medical problems that primarily related to morbid obesity and the use of corticosteroids. That most of the surgical readmissions are for infection and clotting issues is not surprising. It is surprising that instability of the hip does not show up here, despite the 3% or greater frequency. This is, one might assume, because the hip is reduced without an admission. What has been shown in the past and confirmed here is that obesity causes relatively little problem until the body mass index reaches 40, which defines morbid obesity.

B. F. Morrey, MD

Does Obesity Affect Outcomes After Hip Arthroscopy? A Cohort Analysis
Gupta A, Redmond JM, Hammarstedt JE, et al (American Hip Inst, Westmont, IL)
J Bone Joint Surg Am 97:16-23, 2015

Background.—Obesity presents a challenging problem in surgical treatment and has led to poorer postoperative outcomes. The purpose of this study was to evaluate whether hip arthroscopy in the obese patient influences postoperative clinical and patient-reported outcome scores.

Methods.—From February 2008 to February 2012, data were collected prospectively on all patients undergoing primary hip arthroscopy. A total of 680 patients were included. All patients were assessed preoperatively and postoperatively with four patient-reported outcome measures. Pain was estimated on the visual analog scale. The patient satisfaction score was measured. Three groups were stratified by body mass index. The non-obese group, those with a body mass index of <30 kg/m^2 (mean, 23.61 kg/m^2), included 562 patients with a mean age of 34.78 years. The class-I obese group, those with a body mass index of $\geq$30 to 34.9 kg/m^2 (mean, 33.85 kg/m^2), included ninety-four patients with a mean age of 44.02 years. The class-II obese group, those with a body mass index of $\geq$35 to 39.9 kg/m^2 (mean, 39.11 kg/m^2), included twenty-four patients with a mean age of 39.33 years.

Results.—In the non-obese group, the score improvement from the preoperative assessment to the two-year follow-up visit was 63.41 to 83.81 points for the modified Harris hip score, 60.86 to 83.62 points for the Non-Arthritic Hip Score, 66.24 to 86.24 points for the Hip Outcome Score Activities of Daily Living, and 44.01 to 73.26 points for the Hip Outcome Score Sport-Specific Subscale. In the class-I obese group, the score improvement from the preoperative assessment to the two-year follow-up visit was 54.81 to 75.95 points for the modified Harris hip score, 48.98 to 72.51 points for the Non-Arthritic Hip Score, 53.22 to 72.99 points for the Hip Outcome Score Activities of Daily Living, and 30.56 to 60.75 points for the Hip Outcome Score Sport-Specific Subscale. In the class-II obese group, the score improvement from the preoperative assessment to the two-year follow-up visit was 50.81 to 80.01 points for the modified Harris hip score, 42.36 to 72.50 points for the Non-Arthritic Hip Score, 48.11 to 74.73 points for the Hip Outcome Score Activities of Daily Living, and 28.25 to 62.56 points for the Hip Outcome Score Sport-Specific Subscale. Traction time did not vary significantly between groups ($p < 0.05$).

Conclusions.—Our study demonstrated that obese patients started with lower absolute scores preoperatively and ended with lower overall absolute postoperative scores. However, obese patients showed substantial benefit from hip arthroscopy and demonstrated a degree of improvement that was similar to that of the control non-obese group.

Level of Evidence.—Therapeutic Level III. See Instructions for Authors for a complete description of levels of evidence.

▶ I confess that I am drawn to obesity studies like a moth to a flame. This study from a well-respected private practice, with which I am quite familiar, addresses a focused question. The stratification of patients' body mass index into the categories of < 30, 30–35, and 35–40 is a little unconventional but is effective to demonstrate the lower function of the more obese patients. The major finding is that the incremental improvement in pain and function is no different among the 3 groups. This confirms previous observations. The major concern of increased complications and poorer longevity of the grossly obese (BMI > 40) still obtains.

B. F. Morrey, MD

High Early Failure Rate After Cementless Hip Replacement in the Octogenarian
Jämsen E, Eskelinen A, Peltola M, et al (Coxa, Hosp for Joint Replacement, Tampere, Finland; Natl Inst for Health and Welfare, Helsinki, Finland; et al)
Clin Orthop Relat Res 472:2779-2789, 2014

Background.—Use of cementless hip replacements is increasing in many countries, but the best method for fixation for octogenarian patients remains unknown.

Questions/Purposes.—We studied how fixation method (cemented, cementless, hybrid) affects the survival of primary hip replacements and mortality in patients 80 years or older. Specifically, we asked if fixation method affects (1) the risk of revision; (2) the reasons for revision; and (3) the mortality after contemporary primary hip replacement in octogenarian patients.

Methods.—A total of 4777 primary total hip replacements were performed in 4509 octogenarian patients with primary osteoarthritis in Finland between 1998 and 2009 and were registered in the Finnish Arthroplasty Register. Comorbidity data were collected from a nationwide quality register. Survival of hip replacements, using any revision as the end point, and mortality were analyzed using competing risks survival analysis and Cox regression analysis. The average followup was 4 years (range, 1–13 years).

Results.—Cementless hip replacements were associated with a higher rate of early (within 1 year) revision compared with cemented hip replacements (hazard ratio, 2.9; 95% CI, 1.7–5.1), particularly in women. The difference was not explained by comorbidity or provider-related factors. Periprosthetic fracture was the leading mode of failure of cementless hip replacements. After 1 year, there were no differences in the survival rates although 10-year survival was slightly lower for cementless than cemented and hybrid hip replacements (93.9% [95% CI, 91.1%–96.7%] versus 97.4% [95% CI, 96.9%–98.0%] and 98.1% [95% CI, 96.9%–99.4%], respectively). Fixation method was not associated with mortality.

Conclusions.—Cementless fixation was associated with an increased risk of revision and did not provide any benefit in terms of lower mortality in octogenarian patients.

Level of Evidence.—Level II, therapeutic study. See the Instructions for Authors for a complete description of levels of evidence (Figs 1 and 2).

▶ I never cease to be amazed at the ability of surgeons to justify their preferences, even in the face of data. I am not aware of a single publication that demonstrates superiority of the more expensive cementless implants in the older population. Mayo data demonstrated no value in those older than 70 years of age. This Finnish registry analysis reveals the bothersome trend of increasing use of cementless implants in the octogenarian (Fig 1). Sadly, the survival

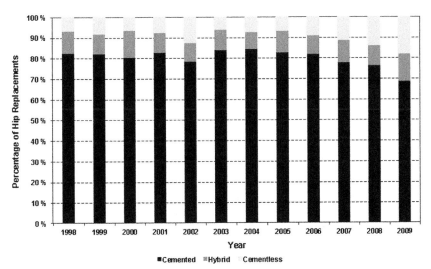

FIGURE 1.—Changes in the use of cemented, hybrid, and cementless fixation in primary hip replacements performed in octogenarian patients with osteoarthritis from 1998 to 2009 are shown. (With kind permission from Springer Science+Business Media: Jämsen E, Eskelinen A, Peltola M, et al. High early failure rate after cementless hip replacement in the octogenarian. *Clin Orthop Relat Res.* 2014;472:2779-2789, with permission from The Association of Bone and Joint Surgeons.)

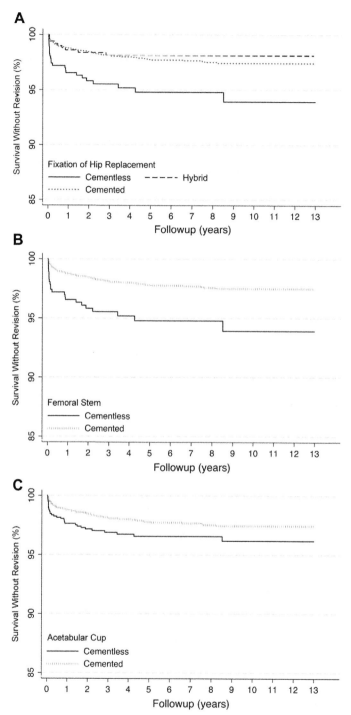

FIGURE 2.—The curves indicate survival without revision after (A) cemented, hybrid, and cementless hip replacement, and (B) in association with the use of cemented and cementless femoral stems and (C) acetabular cups. (With kind permission from Springer Science+Business Media: Jämsen E, Eskelinen A, Peltola M, et al. High early failure rate after cementless hip replacement in the octogenarian. *Clin Orthop Relat Res.* 2014;472:2779-2789, with permission from The Association of Bone and Joint Surgeons.)

data clearly demonstrate the superiority of the cemented implant (Fig 2). These data are clear. One wonders if or when such studies will influence practice. Soon, I hope.

B. F. Morrey, MD

Acetabular Fractures Converted to Total Hip Arthroplasties in the Elderly: How Does Function Compare to Primary Total Hip Arthroplasty?

Schnaser E, Scarcella NR, Vallier HA (Desert Orthopedic Ctr, Rancho Mirage, CA; Case Western Reserve Univ School of Medicine, Cleveland, OH; Case Western Reserve Univ, Cleveland, OH)
J Orthop Trauma 28:694-699, 2014

Objectives.—Little data exist regarding the outcomes of total hip arthroplasty (THA) after acetabular fracture treatment failure. We hypothesize that these patients achieve a lower level of function than those who undergo primary THA for osteoarthritis (atraumatic).

Design.—Retrospective review. Control group consisted of sequential patients who underwent a primary THA for osteoarthritis and were 60 years or older at the time of surgery.

Setting.—Level I Academic Trauma Center.

Patients.—One hundred seventy-one patients older than 60 years when they sustained an acetabular fracture were included in this study. Seventeen (10%) patients were converted to THA. Control patients were treated with primary THA for osteoarthritis.

Main Outcome Measures.—Musculoskeletal function assessment scores and Harris Hip scores were obtained after a minimum followup of 2 years.

Results.—Thirteen patients underwent open reduction and internal fixation, 3 underwent nonoperative treatment, and 1 received an acute THA. The most common fracture patterns converted to THA were associated both column (n = 5) and posterior column with posterior wall (n = 5). The average time to conversion to THA was 35 months. When compared with controls, patients who had THA after an acetabular fracture had significantly higher Musculoskeletal Function Assessment scores and significantly lower Harris Hip scores, indicating worse level of function.

Conclusions.—Patients who undergo THA after acetabular fracture have significantly worse functional outcome scores when compared with patients who undergo a primary THA for osteoarthritis.

Level of Evidence.—Prognostic Level III. See Instructions for Authors for a complete description of levels of evidence.

▶ The observations documented here are not new, nor are they surprising. This is the critical question: What are their significance to the surgeon? The most obvious is the reaffirmation that stiff, painful, previously operated joints do not do as well as replacement for osteoarthritis. The question that has long been asked is whether there are some acetabular fractures that should be treated with primary replacement. Almost all the data to date also reveal poorer outcomes for acetabular fractures treated with acute replacement compared with osteoarthritis. The fact is an acetabular fracture is a high energy soft-tissue injury that has a guarded prognosis at best. The traditional teaching still obtains: Treat the fracture to avoid a nonunion; replace later if you must.

B. F. Morrey, MD

Functional Outcomes After Total Hip Arthroplasty for the Acute Management of Acetabular Fractures: 1- to 14-Year Follow-up
Lin C, Caron J, Schmidt AH, et al (Hennepin County Med Ctr, Minneapolis, MN; Sanford Bemidji Orthopedics, MN; et al)
J Orthop Trauma 29:151-159, 2015

Objective.—This study reports the complications and functional outcomes in patients treated acutely with combined open reduction internal fixation (ORIF) and immediate total hip arthroplasty (THA) for displaced comminuted acetabular fractures.

Design.—Single surgeon retrospective case series.

Setting.—Level 1 trauma center.

Patients.—Thirty-three consecutive patients (18 women; mean age, 66 years) from 1996 to 2011 with an average follow-up of 5.6 years (range, 1—14.3 years) were included in this study.

Intervention.—ORIF and immediate THA.

Main Outcome Measurements.—Oxford Hip Score and reoperation.

Methods.—All patients had at least 1 year of telephone or clinical follow-up. Postoperative complications, reoperations, and available radiographs were reviewed.

Results.—Six patients died of causes unrelated to their injuries or surgery; before death, these patients had well-functioning hips. There was a 15% complication rate. At last follow-up, 94% of hips remained in situ and were functioning well. The average Oxford Hip Score at final follow-up was 17 (range, 12—32), with 93% of patients reporting good to excellent function. There was no statistical association between fracture type, age, or fixation type and outcome.

Conclusions.—Acute ORIF and immediate THA for selected acetabular fractures is a safe viable treatment option with good to excellent functional outcomes and may reduce the need for 2 separate operations in many patients. Functional outcomes are equivalent to those after primary THA for osteoarthritis. This study does not address at which age acute THA is a cost-effective treatment option.

Level of Evidence.—Therapeutic Level IV. See Instructions for Authors for a complete description of levels of evidence.

▶ I found this a very useful contribution because it addresses a true uncertainty in our practice of hip replacement in the setting of the acute acetabular fracture. As such, I see definite similarities with the use of elbow replacement for some C3 fractures in the elderly. In sum, if the fracture is known (guaranteed?) to be associated with arthrosis, even with uneventful healing, then stabilization and replacement is a viable option. In the past, it was suggested the fracture be fixed then replaced. In my opinion, this nicely done clinical study changes this practice. The low 15% complication rate in this complex injury underscores the considerable experience of the surgeon in this practice and may be the best that can be expected.

B. F. Morrey, MD

Acute total hip replacement for acetabular fractures: A systematic review of the literature
De Bellis UG, Legnani C, Calori GM (Istituto Ortopedico G. Pini, Milano, Italy; Università degli Studi di Milano, Milano, Italy)
Injury 45:356-361, 2014

Introduction.—Immediate total hip replacement (THR) in patients with acetabular fractures is controversial because of concerns about high complication rates. The current article is a systematic review of the literature on the use of acute THR for the treatment of acetabular fractures.

Materials and Methods.—This systematic review included studies published in English between 1992 and 2012 of subjects with acetabular fracture undergoing immediate THR. Outcomes of interest included indications; clinical assessment, including walking ability; comparison with control group; associated procedures, and rate of complications, such as loosening or revision surgery.

Results.—This review identified six studies, of which only one included a control group. Acute THR was associated with satisfying outcomes with regard to clinical assessment and walking ability. The comparative study assessed the difference between acute THR and delayed THR in acetabular fractures: improved outcomes were observed in the delayed THR group, although the differences between the two groups were not statistically significant.

Discussion.—According to data reported in the literature, acute primary THR can be successful in patients with poor bone quality, combined acetabular and femoral neck fractures, or pathological fractures and concurrent osteoarthritis of the hip. Relative indications include old age, delayed presentation, substantial medical comorbidities, and pathologic obesity. Clinical outcomes with acute THR were similar to those with delayed THR. Although the results reported in the six studies reviewed here were satisfying overall, there is limited evidence in this area in the existing literature and future prospective investigations are required.

Conclusion.—Data reported in the literature indicate that immediate THR can be successful in appropriately selected elderly patients or patients with extensive osteoporosis, combined acetabular and femoral neck fractures or pathological fractures. There is currently a limited evidence base

TABLE 2.—Clinical Outcomes, Complications and Failure Rates

Author	Harris Hip Score	Complications	Loosening Rate	Dislocation Rate	Revision Rate	Notes
Sermon et al. [12]	21 Excellent 10 Good 15 Fair 7 Bad	18 (28%) Heterotopic ossifications	N/a	0 (0%)	4 (8%)	Reduced revision rate and reduced occurrence of heterotopic ossification in the acute THR group
Mouhsine et al. [13]	N/a	2 (11%) urinary tract infections*	0 (0%)	1 (6%)*	0 (0%)	100% clinically excellent and good result
Mears et al. [14]	89 (range 69–100) 33 (58%) Excellent 12 (21%) Good 9 (16%) Fair 3 (5%) Bad	6 (35%) heterotopic ossifications* 3 (5%) deep venous thrombosis 1 (2%) intolerance to hardware 6 (10%) heterotopic ossifications	0 (0%)	2 (4%)	3 (5%) 1 dislocation 1 hardware removal 1 heterotopic ossification removal	45 (79%) good/excellent Harris Hip Score
Tidemark et al. [15]	85 (range 69–99) 2 (20%) Excellent 4 (40%) Good 3 (30%) Fair 1 (10%) Bad	4 (40%) heterotopic ossifications 1 (10%) deep venous thrombosis	0 (0%)	1 (10%)	0 (0%)	All patients were independent walkers at follow-up with a need for walking aids in 30% of cases

Study	Mean age						Comments
Herscovici et al. [16]	74 (range 42–86)	2 (9%) urinary tract infections 1 (4%) transient ischaemic attack 4 (18%) heterotopic ossifications 1 (4%) wound dehiscence	2 (9%)	3 (14%)	5 (23%)	2 dislocation 2 loosening 1 heterotopic ossification removal	Better results in 19 patients treated using a Kocher-Langenbeck approach compared to ilio-inguinal
Sarkar et al. [17]	N/a	2(10%) recurrent dislocation** 2 (10%) deep infection** 1 (5%) superficial infection** 3 (16%) cup loosening** 1 (5%) stem loosening** 1 (5%) fracture of the ceramic head**	4 (21%)**	2 (10%)**	8 (42%)**	2 dislocation 3 loosening 1 deep infection 1 superficial infection 1 fracture of the ceramic head	Low overall outcomes due to patient's general situation which was frequently compromised by preexisting chronic diseases or by sequelae of concomitant injuries

N/a: Not available.
Editor's Note: Please refer to original journal article for full references.
*Results refer to 17 patients.
**Results refer to 19 patients.
Reprinted from the Injury, International Journal of the Care of the Injured. De Bellis UG, Legnani C, Calori GM. Acute total hip replacement for acetabular fractures: A systematic review of the literature. *Injury.* 2014;45:356-361, Copyright 2014, with permission from Elsevier.

for THR in patients with acetabular fractures; therefore, physicians' practice and expertise are the most useful tools in clinical practice (Table 2).

▶ This topic is relevant to the reconstruction surgeon, trauma surgeon, and the general orthopedist. That only 6 articles were used to draw conclusions is underscored by the authors as a question that needs more clinical data. The important message is that, even in the elderly patient with osteoporosis and concurrent femoral neck fracture, an immediate or subacute hip replacement is an effective option (Table 2). I emphasize, from my experience, the great value of the procedure being done by a trauma surgeon with considerable hip replacement experience. This situation does not exist in all settings.

B. F. Morrey, MD

Hemiarthroplasty using cemented or uncemented stems of proven design: A comparative study
Grammatopoulos G, Wilson HA, Kendrick BJL, et al (JR Hosp, Headley Way Oxford, UK)
Bone Joint J 97-B:94-99, 2015

National Institute of Clinical Excellence guidelines state that cemented stems with an Orthopaedic Data Evaluation Panel (ODEP) rating of > 3B should be used for hemiarthroplasty when treating an intracapsular fracture of the femoral neck. These recommendations are based on studies in which most, if not all stems, did not hold such a rating.

This case-control study compared the outcome of hemiarthroplasty using a cemented (Exeter) or uncemented (Corail) femoral stem. These are the two prostheses most commonly used in hip arthroplasty in the UK.

Data were obtained from two centres; most patients had undergone hemiarthroplasty using a cemented Exeter stem (n = 292/412). Patients were matched for all factors that have been shown to influence mortality after an intracapsular fracture of the neck of the femur. Outcome measures included: complications, re-operations and mortality rates at two, seven, 30 and 365 days post-operatively. Comparable outcomes for the two stems were seen.

There were more intra-operative complications in the uncemented group (13% *vs* 0%), but the cemented group had a greater mortality in the early post-operative period (n = 6). There was no overall difference in the rate of re-operation (5%) or death (365 days: 26%) between the two groups at any time post-operatively.

This study therefore supports the use of both cemented and uncemented stems of proven design, with an ODEP rating of 10A, in patients with an intracapsular fracture of the neck of the femur.

▶ This nicely done case-controlled study using a national database asked an important question that I have been interested in for my entire career. It should be borne in mind that neither of these designs is used to any extent in the United States, but the concept of accepted and proven designs is relevant to US practice. The bottom line is no real difference in any important parameter. It is interesting to note that the increased early mortality of the cemented group is the same between the 2- at 1-year points. So what's the difference? For me, it is the cost.

B. F. Morrey, MD

Hip Resurfacing versus Total Hip Arthroplasty: A Systematic Review Comparing Standardized Outcomes
Marshall DA, Pykerman K, Werle J, et al (Univ of Calgary, Alberta, Canada; et al)
Clin Orthop Relat Res 472:2217-2230, 2014

Background.—Metal-on-metal hip resurfacing was developed for younger, active patients as an alternative to THA, but it remains controversial. Study heterogeneity, inconsistent outcome definitions, and unstandardized outcome measures challenge our ability to compare arthroplasty outcomes studies.

Questions/Purposes.—We asked how early revisions or reoperations (within 5 years of surgery) and overall revisions, adverse events, and postoperative component malalignment compare among studies of metal-on-metal hip resurfacing with THA among patients with hip osteoarthritis. Secondarily, we compared the revision frequency identified in the systematic review with revisions reported in four major joint replacement registries.

Methods.—We conducted a systematic review of English language studies published after 1996. Adverse events of interest included rates of early failure, time to revision, revision, reoperation, dislocation, infection/sepsis, femoral neck fracture, mortality, and postoperative component alignment. Revision rates were compared with those from four national joint replacement registries. Results were reported as adverse event rates per 1000 person-years stratified by device market status (in use and discontinued). Comparisons between event rates of metal-on-metal hip resurfacing and THA are made using a quasilikelihood generalized linear model. We identified 7421 abstracts, screened and reviewed 384 full-text articles, and included 236. The most common study designs were prospective cohort studies (46.6%; n = 110) and retrospective studies (36%; n = 85). Few randomized controlled trials were included (7.2%; n = 17).

Results.—The average time to revision was 3.0 years for metal-on-metal hip resurfacing (95% CI, 2.95–3.1) versus 7.8 for THA (95% CI, 7.2–8.3). For all devices, revisions and reoperations were more frequent with metal-on-metal hip resurfacing than THA based on point estimates and CIs: 10.7 (95% CI, 10.1–11.3) versus 7.1 (95% CI, 6.7–7.6; $p = 0.068$), and 7.9 (95% CI, 5.4–11.3) versus 1.8 (95% CI, 1.3–2.2; $p = 0.084$) per 1000 person-years, respectively. This difference was consistent with three of four national joint replacement registries, but overall national joint replacement registries revision rates were lower than those reported in the literature. Dislocations were more frequent with THA than metal-on-metal hip resurfacing: 4.4 (95% CI, 4.2–4.6) versus 0.9 (95% CI, 0.6–1.2; $p = 0.008$) per 1000 person-years, respectively. Adverse event rates change when discontinued devices were included.

Conclusions.—Revisions and reoperations are more frequent and occur earlier with metal-on-metal hip resurfacing, except when discontinued devices are removed from the analyses. Results from the literature may be misleading without consistent definitions, standardized outcome metrics, and accounting for device market status. This is important when clinicians are assessing and communicating patient risk and when selecting which device is most appropriate for individual patients.

▶ As the question of the resurfacing versus conventional low-friction arthroplasty continues, a detailed analysis of the literature to date is useful. As expected, the findings of the review confirm the higher failure rate of the resurfacing designs. It also confirms the known fact that low-friction arthroplasty is less stable. What I find most important is the stratification based on market acceptance. When considering only those implants available today and deleting those sanctioned by the lack of market acceptance, then the disadvantage lessens. Regardless, the concern regarding the long-term adverse effect of the increased ion burden remains with the metal-on-metal implants.

B. F. Morrey, MD

10-year results of the uncemented Allofit press-fit cup in young patients: 121 hips followed for 10–12 years

Streit MR, Weiss S, Andreas F, et al (Univ of Heidelberg, Germany)
Acta Orthop 85:368-374, 2014

Background and Purpose.—Uncemented acetabular components in primary total hip arthroplasty (THA) are commonly used today, but few studies have evaluated their survival into the second decade in young and active patients. We report on a minimum 10-year follow-up of an uncemented press-fit acetabular component that is still in clinical use.

Methods.—We examined the clinical and radiographic results of our first 121 consecutive cementless THAs using a cementless, grit-blasted, non-porous, titanium alloy press-fit cup (Allofit; Zimmer Inc., Warsaw, IN) without additional screw fixation in 116 patients. Mean age at surgery was 51 (21–60) years. Mean time of follow-up evaluation was 11 (10–12) years.

Results.—At final follow-up, 8 patients had died (8 hips), and 1 patient (1 hip) was lost to follow-up. 3 hips in 3 patients had undergone acetabular revision, 2 for deep infection and 1 for aseptic acetabular loosening.

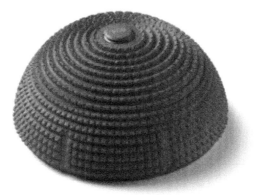

FIGURE 1.—The uncemented Allofit acetabular component with macrotextured surface, hemispherical periphery, and a flattened polar region. (Reprinted from Streit MR, Weiss S, Andreas F, et al. 10-year results of the uncemented Allofit press-fit cup in young patients: 121 hips followed for 10–12 years. *Acta Orthop.* 2014;85:368-374, reprinted by permission of Taylor & Francis Ltd, http://www.informaworld. com.)

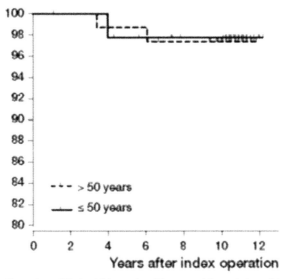

FIGURE 6.—Comparison of Kaplan-Meier survivorship curves with acetabular revision for any reason as endpoint for patients aged ≤ 50 at the time of surgery (n = 45) vs. patients aged > 50 (n = 76) (log-rank test, $p = 0.91$). (Reprinted from Streit MR, Weiss S, Andreas F, et al. 10-year results of the uncemented Allofit press-fit cup in young patients: 121 hips followed for 10–12 years. *Acta Orthop.* 2014;85: 368-374.)

There were no impending revisions at the most recent follow-up. We did not detect periacetabular osteolysis or loosening on plain radiographs in those hips that were evaluated radiographically (n = 90; 83% of the hips available at a minimum of 10 years). Kaplan-Meier survival analysis using revision of the acetabular component for any reason (including isolated inlay revisions) as endpoint estimated the 11-year survival rate at 98% (95% CI: 92—99).

Interpretation.—Uncemented acetabular fixation using the Allofit press-fit cup without additional screws was excellent into early in the second decade in this young and active patient cohort. The rate of complications related to the liner and to osteolysis was low (Figs 1 and 6).

▶ This is a worthwhile contribution because it allows one to realize that we currently have options that almost ensure cup stability with hip replacement. The interesting feature of this almost 99% 10-year survival rate is that the implant was designed to be used without screw supplementation (Fig 1). Furthermore, the sample size averaged approximately 50 years of age, with no difference in survival in those over or under that age (Fig 6). Finally, it is also impressive that the authors found little evidence of osteolysis in the patient sample. In summary, the cup component of hip replacement is extremely reliable, even in the young, for up to 10 years.

B. F. Morrey, MD

Athletic activity after lower limb arthroplasty: A systematic review of current evidence
Jassim SS, Douglas SL, Haddad FS (Univ College London Hosp, UK)
Bone Joint J 96-B:923-927, 2014

In this systematic review, our aim was to explore whether or not patients are able to return to athletic activity following lower limb joint replacement. We also investigated any evidence as to whether participation in athletic activity post-joint replacement increases complications and reduces implant survival.

A PubMed, Embase and Sports Discus search was performed using the MeSH terms 'Sport', 'Athletic', 'Athlete', 'Physical', 'Activity', 'Arthroplasty', 'Total Hip Replacement', 'Hip Resurfacing', 'Total Knee Replacement', 'Unicompartmental Knee Replacement' and 'Unicondylar Knee Replacement'. From this search, duplications were excluded, the remaining abstracts were reviewed and any unrelated to the search terms were excluded. The remaining abstracts had their full papers reviewed.

Following joint replacement, participation in sporting activity is common principally determined by pre-operative patient activity levels, BMI and patient age. The type of joint replaced is of less significance. Total time spent performing activity does not change but tends to be at a lower intensity. There is little evidence in the literature of an association between high activity levels and early implant failure.

▶ This is emerging as one of the most commonly asked questions after hip or knee replacement: What can I do? The answer is changing because of better implants, better technique, and younger, more active patients. We all know that patient compliance is marginal at best, especially in the young. This meta-analysis is comforting in demonstrating that there is no strong evidence that increased activity measurably compromises the intermediate-term outcome. Encouraging. Nonetheless, I continue to recommend that patients "glide" on the implant—that is, walk, swim, cross-country ski, doubles tennis. I still advise against impact loading, such as running and cutting. Maybe I'm wrong, but for now I don't plan on changing my recommendations, realizing many patients will do as they see fit.

B. F. Morrey, MD

Changes in blood ion levels after removal of metal-on-metal hip replacements: 16 patients followed for 0–12 months
Durrani SK, Noble PC, Sampson B, et al (Inst of Orthopedic Res and Education, Houston, TX; Imperial College, London, UK)
Acta Orthop 85:259-265, 2014

Background and Purpose.—In patients with metal-on-metal (MoM) hip prostheses, pain and joint effusions may be associated with elevated blood levels of cobalt and chromium ions. Since little is known about the kinetics of metal ion clearance from the body and the rate of resolution of elevated blood ion levels, we examined the time course of cobalt and chromium ion levels after revision of MoM hip replacements.

Patients and Methods.—We included 16 patients (13 female) who underwent revision of a painful MoM hip (large diameter, modern bearing) without fracture or infection, and who had a minimum of 4 blood metal ion measurements over an average period of 6.1 (0–12) months after revision.

Results.—Average blood ion concentrations at the time of revision were 22 ppb for chromium and 43 ppb for cobalt. The change in ion levels after revision surgery varied extensively between patients. In many cases, over the second and third months after revision surgery ion levels decreased to 50% of the values measured at revision. Decay of chromium levels occurred more slowly than decay of cobalt levels, with a 9% lag in return to normal levels. The rate of decay of both metals followed second-order (exponential) kinetics more closely than first-order (linear) kinetics.

Interpretation.—The elimination of cobalt and chromium from the blood of patients who have undergone revision of painful MoM hip arthroplasties follows an exponential decay curve with a half-life of approximately 50 days. Elevated blood levels of cobalt and chromium ions can persist for at least 1 year after revision, especially in patients with high levels of exposure (Figs 3 and 4).

▶ Today there is less need to point out the concern with metal-on metal-bearings because these are largely avoided in contemporary practice. This interesting study does address a commonly asked question, however: When the

Percentage of initial chromium level

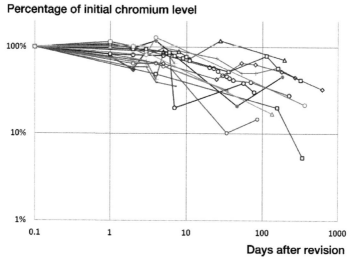

Days after revision

FIGURE 3.—Change in blood chromium as a percentage of the initial value at revision. (Reprinted from Durrani SK, Noble PC, Sampson B, et al. Changes in blood ion levels after removal of metal-on-metal hip replacements: 16 patients followed for 0–12 months. *Acta Orthop.* 2014;85:259-265.)

Percentage of initial cobalt level

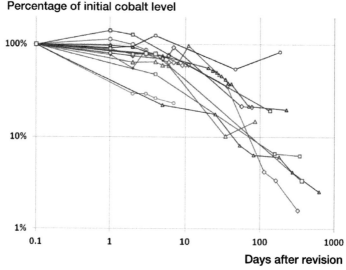

Days after revision

FIGURE 4.—Change in blood cobalt as a percentage of the initial value at revision. (Reprinted from Durrani SK, Noble PC, Sampson B, et al. Changes in blood ion levels after removal of metal-on-metal hip replacements: 16 patients followed for 0–12 months. *Acta Orthop.* 2014;85:259-265, reprinted by permission of Taylor & Francis Ltd, http://www.informaworld.com.)

metallic bearing wear is eliminated, will my blood levels return to normal, and if so, how long does it take? Although this study includes only 16 patients with considerable individual variation, it does provide a basis for an answer. Levels do return toward normal, but the effect is not seen immediately. It will take a year or longer for both chromium and cobalt blood levels to return to near normal (Figs 3 and 4). My concern regarding the ion load in the solid organs remains unanswered by this study.

B. F. Morrey, MD

Can Wear Explain the Histological Variation Around Metal-on-metal Total Hips?
Ebramzadeh E, Campbell P, Tan TL, et al (Orthopaedic Research Ctr, Los Angeles, CA; et al)
Clin Orthop Relat Res 473:487-494, 2014

Background.—There is a general perception that adverse local tissue reactions in metal-on-metal hip arthroplasties are caused by wear, but the degree to which this is the case remains controversial.

Questions/Purposes.—To what extent is the magnitude of wear associated with (1) the histological changes (2) presence of metallosis and (3) likelihood of pseudotumor formation in the periprosthetic tissues?

Methods.—One hundred nineteen metal-on-metal total hip arthroplasties and hip resurfacings were selected from a retrieval collection of over 500 implants (collected between 2004 and 2012) based on the availability of periprosthetic tissues collected during revision, clinical data including presence or absence of pseudotumor or metallosis observed intraoperatively, and wear depth measured using a coordinate measurement machine. Histological features of tissues were scored for aseptic lymphocytic vasculitis-associated lesions (ALVAL). Correlation analysis was performed on the three endpoints of interest.

Results.—With the sample size available, no association was found between wear magnitude and ALVAL score ($\rho = -0.092$, $p = 0.423$). Median wear depth (ball and cup) was greater in hips with metallosis (137 µm range, 8−873 µm) than in those without (18 µm range, 8−174 µm $p < 0.0001$). With the numbers available, no statistically significant association between wear depth and pseudotumor formation could be identified median wear depth was 74 µm in hips with pseudotumors and 26 µm in those without ($p = 0.741$).

Conclusions.—Wear alone did not explain the histopathological changes in the periprosthetic tissues. A larger sample size and more sensitive outcome variable assessments may have revealed a correlation. However, wear depth has been inconsistently associated with pseudotumor formation, perhaps because some patients with hypersensitivity may develop pseudotumors despite low wear.

Clinical Relevance.—Metal wear alone may not explain the histological reactions and pseudotumors around metal-on-metal hip implants (Fig 4).

▶ I selected this article since it is of interest to the orthopedic community, but it is also aligned with our current research efforts at the Mayo Clinic. The fact is, I thought it was well accepted that acute lymphocytic vasculitis-associated

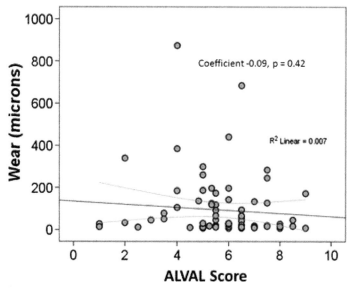

FIGURE 4.—A correlation analysis between ALVAL score and wear depth (μm) is demonstrated. (With kind permission from Springer Science+Business Media: Ebramzadeh E, Campbell P, Tan TL, et al. Can wear explain the histological variation around metal-on-metal total hips? *Clin Orthop Relat Res.* 2014;473:487-494, with permission from The Association of Bone and Joint Surgeons.)

lesion (ALVAL) was an allergic response. As such, it is not "volume dependent." This study confirms this reality, as demonstrated in Fig 4. The severity of the clinical expression, such as development of a periarticular pseudotumor, is probably related to the intensity of the allergic response.

B. F. Morrey, MD

New polyethylenes in total hip replacement: A ten- to 12-year follow-up study

García-Rey E, García-Cimbrelo E, Cruz-Pardos A (Hospital Universitario La Paz, Madrid, Spain)
Bone Joint J 95-B:326-332, 2013

Between 1999 and 2001, 90 patients underwent total hip replacement using the same uncemented acetabular and femoral components with a 28 mm metallic femoral head but with prospective randomisation of the acetabular liner to either Durasul highly cross-linked polyethylene or nitrogen-sterilised Sulene polyethylene. We assessed 83 patients at a minimum follow-up of ten years. Linear penetration of the femoral head was estimated at six weeks, six and 12 months and annually thereafter, using the Dorr method, given the nonspherical shape of the acetabular component.

There was no loosening of any component; only one hip in the Sulene group showed proximal femoral osteolysis. The mean penetration of the femoral head at six weeks was 0.08 mm (0.02 to 0.15) for the Durasul group and 0.16 mm (0.05 to 0.28) for the Sulene group ($p = 0.001$). The mean yearly linear penetration was 64.8% lower for the Durasul group at 0.05 mm/year (SD 0.035) for the Sulene group and 0.02 mm/year (SD 0.016) for the Durasul ($p < 0.001$). Mean linear femoral head penetration at ten years was 61% less in the Durasul than Sulene group. Highly cross-linked polyethylene gives excellent results at ten years.

▶ This retrospective case study is of value despite a very small sample size that would typically be considered inadequate to effectively answer the question. Nonetheless, even with the small sample, the highly cross-linked polyethylene did prove to be superior to traditional polyethylene. The reason this is of value is that cross-linked polyethylene has been well demonstrated to be of theoretical value and is now the standard of practice. Yet there are few clinical studies that demonstrate that this is in fact the case. This study confirms the theory. As is so often the case, however, the industry has moved on, and the vitamin E-treated cross-linked polyethylene appears, at least with wear diminution, to be even more effective to reduce wear particles.

B. F. Morrey, MD

Have cementless and resurfacing components improved the medium-term results of hip replacement for patients under 60 years of age? Patient-reported outcome measures, implant survival, and costs in 24,709 patients
Jameson SS, Mason J, Baker P, et al (Durham Univ, UK; et al)
Acta Orthop 86:7-17, 2015

Background and Purpose.—The optimal hip replacement for young patients remains unknown. We compared patient-reported outcome measures (PROMs), revision risk, and implant costs over a range of hip replacements.

Methods.—We included hip replacements for osteoarthritis in patients under 60 years of age performed between 2003 and 2010 using the commonest brand of cemented, cementless, hybrid, or resurfacing prosthesis (11,622 women and 13,087 men). The reference implant comprised a cemented stem with a conventional polyethylene cemented cup and a standard-sized head (28- or 32-mm). Differences in implant survival were assessed using competing-risks models, adjusted for known prognostic influences. Analysis of covariance was used to assess improvement in PROMs (Oxford hip score (OHS) and EQ5D index) in 2014 linked procedures.

Results.—In males, PROMs and implant survival were similar across all types of implants. In females, revision was statistically significantly higher in hard-bearing and/or small-stem cementless implants (hazard ratio

(HR) = 4) and resurfacings (small head sizes (< 48 mm): HR = 6; large head sizes (≥ 48 mm): HR = 5) when compared to the reference cemented implant. In component combinations with equivalent survival, women reported significantly greater improvements in OHS with hybrid implants (22, $p = 0.006$) and cementless implants (21, $p = 0.03$) (reference, 18), but similar EQ5D index. For men and women, National Health Service (NHS) costs were lowest with the reference implant and highest with a hard-bearing cementless replacement.

Interpretation.—In young women, hybrids offer a balance of good early functional improvement and low revision risk. Fully cementless and resurfacing components are more costly and do not provide any additional benefit for younger patients.

▶ The details of the findings of this national registry study from the United Kingdom are interesting. But the real reason I selected this article is that it once again underscores what has been shown time and time again. In the young patient, in this instance less than 60 years, the reference cemented hip is hard to beat. In spite of theoretical value, hard bearings, resurfacing, and uncemented devices offer no benefit, especially to the female patient. Because they are more costly, one must question the justification of their use.

B. F. Morrey, MD

Do Serologic and Synovial Tests Help Diagnose Infection in Revision Hip Arthroplasty With Metal-on-metal Bearings or Corrosion?

Yi PH, Cross MB, Moric M, et al (Rush Univ Med Ctr, Chicago, IL; Hosp for Special Surgery, NY)
Clin Orthop Relat Res 473:498-505, 2015

Background.—The diagnosis of periprosthetic joint infection (PJI) in patients with failed metal-on-metal (MoM) bearings and corrosion reactions in hip arthroplasties can be particularly difficult, because the clinical presentation of adverse local tissue reactions may mimic that of PJI, because it can also occur concurrently with PJI, and because common laboratory tests used to diagnose PJI may be elevated in patients with MoM THAs.

Questions/Purposes.—We sought to determine the test properties of the serum erythrocyte sedimentation rate (ESR), C-reactive protein (CRP), synovial fluid white blood cell (WBC) count, and synovial fluid differential (percent polymorphonuclear cells [PMNs]) in diagnosing PJI in either MoM hips undergoing revision for a variety of indications or in non-MoM hips undergoing revision for either corrosion reaction or full-thickness wear. Additionally, we sought to describe how MoM bearings, metal debris, and corrosion reactions can confound the analysis of the synovial fluid WBC count and affect its diagnostic use for PJI.

Methods.—We reviewed 150 revision hips meeting specified inclusion criteria (92 MoM total hips, 19 MoM hip resurfacings, 30 non-MoM bearings with corrosion, and nine full-thickness bearing surface wear with metallosis). In our review, we diagnosed 19 patients as infected using Musculoskeletal Infection Society (MSIS) criteria. Mean laboratory values were compared between infected and not infected patients and receiver operator characteristic curves were generated with an area under the curve (AUC) to determine test performance and optimal cutoffs.

Results.—After excluding the inaccurate synovial fluid samples, the synovial fluid WBC count (performed accurately in 102 patients) was the best test for the diagnosis of PJI (AUC = 98%, optimal cutoff 4350 WBC/μL) followed by the differential (performed accurately in 102 patients AUC = 90%, optimal cutoff 85% PMN). The ESR (performed in 131 patients) and CRP (performed in 129 patients) both had good sensitivity (83% and 94%, respectively). Patients meeting MSIS criteria for PJI had higher mean serum ESR, CRP, synovial fluid WBC count, and differential than those not meeting MSIS criteria ($p < 0.05$ for all). An observer blinded to the MSIS diagnosis of the patient assessed the synovial fluid samples for inaccuracy secondary to metal or cellular debris. Synovial fluid sample "inaccuracy" was defined as the laboratory technician noting the presence of metal or amorpous material, fragmented cells, or clots, or the sample having some defect preventing an automated cell count from being performed. Of the 141 patients who had a synovial fluid sample initially available for review, 47 (33%) had a synovial fluid sample deemed to be inaccurate. A synovial fluid WBC count was still reported however, 35 of these 47 hips (75%) and 11 of these 35 (31%) were falsely positive for infection.

Conclusions.—The diagnosis of PJI is extremely difficult in patients with MoM bearings or corrosion and the synovial fluid WBC count can frequently be falsely positive and should be relied on only if a manual count is done and if a differential can be performed. A more aggressive approach to preoperative evaluation for PJI is recommended in these patients to allow for careful evaluation of the synovial fluid specimen, the integration of synovial fluid culture results, and repeat aspiration if necessary.

Level of Evidence.—Level III, diagnostic study. See Guidelines for Authors for a complete description of levels of evidence (Fig 1).

▶ There is a growing awareness of the difficulty in diagnosing prosthetic joint infections at all anatomic sites. The question is made more complicated with the reactive effects of metal-on-metal implants. The conclusion that the issue is complex was known before the article was reviewed. The value is the demonstration of the threshold values for erythrocyte sedimentation rate, C-reactive protein, white cell count on aspiration, and differential count of the aspirate. Fig 1 summarizes the findings with their respective statistical accuracy. However, as the authors point out, there is no one definitive test. We would

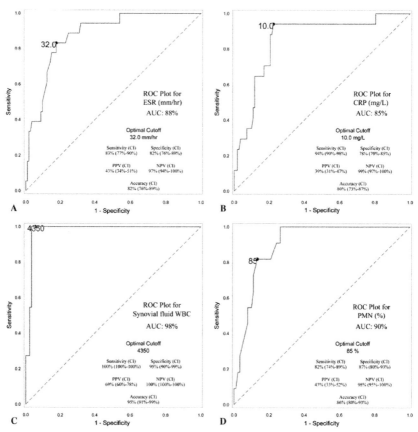

FIGURE 1.—(A) A receiver operating characteristic (ROC) curve for the serum ESR is shown with an AUC of 88%. A cutoff value of 32.0 mm/hr demonstrates 83% sensitivity, 82% specificity, 43% positive predictive value (PPV), 97% negative predictive value (NPV), and 82% accuracy. (B) A ROC curve for the serum CRP is shown with an AUC of 85%. A cutoff value of 10.0 mg/L demonstrates 94% sensitivity, 78% specificity, 39% PPV, 99% NPV, and 80% accuracy. (C) A ROC curve for the synovial fluid WBC count is shown with an AUC of 98%. A cutoff value of 4350 cells/μL demonstrates 100% sensitivity, 95% specificity, 69% PPV, 100% NPV, and 95% accuracy. (D) A ROC curve for the %PMN is shown with an AUC of 90%. A cutoff value of 85% PMNs demonstrates 82% sensitivity, 87% specificity, 43% PPV, 98% NPV, and 86% accuracy. CI = confidence interval. (With kind permission from Springer Science+Business Media: Yi PH, Cross MB, Moric M, et al. Do serologic and synovial tests help diagnose infection in revision hip arthroplasty with metal-on-metal bearings or corrosion? *Clin Orthop Relat Res.* 2015;473:498-505, with permission from The Association of Bone and Joint Surgeons.)

emphasize the importance of the aspirate data, especially the differential count of > 85% polymorphonuclear neutrophils.

B. F. Morrey, MD

Dislocation after the first and multiple revision total hip arthroplasty: comparison between acetabulum-only, femur-only and both component revision hip arthroplasty

Kosashvili Y, Drexler M, Backstein D, et al (Mount Sinai Hosp, Toronto, Ontario, Canada; et al)
Can J Surg 57:e15-e18, 2014

Background.—Dislocation may complicate revision total hip arthroplasty (THA). We examined the correlation between the components revised during hip arthroplasty (femur only, acetabulum only and both components) to the rates of dislocation in the first and multiple revision THA.

Methods.—We obtained data from consecutive revision THAs performed between January 1982 and December 2005. Patients were grouped into femur-only revision, acetabulum-only revision and revision THA for both components.

Results.—A total of 749 revision THAs performed during the study period met our inclusion criteria: 369 first-time revisions and 380 repeated revisions. Dislocation rates in patients undergoing first-time revisions (5.69%) were significantly lower than in those undergoing repeated revisions (10.47%; $p = 0.022$). Within the group of first-time revisions, dislocation rates for acetabulum-only revisions (10.28%) were significantly higher than those for both components (4.61%) and femur-only (0%) reconstructions ($p = 0.025$).

Conclusion.—Although patients undergoing first-time revisions had lower rates of dislocations than those undergoing repeated revisions, acetabulum-only reconstructions performed at first-time revision arthroplasty entailed an increased risk for instability.

▶ It has been a while since we have included articles regarding hip instability. There are few studies of instability after revision. This Toronto experience provides some interesting information. Essentially, the likelihood of a dislocation after the first revision is about 5%, which is about half the 10% seen after multiple revisions. Furthermore, it is noteworthy that revision of the acetabular component alone is more likely to lead to instability than revision of the femoral or of both components (Fig 1 in the original article). Because the study covered several decades, the trend of instability as a function of time is an important consideration. Despite improved understanding and technique, there was really no lessening of these instability percentages over time (Fig 2 in the original article). It would be interesting to compare these findings with those of other centers.

B. F. Morrey, MD

Functional and radiological outcome of periprosthetic femoral fractures after hip arthroplasty

Moreta J, Aguirre U, de Ugarte OS, et al (Hosp Galdakao-Usansolo, Bizkaia, Spain)
Injury 46:292-298, 2015

Background.—The aim of this study was to determine the functional and radiological results of the treatment of periprosthetic femoral fractures.

Materials and Methods.—A review was performed of all periprosthetic femur fractures after a total hip arthroplasty (THA) or hemiarthroplasty (HA) treated at our institution from 1995 to 2011. Functional outcome was assessed in terms of the Harris Hip Score and ambulatory status. Radiological findings were classified using Beals and Tower's criteria.

Results.—A total of 59 periprosthetic fractures were identified in 58 patients. The mean age of patients was 79 years old and the mean follow-up time was 33.6 months. Local risk factors were identified in 71% of the patients, principally osteoporosis (59%), followed by osteolysis (24%) and loosening of the stem (19%). In the multivariable analysis, the presence of local risk factors was associated with worsening of patients' ambulatory status. According to the Vancouver classification, there were 8 type A, 46 type B and 5 type C fractures. Of the type B fractures 24 were B1, 14 were B2 and 8 were B3.

Fracture union was achieved in 54 fractures, with a mean union time of 6 months. Applying Beals and Tower's criteria, radiological results were excellent in 20 patients (34%), good in 22 (37%), and poor in 17 (29%). None of the patients improved their ability to walk after these fractures and 31 patients (52%) did not regain their prefracture walking status. The mean Harris Hip Score postoperatively was 67.9.

There were major or minor complications in 33 patients (56%) and 11 patients (19%) required further operations.

Conclusion.—Although this study shows good radiological results following methods of treatment in accordance with the Vancouver classification, there was marked functional deterioration in many patients and a high rate of complications. Local risk factors were associated with poorer ambulatory status (Fig 1).

▶ I anticipated the findings of this study would be similar to the impact of infected joints or of femoral neck fractures in the elderly—successful management of the primary problem is accompanied by a worsening in the premorbid state. This nicely done study shows this is clearly the case. However, unlike the data in the other 2 conditions, which indicated a lower than desired successful management of the primary condition, healing of the facture was successfully achieved. Only 70% achieved definite healing, and there was a greater than 50% complication rate. Hence, the functional outcome summarized with

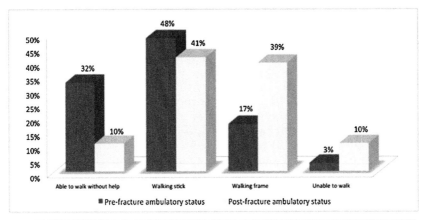

	Pre-fracture ambulatory status of the patients	Post-fracture ambulatory status of the patients	p- value
Able to walk withot help	19 (32 %)	6 (10%)	<0.001
Walking stick	28 (48%)	24 (41%)	0.45
2 Crutches / Walking frame	10 (17%)	23 (39%)	< 0.001
Unable to walk	2 (3%)	6 (10%)	0.45

FIGURE 1.—Pre and post-fracture ambulatory status stratified by patient's mobility classification. (Reprinted from the Injury, International Journal of the Care of the Injured. Moreta J, Aguirre U, de Ugarte OS, et al. Functional and radiological outcome of periprosthetic femoral fractures after hip arthroplasty. *Injury.* 2015;46:292-298, Copyright 2015, with permission from Elsevier.)

worsening of the ambulatory state is not surprising (Fig 1). These are important data when discussing this problem before surgery with the family.

B. F. Morrey, MD

Autologous wound drains have no effect on allogeneic blood transfusions in primary total hip and knee replacement: a three-arm randomised trial
Thomassen BJW, den Hollander PHC, Kaptijn HH, et al (Orthopaedic Surgeon Med Ctr Haaglanden, The Netherlands; The Lange Land Hosp, The Netherlands; et al)
Bone Joint J 96-B:765-771, 2014

We hypothesised there was no clinical value in using an autologous blood transfusion (ABT) drain in either primary total hip (THR) or total knee replacement (TKR) in terms of limiting allogeneic blood transfusions when a modern restrictive blood management regime was followed. A total of 575 patients (65.2% men), with a mean age of 68.9 years (36 to 94) were randomised in this three-arm study to no drainage (group A), or to wound drainage with an ABT drain for either six hours (group B) or 24 hours (group C). The primary outcome was the number of patients receiving allogeneic blood transfusion. Secondary outcomes were postoperative haemoglobin (Hb) levels, length of hospital stay and adverse events.

This study identified only 41 transfused patients, with no significant difference in distribution between the three groups ($p = 0.857$). The mean pre-operative haemoglobin (Hb) value in the transfused group was 12.8 g/dL (9.8 to 15.5) *versus* 14.3 g/dL (10.6 to 18.0) in the non-transfused group ($p < 0.001$, 95% confidence interval: 1.08 to 1.86). Post-operatively, the median of re-transfused shed blood in patients with a THR was 280 mL (Interquartile range (IQR) 150 to 400) and in TKR patients 500 mL (IQR 350 to 650) ($p < 0.001$). ABT drains had no effect on the proportion of transfused patients in primary THR and TKR. The secondary outcomes were also comparable between groups.

▶ This is an excellent prospective randomized trial addressing a significant issue: What is the value of postoperative blood drainage salvage and retransfusion? This question is further stratified into early retransfusion, group B, and late, 24-hour, retransfusion.

The study requires little comment because the data are clear. This adequately powered and carefully performed study reveals no advantage for retransfusion early or late in the primary hip or knee patient (Table 3 in the original article). One may suggest that drainage lessens other wound-related problems. This is not the case (Table 4 in the original article). I personally have discontinued routine wound drainage for more than 25 years and discontinued routine reinfusion for more than 20 years. This study would seem to justify this clinical practice. However, as is well known, practices change slowly, even in the face of hard evidence.

B. F. Morrey, MD

8   Total Knee Arthroplasty

Introduction

Total knee is arguably the most successful joint replacement, with the possible exception of hip replacement. Therefore, I find it very interesting that several articles concentrate on that residual group of patients who do not do well after knee joint replacement. I am surprised that the percentages of residual pain quoted in these articles are considerably higher than what is generally accepted by our profession. A 20% incidence of residual pain seems incongruous with an often quoted 95% early success rate. As we move forward, it appears as though patients are becoming more discriminating, and what was considered possibly a satisfactory result in the past may not be considered the same with current outcome tools. Fortunately, the science and practice of total knee replacement is quite refined. Most surgeons can demonstrate very satisfactory outcomes. There are truly no real technological advances, in my opinion, even though the profession continues to investigate navigation (which was not covered this year), instrumentation accuracy, and specific design features. On the whole, these investigations have not been fruitful. However, I do think the analysis of why the knee fails is important, and articles relating to this topic have been included this year.

Bernard F. Morrey, MD

Dramatic Increase in Total Knee Replacement Utilization Rates Cannot Be Fully Explained by a Disproportionate Increase Among Younger Patients
Bernstein J, Derman P (Univ of Pennsylvania, Philadelphia; Hosp for Special Surgery, NY)
Orthopedics 37:e656-e659, 2014

The incidence of total knee replacement in the United States more than doubled between 1999 and 2008, increasing from approximately 263,000 to 616,000 cases. The purpose of this study is to evaluate the claim that there has been a disproportionate increase in knee replacements among younger patients owing to expanding indications for the procedure in this group. Data on the US population for individuals 18 to 44 years old, 45 to 64 years old, and 65 years and older were obtained from census data; the number of total knee replacements performed annually in each age group was acquired from the Agency for Healthcare Research and Quality and per-capita incidence rates were calculated. Applying the 1999 rates to the 2008 population, the number of knee replacements anticipated on the basis of population growth for each cohort was determined and compared with the number observed, yielding the unexplained growth. The data revealed that in 2008, approximately 305,000 knee replacements were performed beyond the number predicted by population growth alone. The largest segment of growth (151,000 cases) was among patients 65 years and older; the per-capita growth rate was highest in this cohort as well, increasing from 5.2 to 9.1 procedures per 1,000 individuals. The data show conclusively that a disproportionate increase in knee replacements among younger patients is not a full explanation for the growth in utilization. In fact, it is not even the best among alternative explanations. The main locus of growth was among traditional patients 65 years and older.

▶ The growing number of knee replacements is one of the most significant features in the spiraling cost of health care in the United States. In fact, one may question whether the growing frequency of this procedure is sustainable. Hence, if this trend needs to be controlled, the issue must be understood, and studies such as this are critical. It has been hypothesized that the rapid increase in the rate of this procedure is due to an increasing rate of surgery being performed in the younger age group. This analysis clearly shows this is not the case. What is the alternate explanation? We would offer 2. The first is a greater unwillingness from our patient population to tolerate pain—any pain. The second is the willingness of the surgeon to alter the traditional indications for this surgery and performing procedures on patients with less severe symptoms. Finally, notice the data are from 2008. Since then, the trend has only increased, so the problem is worse than this study demonstrates.

B. F. Morrey, MD

Intermediate and Long-Term Quality of Life After Total Knee Replacement: A Systematic Review and Meta-Analysis

Shan L, Shan B, Suzuki A, et al (The Univ of Melbourne, Victoria, Australia; Monash Univ, Victoria, Australia; Wollongong Hosp, New South Wales, Australia)
J Bone Joint Surg Am 97:156-168, 2015

Background.—Total knee replacement is a highly successful and frequently performed operation. Technical outcomes of surgery are excellent, with favorable early postoperative health-related quality of life. This study reviews intermediate and long-term quality of life after surgery.

Methods.—A systematic review and meta-analysis of all studies published from January 2000 onward was performed to evaluate health-related quality of life after primary total knee replacement for osteoarthritis in patients with at least three years of follow-up. Key outcomes were postoperative quality of life, function, and satisfaction compared with the preoperative status. Strict inclusion and exclusion criteria were applied. Quality appraisal and data tabulation were performed with use of predefined criteria. Data were synthesized by narrative review and random-effects meta-analysis utilizing standardized mean differences. Heterogeneity was assessed with the tau^2 and I^2 statistics.

Results.—Nineteen studies were included in the review. Intermediate and long-term postoperative quality of life was superior to the preoperative level in qualitative and quantitative analyses. The pooled effect in combined WOMAC (Western Ontario and McMaster Universities Osteoarthritis Index) and KSS (Knee Society Score) outcomes was a marked improvement from baseline with respect to the total score (2.17; 95% CI [confidence interval], 1.13 to 3.22; $p < 0.0001$) and the pain (1.72; 95% CI, 0.97 to 2.46; $p < 0.00001$) and function (1.26; 95% CI, 0.87 to 1.64; $p < 0.00001$) domains. Most patients were satisfied with the surgery and derived substantial benefits for daily functional activities. Tau^2 (0.20 to 1.10) and I^2 (90% to 98%) values implied significant clinical and statistical heterogeneity.

Conclusions.—Total knee replacement confers significant intermediate and long-term benefits with respect to both disease-specific and generic health-related quality of life, especially pain and function, leading to positive patient satisfaction. Recommendations for necessary future studies are provided.

Level of Evidence.—Therapeutic Level II. See Instructions for Authors for a complete description of levels of evidence.

▶ One might conclude that this article shows the obvious. Total knee replacement improves the quality of life (QoL). Actually, I agree that it does demonstrate the obvious. This conclusion was made after an exhaustive process in which 19 articles with 5110 patients were reviewed. Importantly, it studies the currency of the realm, QoL. This report does demonstrate that improvement is measured as early as 6 months and persists throughout life. It further shows that the QoL is recognized with both general and disease-specific tools. I do have a problem with the final thought that, to be absolutely definitive, a randomized, controlled trial would be helpful. I disagree. Enough is enough.

B. F. Morrey, MD

Chronic Postoperative Pain After Primary and Revision Total Knee Arthroplasty

Petersen KK, Simonsen O, Laursen MB, et al (Aalborg Univ Hosp, Denmark)
Clin J Pain 31:1-6, 2015

Objectives.—Clinical experience suggests that patients with osteoarthritis (OA) undergoing revision total knee arthroplasty (TKA) experience more chronic complications after surgery compared with patients receiving primary TKA. This study aimed to investigate the difference in pain, mobility, and quality of life (QoL) in patients after revision TKA compared with patients after primary TKA.

Methods.—A total of 99 OA patients after revision TKA surgery and 215 patients after primary TKA surgery were investigated in a cross-sectional study using: a pain description of current pain (nonexistent, mild, moderate, severe, or unbearable), the pain intensity visual analogue scale, the Knee Society Score, and the Osteoarthritis Research Society International questionnaire.

Results.—Nineteen percent after primary TKA surgery and 47% after revision TKA surgery experienced severe to unbearable chronic postoperative pain. After revision TKA surgery patients reported higher pain

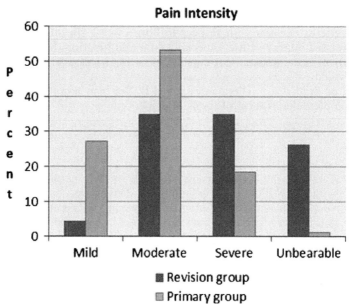

FIGURE 1.—Pain intensities for patients after primary and revision TKA surgery. After revision TKA surgery patients had increased pain intensity ($P = 0.006$) compared with patients after primary surgery. A total of 19% of the primary patients and 47% of the revision TKA patients reported severe to unbearable pain 3 years after surgery. TKA indicates total knee arthroplasty. (Reprinted from Petersen KK, Simonsen O, Laursen MB, et al. Chronic postoperative pain after primary and revision total knee arthroplasty. *Clin J Pain.* 2014;31:1-6, with permission from Lippincott Williams & Wilkin.)

intensities during rest ($P = 0.039$), while walking ($P = 0.008$), and on average over the last 24 hours ($P = 0.050$) compared with the patients after primary TKA surgery. Patients after revision TKA surgery had reduced walking distance ($P = 0.001$), increased use of walking aids ($P = 0.015$), and showed an overall decreased QoL ($P < 0.001$) compared with patients after primary TKA surgery. No significant improvement was found in walking distance ($P = 0.448$) for patients before revision TKA surgery compared with after revision TKA surgery.

Discussion.—More than twice as many patients have pain after revision surgery compared with patients after primary TKA. Patients after revision TKA surgery have reduced function, poorer QoL, and higher pain intensity compared with patients after primary TKA surgery (Fig 1).

▶ This article was selected for an unusual reason: I don't understand the data. Coming from a reliable national registry, on which we have come to rely, further enhances the problem. At 3 years in Denmark, almost 20% of patients with primary replacement still had considerable pain. The thrust of the article is that almost 50% of patients undergoing revision also had moderate or worse pain and were worse than those with primary replacement. This is no surprise and is well documented. What is just unthinkable is the astronomical rate of residual pain in the primary replacement group (Fig 1). It is also noted the revisions occurred on average less than 3 years after primary replacement, and 30% were for unexplained reasons, including unexplained pain. This is not my practice. Still, these baseline numbers are extremely high based on an honest assessment of my own practice.

B. F. Morrey, MD

Dissatisfied patients after total knee arthroplasty: A registry study involving 114 patients with 8–13 years of follow-up

Ali A, Sundberg M, Robertsson O, et al (Lund Univ and Skåne Univ Hosp, Sweden; et al)
Acta Orthop 85:229-233, 2014

Background and Purpose.—In 2003, an enquiry by the Swedish Knee Arthroplasty Register (SKAR) 2—7 years after total knee arthroplasty (TKA) revealed patients who were dissatisfied with the outcome of their surgery but who had not been revised. 6 years later, we examined the dissatisfied patients in one Swedish county and a matched group of very satisfied patients.

Patients and Methods.—118 TKAs in 114 patients, all of whom had had their surgery between 1996 and 2001, were examined in 2009—2010. 55 patients (with 58 TKAs) had stated in 2003 that they were dissatisfied with their knees and 59 (with 60 TKAs) had stated that they were very satisfied with their knees. The patients were examined clinically and radiographically, and performed functional tests consisting of the 6-minute walk

TABLE 2.—Patient Characteristics

Variables	Dissatisfied n = 55	Very Satisfied n = 59	RR[a]	Mean Diff.[b]	p-Value	95% CI
Mean age	78 (SD 8)	79 (SD 7)				
Gender (female)	39	43				
Mean follow-up, years	10.5 (SD 2.5)	10.5 (SD 2.5)				
Mean VAS score (0–100)	52	22		31	< 0.001	23 to 39
HAD[c], no. patients	23	6	4.1		0.001	2 to 9
Mean ROM, degrees	97	108		−13	< 0.001	−18 to −7
Mean 6MW test result, m	295	318		−35	0.07	−74 to 3
Mean chair test result, s	19	17		2.7	0.1	−0.5 to 6
Mean BMI	32	30		1.4	0.2	−0.7 to 3
Smokers	2	4	0.8		0.3	0.6 to 1
Increased knee laxity	3	5	0.6		0.4	0.1 to 2
Patella tenderness	8	6	0.8		0.8	0.2 to 4

[a]RR: relative risk, dissatisfied vs. very satisfied.
[b]Mean difference, dissatisfied vs. very satisfied.
[c]Anxiety and/or depression according to the Hospital Anxiety and Depression scale.
Reprinted from Ali A, Sundberg M, Robertsson O, et al. Dissatisfied patients after total knee arthroplasty: A registry study involving 114 patients with 8e13 years of follow-up. *Acta Orthop.* 2014;85:229–233, reprinted by permission of Taylor & Francis Ltd, http://www.informaworld.com.

and chair-stand test. All the patients filled out a visual analog scale (VAS, 0–100 mm) regarding knee pain and also the Hospital and Anxiety and Depression scale (HAD).

Results.—Mean VAS score for knee pain differed by 30 mm in favor of the very satisfied group (p < 0.001). 23 of the 55 patients in the dissatisfied group and 6 of 59 patients in the very satisfied group suffered from anxiety and/or depression (p = 0.001). Mean range of motion was 11 degrees better in the very satisfied group (p < 0.001). The groups were similar with regard to clinical examination, physical performance testing, and radiography.

Interpretation.—The patients who reported poor response after TKA continued to be unhappy after 8–13 years, as demonstrated by VAS pain and HAD, despite the absence of a discernible objective reason for revision (Table 2).

▶ We are once again indebted not only to a national database but also to the ingenuity of the investigators. What an interesting and insightful question. We are all faced with the knee replacement that looks good to excellent radiographically and clinically in a patient with nagging or bitter pain. Although this is a frustrating experience, these data indicate that a reoperation without a clear basis is unwise. No surprise there. But the study also provides some important objective insights. The dissatisfaction is primarily based on persistent pain, and this most strongly relates to depression. But the dissatisfied individual also has less motion (Table 2). These findings underscore a lesson I was taught in the first year of my training: You can't cure psychological conditions with a scalpel.

B. F. Morrey, MD

45-day mortality after 467 779 knee replacements for osteoarthritis from the National Joint Registry for England and Wales: An observational study
Hunt LP, on behalf of the National Joint Registry for England and Wales (Univ of Bristol, UK; et al)
Lancet 384:1429-1436, 2014

Background.—Understanding the risk factors for early death after knee replacement could help to reduce the risk of mortality after this procedure. We assessed secular trends in death within 45 days of knee replacement for osteoarthritis in England and Wales, with the aim of investigating whether any change that we recorded could be explained by alterations in modifi able perioperative factors.

Methods.—We took data for knee replacements done for osteoarthritis in England and Wales between April 1, 2003, and Dec 31, 2011, from the National Joint Registry for England and Wales. Patient identifiers were used to link these data to the national mortality database and the Hospital Episode Statistics database to obtain details of death, sociodemographics, and comorbidity. We assessed mortality within 45 days by Kaplan-Meier analysis and assessed the role of patient and treatment factors by Cox proportional hazards models.

Findings.—467 779 primary knee replacements were done to treat osteoarthritis during 9 years. 1183 patients died within 45 days of surgery, with a substantial secular decrease in mortality from 0·37% in 2003 to 0·20% in 2011, even after adjustment for age, sex, and comorbidity. The use of unicompartmental knee replacement was associated with substantially lower mortality than was total knee replacement (hazard ratio

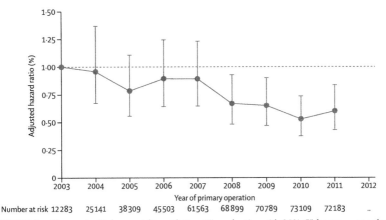

FIGURE 2.—Changes in 45-day mortality with time. Hazard ratios with 95% CI for every year of primary after adjustment for sex and age. *Numbers shown underneath the plotted values are the number of primary operations done that year. (Reprinted from The Lancet. Hunt LP, on behalf of the National Joint Registry for England and Wale. 45-day mortality after 467 779 knee replacements for osteoarthritis from the National Joint Registry for England and Wales: an observational study. *Lancet.* 2014;384:1429-1436 Copyright 2014, with permission from Elsevier.)

[HR] $0 \cdot 32$, 95% CI $0 \cdot 19 - 0 \cdot 54$, $p < 0 \cdot 0005$). Several comorbidities were associated with increased mortality: myocardial infarction (HR $3 \cdot 46$, 95% CI $2 \cdot 81 - 4 \cdot 14$, $p < 0 \cdot 0005$), cerebrovascular disease ($3 \cdot 35$, $2 \cdot 7 - 4 \cdot 14$, $p < 0 \cdot 0005$), moderate/severe liver disease ($7 \cdot 2$, $3 \cdot 93 - 13 \cdot 21$, $p < 0 \cdot 0005$), and renal disease ($2 \cdot 18$, $1 \cdot 76 - 2 \cdot 69$, $p < 0 \cdot 0005$). Modifiable perioperative risk factors, including surgical approach and thromboprophylaxis were not associated with mortality.

Interpretation.—Postoperative mortality after knee replacement has fallen substantially between 2003 and 2011. Efforts to further reduce mortality should concentrate more on older patients, those who are male and those with specific comorbidities, such as myocardial infarction, cerebrovascular disease, liver disease, and renal disease (Fig 2).

▶ With the increasing incidence of joint replacements, especially at the knee, these data are of some value. The denominator of almost 500 000 is impressive, and a national registry is the only source of such numbers, which are required to study an event that occurs less than 1% of the time. The impressive trend for me was the considerable reduction in the mortality from 2003 to 2011 from .37% to .2% (Fig 2). I was surprised to find that the hemi-replacement had a lower incidence of mortality than the 3-compartment replacement. It is not surprising that medical comorbidities involving the cardiovascular system were associated with a higher 45-day mortality rate and that surgical approach had no such influence. However, it was surprising that thromboembolic prophylaxis had no influence on the mortality incidence.

B. F. Morrey, MD

Adverse outcomes after total and unicompartmental knee replacement in 101 330 matched patients: A study of data from the National Joint Registry for England and Wales
Liddle AD, Judge A, Pandit H, et al (Univ of Oxford, UK; Univ of Southampton, UK)
Lancet 384:1437-1445, 2014

Background.—Total knee replacement (TKR) or unicompartmental knee replacement (UKR) are options for end-stage osteoarthritis. However, comparisons between the two procedures are confounded by differences in baseline characteristics of patients undergoing either procedure and by insufficient reporting of endpoints other than revision. We aimed to compare adverse outcomes for each procedure in matched patients.

Methods.—With propensity score techniques, we compared matched patients undergoing TKR and UKR in the National Joint Registry for England and Wales. The National Joint Registry started collecting data in April 1, 2003, and is continuing. The last operation date in the extract of data used in our study was Aug 28, 2012. We linked data for multiple potential confounders from the National Health Service Hospital Episode

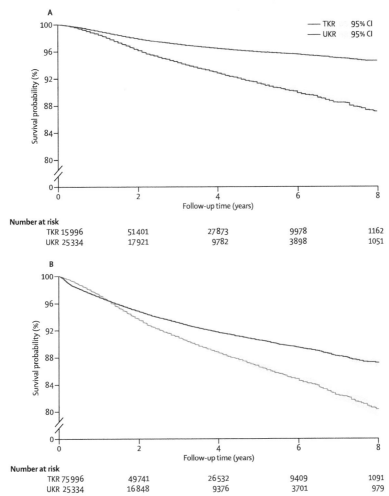

FIGURE 1.—Kaplan-Meier curve of revision (A) and revision/reoperation (B) to 8 years in matched patients. UKR = unicompartmental knee replacement. TKR = total knee replacement. (Reprinted from The Lancet. Liddle AD, Judge A, Pandit H, et al. Adverse outcomes after total and unicompartmental knee replacement in 101 330 matched patients: A study of data from the National Joint Registry for England and Wales. *Lancet.* 2014;384:1437-1445, Copyright 2014, with permission from Elsevier.)

Statistics database. We used regression models to compare outcomes including rates of revision, revision/reoperation, complications, readmission, mortality, and length of stay.

Findings.—25 334 UKRs were matched to 75 996 TKRs on the basis of propensity score. UKRs had worse implant survival both for revision (subhazard ratio [SHR] 2·12, 95% CI 1·99–2·26) and for revision/reoperation (1·38, 1·31–1·44) than TKRs at 8 years. Mortality was significantly higher for TKR at all timepoints than for UKR (30 day: hazard

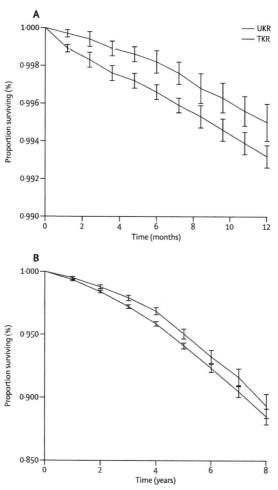

FIGURE 2.—Survival curves showing comparison of mortality at 1 year (A) and 8 years (B). UKR = unicompartmental knee replacement. TKR = total knee replacement. Error bars show 95% CI. (Reprinted from The Lancet. Liddle AD, Judge A, Pandit H, et al. Adverse outcomes after total and uni-compartmental knee replacement in 101 330 matched patients: A study of data from the National Joint Registry for England and Wales. *Lancet.* 2014;384:1437-1445, Copyright 2014, with permission from Elsevier.)

ratio 0·23, 95% CI 0·11−0·50; 8 year: 0·85, 0·79−0·92). Length of stay, complications (including thromboembolism, myocardial infarction, and stroke), and rate of readmission were all higher for TKR than for UKR.

Interpretation.—In decisions about which procedure to offer, the higher revision/reoperation rate of UKR than of TKR should be balanced against a lower occurrence of complications, readmission, and mortality, together with known benefits for UKR in terms of postoperative function.

If 100 patients receiving TKR received UKR instead, the result would be around one fewer death and three more reoperations in the first 4 years after surgery (Figs 1 and 2).

▶ This contribution from the UK national database provides interesting insights regarding the outcomes of total and unicompartment knee replacement. Conflicting data make it difficult to develop a clear perspective of the risk and benefits when comparing the 2 procedures. The large database of more than 100 000 procedures provides credibility to data and conclusion. Simply stated, as is generally accepted, the unicompartment replacement is associated with a higher revision rate at 1 and 8 years (Fig 1). However, the 1-year mortality is less for unicompartment knee replacement (Fig 2). The article offers a reasonable perspective that the unicompartment procedure has sufficient advantages to allow one to accept the higher revision rate in some patients.

B. F. Morrey, MD

Implant design influences patient outcome after total knee arthroplasty: a prospective double-blind randomised controlled trial
Hamilton DF, Burnett R, Patton JT, et al (Univ of Edinburgh, UK)
Bone Joint J 97-B:64-70, 2015

Total knee arthroplasty (TKA) is an established and successful procedure. However, the design of prostheses continues to be modified in an attempt to optimise the functional outcome of the patient.

The aim of this study was to determine if patient outcome after TKA was influenced by the design of the prosthesis used.

A total of 212 patients (mean age 69; 43 to 92; 131 female (62%), 81 male (32%)) were enrolled in a single centre double-blind trial and randomised to receive either a Kinemax (group 1) or a Triathlon (group 2) TKA.

Patients were assessed pre-operatively, at six weeks, six months, one year and three years after surgery. The outcome assessments used were the Oxford Knee Score; range of movement; pain numerical rating scales; lower limb power output; timed functional assessment battery and a satisfaction survey. Data were assessed incorporating change over all assessment time points, using repeated measures analysis of variance longitudinal mixed models. Implant group 2 showed a significantly greater range of movement ($p = 0.009$), greater lower limb power output ($p = 0.026$) and reduced report of 'worst daily pain' ($p = 0.003$) over the three years of follow-up. Differences in Oxford Knee Score ($p = 0.09$), report of 'average daily pain' ($p = 0.57$) and timed functional performance tasks ($p = 0.23$) did not reach statistical significance. Satisfaction with outcome was significantly better in group 2 ($p = 0.001$).

These results suggest that patient outcome after TKA can be influenced by the prosthesis used.

▶ Frankly, I have become somewhat cynical over the years when observing the numerous minor design modifications of hip and knee implants that represent change but not progress. I was expecting this study to confirm this perception, which is based on previous studies. So I was surprised to see the modified design of the manufacturer actually did improve the short-term Oxford score as well as knee flexion by a statistically significant amount (Fig 2a and b in the original article). Although patient satisfaction was not statistically different, it did approach significance, *P* < .09, which of course may well represent the underpowered nature of the study.

B. F. Morrey, MD

A systematic review and meta-analysis of patient-specific instrumentation for improving alignment of the components in total knee replacement
Thienpont E, Schwab PE, Fennema P (Univ Hosp Saint Luc-UCL, Brussels, Belgium; AMR Advanced Med Res, Männedorf, Switzerland)
Bone Joint J 96-B:1052-1061, 2014

We conducted a meta-analysis, including randomised controlled trials (RCTs) and cohort studies, to examine the effect of patient-specific instruments (PSI) on radiological outcomes after total knee replacement (TKR) including: mechanical axis alignment and malalignment of the femoral and tibial components in the coronal, sagittal and axial planes, at a threshold of >3° from neutral. Relative risks (RR) for malalignment were determined for all studies and for RCTs and cohort studies separately.

Of 325 studies initially identified, 16 met the eligibility criteria, including eight RCTs and eight cohort studies. There was no significant difference in the likelihood of mechanical axis malalignment with PSI versus conventional TKR across all studies (RR = 0.84, $p = 0.304$), in the RCTs (RR = 1.14, $p = 0.445$) or in the cohort studies (RR = 0.70, $p = 0.289$). The results for the alignment of the tibial component were significantly worse using PSI TKR than conventional TKR in the coronal and sagittal planes (RR = 1.75, $p = 0.028$; and RR = 1.34, $p = 0.019$, respectively, on pooled analysis). PSI TKR showed a significant advantage over conventional TKR for alignment of the femoral component in the coronal plane (RR = 0.65, $p = 0.028$ on pooled analysis), but not in the sagittal plane (RR = 1.12, $p = 0.437$). Axial alignment of the tibial ($p = 0.460$) and femoral components ($p = 0.127$) was not significantly different.

We conclude that PSI does not improve the accuracy of alignment of the components in TKR compared with conventional instrumentation (Fig 1).

▶ I read this article in amazement. Fortunately, total knee replacement is so successful that it is difficult to improve our current outcomes, try as we may.

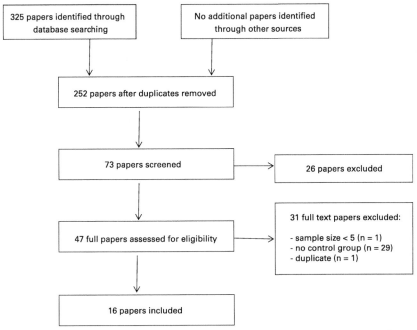

FIGURE 1.—Flowchart of randomised controlled trials (RCTs) and cohort studies identified for the meta-analysis. (Reprinted from Thienpont E, Schwab PE, Fennema P. A systematic review and meta-analysis of patient-specific instrumentation for improving alignment of the components in total knee replacement. *Bone Joint J*. 2014;96-B:1052-1061, with permission from The British Editorial Society of Bone & Joint Surgery.)

Not all would be familiar with patient-specific instrumentation. This costly process requires expensive magnetic resonance imaging and computed tomography imaging to create disposable patient-specific cutting blocks. I think there is merit to document the extent to which the investigators went to adequately address the issue (Fig 1). The analysis is primarily a statistical comparison of this methodology, navigation, and conventional instrumentation and technique. Would one be able to guess the outcome?

There is no difference in any of these preparation systems, which leaves me with one simple conclusion: Do what works and is least costly.

B. F. Morrey, MD

A comparison of patient-specific and conventional instrumentation for total knee arthroplasty: a multicentre randomised controlled trial
Abane L, Anract P, Boisgard S, et al (Centre Hospitalier Régional Universitaire de Clermont Ferrand, France)
Bone Joint J 97-B:56-63, 2015

In this study we randomised 140 patients who were due to undergo primary total knee arthroplasty (TKA) to have the procedure performed using either patient-specific cutting guides (PSCG) or conventional instrumentation (CI).

The primary outcome measure was the mechanical axis, as measured at three months on a standing long-leg radiograph by the hip–knee–ankle (HKA) angle. This was undertaken by an independent observer who was blinded to the instrumentation. Secondary outcome measures were component positioning, operating time, Knee Society and Oxford knee scores, blood loss and length of hospital stay.

A total of 126 patients (67 in the CI group and 59 in the PSCG group) had complete clinical and radiological data. There were 88 females and 52 males with a mean age of 69.3 years (47 to 84) and a mean BMI of 28.6 kg/m^2 (20.2 to 40.8). The mean HKA angle was 178.9° (172.5 to 183.4) in the CI group and 178.2° (172.4 to 183.4) in the PSCG group ($p = 0.34$). Outliers were identified in 22 of 67 knees (32.8%) in the CI group and 19 of 59 knees (32.2%) in the PSCG group ($p = 0.99$). There was no significant difference in the clinical results ($p = 0.95$ and 0.59, respectively). Operating time, blood loss and length of hospital stay were not significantly reduced ($p = 0.09$, 0.58 and 0.50, respectively) when using PSCG.

The use of PSCG in primary TKA did not reduce the proportion of outliers as measured by post-operative coronal alignment.

▶ This French prospective randomized study needs no commentary. The reason to select it is to simply reinforce the finding that patient-specific instrumentation has not added value to traditional instrumentation. We know the only difference is that it does add cost. Enough said.

B. F. Morrey, MD

All-Polyethylene Versus Metal-Backed Tibial Components—An Analysis of 27,733 Cruciate-Retaining Total Knee Replacements from the Swedish Knee Arthroplasty Register

Gudnason A, Hailer NP, W-Dahl A, et al (Uppsala Univ Hosp, Sweden; Lund Univ, Sweden)
J Bone Joint Surg Am 96:994-999, 2014

Background.—Currently, the use of metal-backed tibial components is more common than the use of all-polyethylene components in total knee arthroplasty. However, the available literature indicates that all-polyethylene tibial components are not inferior to the metal-backed design. We hypothesized that there would be no difference in the ten-year survival rate between all-polyethylene and metal-backed tibial components of a specific design in a large nationwide cohort.

Methods.—In the Swedish Knee Arthroplasty Register, we identified 27,733 cruciate-retaining total knee replacements using the press-fit condylar prosthesis with either metal-backed or all-polyethylene tibial components inserted from 1999 to 2011. Unadjusted survival functions were calculated with the end points of revision for any reason, revision due to infection, and revision due to reasons other than infection, and the differences between the groups were investigated with the log-rank test. Cox proportional hazard models were fitted to analyze the influence of various covariates on the adjusted relative risk of revision.

Results.—The median duration of follow-up was 4.5 years (range, zero to 12.9 years). Of all total knee replacements, 16,896 (60.9%) were in women and 10,837 (39.1%) were in men. Metal-backed components were used in 16,011 total knee arthroplasties (57.7%) and all-polyethylene in 11,722 total knee arthroplasties (42.3%). With revision for any reason as the end point, the all-polyethylene tibial component had slightly superior, unadjusted ten-year survival compared with the metal-backed component: 97.2% (95% confidence interval [CI], 96.7% to 97.7%) compared with 96.6% (95% CI, 96.2% to 96.9%; p = 0.002). Cox multiple regression analysis adjusting for age group, sex, and patellar resurfacing showed that all-polyethylene components had a reduced risk of revision for any reason (relative risk = 0.75; 95% CI, 0.64 to 0.89) and a reduced risk of revision due to infection (relative risk = 0.63; 95% CI, 0.46 to 0.86). Patellar resurfacing and male sex increased the risk of revision due to infection (relative risk = 2.22 [95% CI, 1.37 to 3.62] and 2.21 [95% CI, 1.66 to 2.94], respectively).

Conclusions.—These all-polyethylene tibial components were at least as good as or superior to metal-backed tibial components with respect to implant survivorship at ten years in cruciate-retaining total knee replacements. We concluded that these less expensive all-polyethylene tibial components can be safely and effectively used in total knee arthroplasty.

Level of Evidence.—Therapeutic Level III. See Instructions for Authors for a complete description of levels of evidence.

▶ I must admit that I have a clear bias to include material that supports my own views.

This report from the Swedish registry addresses an important and debated issue among knee surgeons: Which is superior, metal-backed modular or monoblock all-polyethylene tibial components? The survival curves in Fig 1 in the original article clearly demonstrate a statistical advantage for the all-polyethylene component, especially after the 5-year mark. I have used the all-polyethylene tibial component with a cruciate-retaining design for 20 years when documentation revealed that modularity was of no value to improve stability, improve motion, or simplify revisions. An additional assessment studying cruciating substitution designs would be of interest. Finally, when we really do become responsible for cost containment, which must happen, these data will be acted on. Sadly, I suspect few will change their preference, despite these data.

B. F. Morrey, MD

Comparative Survivorship of Different Tibial Designs in Primary Total Knee Arthroplasty

Kremers HM, Sierra RJ, Schleck CD, et al (Mayo Clinic, Rochester, MN)

J Bone Joint Surg Am 96:e121(1-7), 2014

Background.—Few registry-based studies in the United States have compared the survivorship of different knee implant designs in total knee arthroplasty. The purpose of this study was to compare differences in survivorship of commonly used tibial implant designs in primary total knee arthroplasty.

Methods.—A total of 16,584 primary total knee arthroplasties in 11,992 patients were performed at a single institution from 1985 to 2005. Patients were prospectively followed at regular intervals to ascertain details of subsequent revisions. Overall revision rates and revisions for aseptic loosening, wear, and osteolysis were compared across twenty-two tibial implant designs using Cox proportional hazards regression models adjusting for age, sex, calendar year, and body mass index.

Results.—In comparison with metal-backed modular implants, all-polyethylene tibial components had a significantly lower risk of revision (hazard ratio, 0.3; 95% confidence intervals: 0.2, 0.5 [$p < 0.0001$]). The risk reduction with all-polyethylene tibial components was not affected by age, sex, or body mass index. With metal-backed modular tibial designs, cruciate-retaining knees performed better than the posterior-stabilized knees ($p = 0.002$), but this finding was limited to one specific metal-backed modular tibial component, the Press Fit Condylar design. With all-polyethylene tibial components, there was no survivorship difference between cruciate-retaining and posterior-stabilized designs.

Conclusions.—All-polyethylene tibial components were associated with better outcomes than metal-backed modular components. Cruciate-retaining and posterior-stabilized designs performed equally well, except with the Press Fit Condylar design. Obese patients may have superior results with all-polyethylene and posterior-stabilized components.

Level of Evidence.—Therapeutic Level III. See Instructions for Authors for a complete description of levels of evidence.

▶ To be honest, I was unaware of the origin of this study when I selected it for review. Yet I am proud of my partners for this analysis and contribution. At the Mayo Clinic, assessment of more than 16 000 knee replacements revealed that the all-polyethylene tibial component offers superior outcomes, *P* < .0001. Furthermore, the cruciate-retaining cruciate option outperformed the modular replacement, *P* < .002 (Figs 1-4 in the original article). That I have resorted to an all-polyethylene cruciate-retaining design for the past 20 years is comforting personally, but does not change the reality; this appears to be the optimal design, and, in fact, is the less expensive option as well.

B. F. Morrey, MD

Does the length of incision in the quadriceps affect the recovery of strength after total knee replacement? a prospective randomised clinical trial

Chareancholvanich K, Pornrattanamaneewong C (Mahidol Univ, Bangkok, Thailand)
Bone Joint J 96-B:902-906, 2014

We have compared the time to recovery of isokinetic quadriceps strength after total knee replacement (TKR) using three different lengths of incision in the quadriceps. We prospectively randomised 60 patients into one of the three groups according to the length of incision in the quadriceps above the upper border of the patella (2 cm, 4 cm or 6 cm). The strength of the knees was measured pre-operatively and every month post-operatively until the peak quadriceps torque returned to its pre-operative level.

There was no significant difference in the mean operating time, blood loss, hospital stay, alignment or pre-operative isokinetic quadriceps strength between the three groups. Using the Kaplan—Meier method,

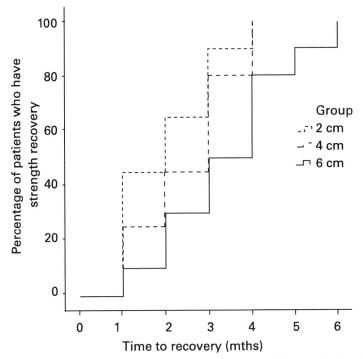

FIGURE 3.—Cumulative percentage of patients who have recovery of the strength of quadriceps. (Reprinted from Chareancholvanich K, Pornrattanamaneewong C. Does the length of incision in the quadriceps affect the recovery of strength after total knee replacement? a prospective randomised clinical trial. *Bone Joint J*. 2014;96-B:902-906, with permission from The British Editorial Society of Bone & Joint Surgery.)

group A had a similar mean recovery time to group B (2.0 ± 0.2 vs 2.5 ± 0.2 months, $p = 0.176$). Group C required a significantly longer recovery time (3.4 ± 0.3 months) than the other groups ($p < 0.03$). However, there were no significant differences in the mean Oxford knee scores one year post-operatively between the groups.

We conclude that an incision of up to 4 cm in the quadriceps does not delay the recovery of its isokinetic strength after TKR (Fig 3).

▶ This study has all the ingredients one might desire. It addresses a clinically relevant issue with a prospective randomized and controlled study. The data clearly demonstrate that incisions extending more than 4 cm into the quadriceps tendon proximal to the superior pole of the patella have a longer short-term recovery of strength (Fig 3).

There are several points to consider. The technique itself is that of a rather limited exposure without inverting the patella. The experienced surgeon was able to execute a similarly effective procedure in any of the 3 exposures. Finally, at 1 year there was no difference in function. So the take-home message is that extended incisions into the quadriceps tendon in excess of 4 cm increase the morbidity of the recovery process.

B. F. Morrey, MD

Symptomatic Flexion Instability in Posterior Stabilized Primary Total Knee Arthroplasty

Deshmane PP, Rathod PA, Deshmukh AJ, et al (Insall Scott Kelly Inst, NY; North Shore LIJ/Lenox Hill Hosp, NY; et al)
Orthopedics 37:e768-e774, 2014

Flexion instability in posterior-stabilized total knee arthroplasty is a relatively uncommon but distinct problem that is often underdiagnosed and may require surgical management. This retrospective study evaluated the authors' management strategy and assessed the results of revision surgery. The authors identified 19 knees that underwent revision for isolated flexion instability after primary posterior-stabilized total knee arthroplasty. All patients had typical symptoms and signs of flexion instability, which include diffuse pain, especially when negotiating stairs, a sense of instability without giving way, recurrent joint effusions, and diffuse periarticular tenderness. Knee Society scores were used to assess pain and function. Complete revision was performed in 11 knees, femoral revision with a thicker insert was performed in 1 knee, and isolated tibial polyethylene insert exchange was performed in 7 knees. Postoperatively, all patients reported improvement in instability symptoms and signs associated with improvement in mean Knee Society scores. Revision surgery with careful gap balancing is successful in the management of isolated flexion instability in posterior-stabilized total knee arthroplasty. Isolated tibial polyethylene insert exchange may have a role in selected patients where component malalignment and malrotation is ruled out and a thicker and/or semicon-strained insert can be used, while limiting the resultant flexion contracture to less than 5°.

▶ Although small, this case series is useful for 2 reasons. First, it calls attention to an uncommon but real problem after replacement—that of flexion insta-bility—that has a relatively easy solution. The diagnosis is suspected with complaints of pain or insecurity going up, and especially down the stairs. The problem is confirmed by lateral imaging demonstrating excessive distraction or excursion of the tibia referable to the femur. Fortunately, the solution is simply that of replacing the tibial with a thicker insert. In fact, often as little as an addi-tional 2 mm is adequate to solve the problem. This information should prove use-ful in the occasional patient with this problem.

B. F. Morrey, MD

CORR Insights®: Rotating-platform TKA No Different from Fixed-bearing TKA Regarding Survivorship or Performance: A Meta-analysis
Kim TK (Seoul Natl Univ Bundang Hosp, Gyeonggi-do, South Korea)
Clin Orthop Relat Res 472:2194-2196, 2014

Background.—The choice of knee replacement for a patient is a valid concern for arthroplastic surgeons. Many possibilities are available and the claims for superior performance or special characteristics are many. However, not all of them will deliver on their claims. The major types between which surgeons must choose are those with mobile or fixed bear-ings. Mobile bearings have the advantages of increased conformity that may improve longevity because of reduced wear, potentially better kine-matics, and possibly better function because they self-adjust in rotational alignment. Although much evidence shows reduced pain, better function, and improved durability, the superiority of mobile bearings has not been proven through meta-analyses. To complicate matters, not all mobile bear-ing designs are the same, but they are often considered as a single group in comparisons against fixed-bearing implants. The performances of rotating platform knees may be better than those of fixed-bearing devices if the com-parisons are limited to a single type.

Analysis.—A meta-analysis was undertaken to determine how the performance of a rotating platform knee compares to that of a fixed-bearing design. The comparison looked at four specific areas: clinical per-formance, component alignment, adverse event rates, and revision rates. A review of studies published between 2001 and 2013 identified 17 studies (930 contemporary rotating platform implants and 904 fixed-bearing implants) for analysis. Only in respect to the tibial component coronal alignment was there a difference between the two and it favored the fixed design. The small effect size did not appear to have clinical relevance, although the difference was statistically significant. The conclusion was that neither the rotating platform nor the fixed-bearing prosthesis was superior. As a result, implant choice should be based on factors other than performance. Among these factors are cost and the surgeon's experience.

Limitations.—The study, because it is a meta-analysis, has several limitations. Fourteen of the 17 original studies analyzed were small series with fewer than 100 TKAs in each study group. Study numbers analyzed for specific variables were also small. Most of the rotating-platform products were manufactured by one company. Seven of the 17 studies had a high proportion of cases that used a product from a different company for comparison, which may have introduced confounding factors other than the design of the device.

The outcome scales used in comparisons between mobile and fixed devices were objective scores, which tend to be insensitive to what patients care about in their replacement knees. None of the scales measured patient outcomes or satisfaction. Follow-up periods were also short, with none reaching 10 years.

Conclusions.—The success of a knee replacement depends on a number of factors. Further research is needed to develop additional designs, such as those with dual articulation of the mobile bearings. Studies should continue to investigate the efficacy of mobile bearing knees or specific types of mobile bearing devices with respect to pain, function, and durability in patients and for a longer period of time.

▶ I could kick myself for including this article, but in case you missed previous editions at a time when this was a legitimate question, numerous comparative studies were reviewed in the YEAR BOOK, showing no difference with fixed and mobile bearing total knee arthroplasty. This meta-analysis simply summarizes these data. NO DIFFERENCE. This is the last time this topic will be reviewed in the YEAR BOOK, I promise.

B. F. Morrey, MD

In-Hospital Complication Rates and Associated Factors After Simultaneous Bilateral Versus Unilateral Total Knee Arthroplasty
Odum SM, Springer BD (OrthoCarolina Res Inst, Inc, Charlotte, NC; OrthoCarolina Hip and Knee Ctr, Charlotte, NC)
J Bone Joint Surg Am 96:1058-1065, 2014

Background.—Data comparing complication rates following simultaneous bilateral total knee arthroplasty with those of unilateral total knee arthroplasty are conflicting. The purpose of this study was to compare in-hospital complication rates following simultaneous bilateral versus unilateral total knee arthroplasty and to determine factors associated with in-hospital complication rates in a large cohort of patients identified from the Nationwide Inpatient Sample (NIS).

Methods.—The 2004 to 2007 NIS data set was used to identify 407,070 total knee arthroplasties: 24,574 simultaneous bilateral and 382,496 unilateral total knee arthroplasties. Complications, based on International Classification of Diseases, Ninth Revision, Clinical Modification (ICD-9-CM) codes, were categorized as none, minor, major, or mortality. Covariates included comorbidities, demographic information, payer type, and hospital total knee arthroplasty volume. Multiple logistic regression was used to calculate odds ratios (ORs) and 95% confidence intervals (CIs).

Results.—Simultaneous bilateral total knee arthroplasty was associated with significantly higher odds of an in-hospital complication compared with unilateral total knee arthroplasty: OR, 1.51 (95% CI, 1.42 to 1.62) for minor complication; OR, 1.30 (95% CI, 1.14 to 1.47) for major complication; and OR, 2.51 (95% CI, 1.66 to 3.80) for mortality. Patients with greater numbers of medical comorbidities were more likely to have an in-hospital complication. Compared with whites, African-American and Asian/Pacific Islander groups had significantly higher odds of a minor complication. Female patients were less likely than male patients to have an in-hospital complication. Patients who were less than sixty-five years old at the time of surgery had significantly reduced odds of a minor complication and mortality compared with patients who were seventy-five years of age or older. Compared with hospitals with a very-high volume of total knee arthroplasty procedures performed ($\geq$850), lower-volume hospitals had significantly increased odds of minor complications and mortality.

Conclusions.—While complication rates following either unilateral or simultaneous bilateral total knee arthroplasty are low, simultaneous bilateral total knee arthroplasty was associated with higher odds of in-hospital complications, including mortality, compared with unilateral total knee arthroplasty. Patient demographic information, preoperative health status, payer type, and hospital total knee arthroplasty volume were all significant factors in complication rates following bilateral total knee arthroplasty.

Level of Evidence.—Therapeutic Level III. See Instructions for Authors for a complete description of levels of evidence.

▶ The question of staged or simultaneous bilateral replacements remains a source of debate within the arthroplasty community. To be honest, this study does not provide any new information but does confirm what is known. Bilateral simultaneous knee replacement places the older patient at increased risk, especially if there is a preexisting cardiac condition. It is for this reason that we would emphasize that this is and should be recognized as a contraindication. It should also be pointed out that with the large database, the statistical differences are present, and the absolute risk is small. Furthermore, previous studies have demonstrated the increased satisfaction that exists in those having had the simultaneous procedure. So, although it is a matter of surgeon perspective, clear information to the patient resolves the issue.

B. F. Morrey, MD

Morbid Obesity: A Significant Risk Factor for Failure of Two-Stage Revision Total Knee Arthroplasty for Infection

Watts CD, Wagner ER, Houdek MT, et al (Mayo Clinic, Rochester, MN)
J Bone Joint Surg Am 96:e154(1-7), 2014

Background.—Obese patients have a higher risk of complications following primary total knee arthroplasty, including periprosthetic joint infection. However, there is a paucity of data concerning the efficacy of two-stage revision arthroplasty in obese patients.

Methods.—We performed a two-to-one matched cohort study to compare the outcomes of thirty-seven morbidly obese patients (those with a body mass index of ≥ 40 kg/m^2) who underwent two-stage revision total knee arthroplasty for periprosthetic joint infection following primary total knee arthroplasty with the outcomes of seventy-four non-obese patients (those with a body mass index of < 30 kg/m^2). Groups were matched by sex, age, and date of reimplantation. Outcomes included subsequent revision, reinfection, reoperation, and Knee Society pain and function scores. The minimum follow-up time was five years.

Results.—Morbidly obese patients had a significantly increased risk for revision surgery (32% compared with 11%; $p < 0.01$), reinfection (22% compared with 4%; $p < 0.01$), and reoperation (51% compared with 16%; $p < 0.01$). Implant survival rates were 80% for the morbidly obese group and 97% for the non-obese group at five years and 55% for the morbidly obese group and 82% for the non-obese group at ten years. Knee Society pain scores improved significantly following surgery in both groups; the mean scores (and standard deviation) were 50 ± 5 points for the morbidly obese group and 55 ± 2 points for the non-obese group ($p = 0.06$) preoperatively, 74 ± 5 points for the morbidly obese group and 89 ± 2 points for the non-obese group ($p < 0.0001$) at two years, 72 ± 6 points for the morbidly obese group and 88 ± 3 points for the non-obese group ($p < 0.0001$) at five years, and 56 ± 9 points for the morbidly obese group and 84 ± 3 points for the non-obese group ($p = 0.01$) at ten years.

Conclusions.—Morbid obesity significantly increased the risk of subsequent revision, reoperation, and reinfection following two-stage revision total knee arthroplasty for infection. In addition, these patients had worse pain relief and overall function at intermediate-term clinical follow-up. Although two-stage revision should remain a standard treatment for chronic periprosthetic joint infection in morbidly obese patients, increased failure rates and poorer outcomes should be anticipated.

Level of Evidence.—Prognostic Level III. See Instructions for Authors for a complete description of levels of evidence.

▶ This is a well-done study that characterizes the markedly negative impact of morbid obesity, body mass index (BMI) > 40, in those with a 2-staged reimplantation for infection. First, I noticed with some amusement and even more sadness that we now consider a BMI < 30 to be nonobese. Regardless, the careful analysis is of a cohort of more than 2400 patients followed for at least 5 years and it lends great credibility to the conclusions well summarized in the abstract. As might be expected, every parameter is adversely compromised by morbid obesity. Sadly, in reality there is not much we can do about it, except be aware of these increased risks and convey them to our patients.

B. F. Morrey, MD

Arthrodesis Should Be Strongly Considered After Failed Two-stage Reimplantation TKA
Wu CH, Gray CF, Lee G-C (Univ of Pennsylvania, Philadelphia)
Clin Orthop Relat Res 472:3295-3304, 2014

Background.—A two-stage reimplantation procedure is a well-accepted procedure for management of first-time infected total knee arthroplasty (TKA). However, there is a lack of consensus on the treatment of subsequent reinfections.

Questions/Purposes.—The purpose of this study was to perform a decision analysis to determine the treatment method likely to yield the highest quality of life for a patient after a failed two-stage reimplantation.

Methods.—We performed a systematic review to estimate the expected success rates of a two-stage reimplantation procedure, chronic suppression, arthrodesis, and amputation for treatment of infected TKA. To determine utility values of the various possible health states that could arise after two-stage revision, we used previously published values and methods to determine the utility and disutility tolls for each treatment option and performed a decision tree analysis using the TreeAgePro 2012 software suite (Williamstown, MA, USA). These values were subsequently varied to perform sensitivity analyses, determining thresholds at which different treatment options prevailed.

Results.—Overall, the composite success rate for two-stage reimplantation was 79.1% (range, 33.3%−100%). The utility (successful outcome) and disutility toll (cost for treatment) for two-stage reimplantation were determined to be 0.473 and 0.20, respectively the toll for undergoing chronic suppression was set at 0.05 the utility for arthrodesis was 0.740 and for amputation 0.423. We set the utilities for subsequent two-stage revision and other surgical procedures by subtracting the disutility toll from the utility each time another procedure was performed. The two-way sensitivity analysis varied the utility status after an additional two-stage reimplantation (0.47−0.99) and chance of a successful two-stage reimplantation (45%−95%). The model was then extended to a three-way sensitivity analysis twice: once by setting the variable arthrodesis utility at a value of 0.47 and once more by setting utility of two-stage reimplantation at 0.05 over the same range of values on both axes. Knee arthrodesis emerged as the treatment most likely to yield the highest expected utility (quality of life) after initially failing a two-stage revision. For a repeat two-stage revision to be favored, the utility of that second

TABLE 1.—Summary of Important Values for Decision Tree

Variable Name	Utility	Probability of Success	Utility Toll
Amputation	0.423	1.00	
Fusion	0.74	0.786	
Two-stage reimplantation	0.473	0.791	
Chronic suppression		0.52	
Revision toll			0.2
Chronic suppression toll			0.05

With kind permission from Springer Science+Business Media: Wu CH, Gray CF, Lee G-C. Arthrodesis Should Be Strongly Considered After Failed Two-stage Reimplantation TKA. *Clin Orthop Relat Res.* 2014;472:3295-3304.

two-stage revision had to substantially exceed the published utility of primary TKA of 0.84 and the probability of achieving infection control had to exceed 90%.

Conclusions.—Based on best available evidence, knee arthrodesis should be strongly considered as the treatment of choice for patients who have persistent infected TKA after a failed two-stage reimplantation procedure. We recognize that particular circumstances such as severe bone loss can preclude or limit the applicability of fusion as an option and that individual clinical circumstances must always dictate the best treatment, but where arthrodesis is practical, our model supports it as the best approach (Table 1).

▶ This is a really interesting study not just because the question is of growing interest and value but also because it introduces a methodology and lexicon not familiar to the orthopedic surgeon (Table 1). We have all encountered the failed staged reimplantation for an infected knee replacement. Our instinct is to try again, at least that is what I do because the technical difficulty of fusion and the presumed functional loss justifies another try. This analysis of 204 articles on staged reimplantation allowed retention of 18 for analysis; of 141 studies dealing with arthrodesis, 17 were worthy of further study. Using quality-of-life metrics, the conclusion is that, assuming the bone is of adequate quality, arthrodesis affords a more reliable control of the infection and—surprise—a higher quality of life. Emotionally, I'm not quite sure this is true. However, the methodology is convincing.

B. F. Morrey, MD

Failure of aseptic revision total knee arthroplasties: 145 revision failures from the Norwegian Arthroplasty Register, 1994-2011
Leta TH, Lygre SHL, Skredderstuen A, et al (Haukeland Univ Hosp, Bergen, Norway; et al)
Acta Orthop 86:48-57, 2015

Background and Purpose.—In Norway, the proportion of revision knee arthroplasties increased from 6.9% in 1994 to 8.5% in 2011. However, there is limited information on the epidemiology and causes of subsequent failure of revision knee arthroplasty. We therefore studied survival rate and determined the modes of failure of aseptic revision total knee arthroplasties.

Method.—This study was based on 1,016 aseptic revision total knee arthroplasties reported to the Norwegian Arthroplasty Register between 1994 and 2011. Revisions done for infections were not included. Kaplan-Meier and Cox regression analyses were used to assess the survival rate and the relative risk of re-revision with all causes of re-revision as endpoint.

Results.—145 knees failed after revision total knee arthroplasty. Deep infection was the most frequent cause of re-revision (28%), followed by instability (26%), loose tibial component (17%), and pain (10%). The cumulative survival rate for revision total knee arthroplasties was 85% at 5 years, 78% at 10 years, and 71% at 15 years. Revision total knee arthroplasties with exchange of the femoral or tibial component exclusively had a higher risk of re-revision (RR = 1.7) than those with exchange of the whole prosthesis. The risk of re-revision was higher for men (RR = 2.0) and for patients aged less than 60 years (RR = 1.6).

Interpretation.—In terms of implant survival, revision of the whole implant was better than revision of 1 component only. Young age and male sex were risk factors for re-revision. Deep infection was the most

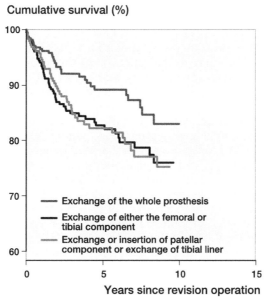

FIGURE 2.—(D) With all causes of re-revision as the endpoint. (Reprinted from Leta TH, Lygre SHL, Skredderstuen A, et al. Failure of aseptic revision total knee arthroplasties: 145 revision failures from the norwegian arthroplasty register, 1994-2011. *Acta Orthop.* 2015;86:48-57, reprinted by permission of Taylor & Francis Ltd, http://www.informaworld.com.)

frequent cause of failure of revision of aseptic total knee arthroplasties (Fig 2D).

▶ The authors introduce the topic with the recognition of the increased frequency with which the knee is being replaced and the incumbent expectation of an increased number of revisions. I found the 85% success of the revision at 5 years roughly similar to what I have advised my patients: approximately 88% for more than 5 years. The reason for a failed revision is most commonly infection (28%), but it is surprising to see that instability accounts for almost the same number of failed revisions (25%). One additional point of which I have been aware was reinforced by this study. The survival of revising both implants is greater than that of a single component revision (Fig 2D).

B. F. Morrey, MD

Porous Tantalum Metaphyseal Cones for Severe Tibial Bone Loss in Revision Knee Arthroplasty: A Five to Nine-Year Follow-up

Kamath AF, Lewallen DG, Hanssen AD (Mayo Clinic, Rochester, MN)
J Bone Joint Surg Am 97:216-223, 2015

Background.—Severe metaphyseal and meta-diaphyseal bone loss poses important challenges in revision total knee arthroplasty. The best strategy for addressing massive tibial bone loss has not been determined. The purpose of this study was to assess the intermediate-term clinical and radiographic results of porous tibial cone implantation.

Methods.—Sixty-six porous tantalum tibial cones (sixty-three patients) were reviewed at a mean follow-up time of seventy months (range, sixty to 106 months). According to the Anderson Orthopaedic Research Institute bone defect classification, twenty-four knees had a Type-3 defect, twenty-five knees had a Type-2B defect, and seventeen knees had a Type-2A defect.

Results.—The mean age at the time of the index revision was sixty-seven years (range, forty-one to eighty-three years), and 57% of patients were female. The mean American Society of Anesthesiologists Physical Status was 2.4 (range, 2 to 3), and the mean body mass index was 33 kg/m^2 (range, 25 to 53 kg/m^2). Fifteen patients (24%) were on immunosuppressant medications, and eight patients (13%) were current smokers. The patients underwent a mean number of 3.4 prior knee surgical procedures (range, one to twenty procedures), and 49% of patients (thirty-one patients) had a history of periprosthetic infection. The mean Knee Society Scores improved significantly from 55 points preoperatively (range, 4 to 97 points) to 80 points (range, 28 to 100 points) at the time of the latest follow-up ($p < 0.0001$). One patient had progressive radiolucencies about the tibial stem and cone on radiographs. One patient had complete radiolucencies about the tibial cone, concerning for fibrous ingrowth. Three other cones were revised: one for infection, one for aseptic loosening, and one for periprosthetic fracture. Revision-free survival of the tibial cone component was >95% at the time of the latest follow-up.

Conclusions.—Porous tantalum tibial cones offer a promising management option for severe tibial bone loss. At the intermediate-term follow-up (five to nine years), porous tantalum tibial cones had durable clinical results and radiographic fixation. The biologic ingrowth of these implants offers the potential for successful long-term structural support in complex knee reconstruction.

Level of Evidence.—Therapeutic Level IV. See Instructions for Authors for a complete description of levels of evidence (Fig 3).

▶ I generally do not include reports that I feel have little use to the surgeon with a less specialized practice. Yet, I have included this report because it provides some clinical context to a promising technology that I and others considered a real breakthrough 15 years ago—porous tantalum. Hence, this long-term surveillance study of the use of tantalum cones for difficult revision knee surgery provides clinical justification to the optimism generated by this technology. The group of 66 procedures is characterized as true salvage procedures with more

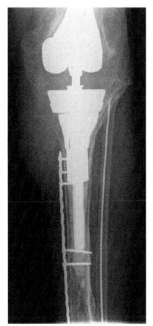
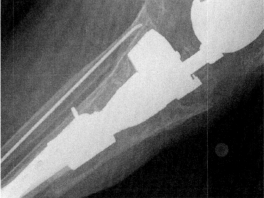

FIGURE 3.—Anteroposterior (**A**) and lateral (**B**) radiographs of the left knee in a sixty-five-year-old female patient nine years after knee reconstruction with tibial porous metal cylinder cone, femoral cone use in the tibia and femur, and stacked tibial baseplate augments. The patient had a history of multiple failed attempts at eradicating infection preoperatively, gastrocnemius flap coverage, fixation of tibial shaft fracture, and prior extensor mechanism deficiency with patellar nonunion. (Reprinted from Kamath AF, Lewallen DG, Hanssen AD. Porous tantalum metaphyseal cones for severe tibial bone loss in revision knee arthroplasty: a five to nine-year follow-up. *J Bone Joint Surg Am.* 2015;97:216-223, with permission from The Journal of Bone and Joint Surgery, Incorporated.)

than 90% having type 2B or 3 defects and with an average of almost 3.5 previous knee procedures. Nonetheless, the authors report the amazing result that more than 90% of the cohort is free of revision at a minimum of 5 years' surveillance. The difficulty of the revisions justifies these being classified as true salvage procedures, which further provides credibility to this reconstructive strategy and to the clinical competency of the authors (Fig 3).

B. F. Morrey, MD

9 Foot and Ankle

Introduction

The foot and ankle is arguably the most complex and diverse anatomic region reviewed in this YEAR BOOK. I spent seven years in the foot clinic at the Mayo Clinic and thus continue to enjoy reviewing this material and observing the progress that has been made over the years.

This year I have attempted to include material that reflects the spectrum of the practice, from the diabetic foot to the surgical techniques of bunionectomy. I am aware of my bias for certain topics and have tried not to include an excessive number of articles reflecting my personal interests, such as the management of Achilles tendinopathy and rupture, long-term benefit of ankle fusion, and diabetic foot ulcers. I hope this section reflects the balance and advances being made in the management of foot and ankle problems.

Bernard F. Morrey, MD

Autologous Chondrocyte Implantation of the Ankle: 2- to 10-Year Results
Kwak SK, Kern BS, Ferkel RD, et al (North Jersey Orthopaedic Specialists, Teaneck, NJ; The Orthopaedic Inst of Western Kentucky, Paducah, KY; Southern California Orthopedic Inst, Van Nuys, CA; et al)
Am J Sports Med 42:2156-2164, 2014

Background.—The treatment of osteochondral lesions of the talus after failed surgery is challenging, with no clear solution. Shortterm results using autologous chondrocyte implantation have been promising.

Purpose.—To report the long-term outcomes of patients who underwent autologous chondrocyte implantation (ACI) of the talus after failed marrow stimulation techniques for osteochondral lesions of the talus (OLTs).

Study Design.—Case series; Level of evidence, 4.

Methods.—Thirty-two consecutive patients underwent ACI of the talus, and 29 patients (15 male, 14 female; mean age, 34 years [range, 16-54 years]) were available for follow-up. There were 23 medial and 6 lateral lesions, with a mean size of 18×11 mm (198 mm^2; range, 80-500 mm^2). Twenty patients underwent ACI of the talus alone; 9 underwent ACI with bone grafting of underlying cysts. Follow-up was performed

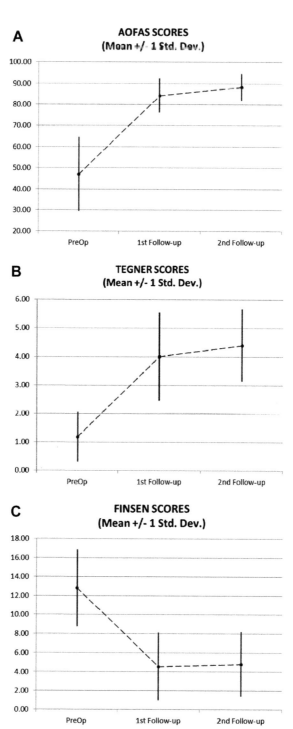

FIGURE 3.—First 11 patients. No significant differences were seen in the first 11 patients from initial to subsequent follow-up on American Orthopaedic Foot and Ankle Society (AOFAS), Tegner, or Finsen scores. (A) AOFAS scores in the first 11 patients. (B) Tegner scores in the first 11 patients. (C) Finsen scores in the first 11 patients. (Reprinted from Kwak SK, Kern BS, Ferkel RD, et al. Autologous chondrocyte implantation of the ankle: 2- to 10-year results. *Am J Sports Med.* 2014;42:2156-2164, with permission from The Author(s).)

at a mean of 70 months (range, 24-129 months). Patient outcomes were evaluated using the simplified symptomatology score, Tegner activity score, Finsen score, and American Orthopaedic Foot and Ankle Society (AOFAS) ankle-hindfoot score. Twenty-five patients (86%) underwent second-look arthroscopic surgery at the time of hardware removal and were assessed with the International Cartilage Repair Society (ICRS) score. Postoperative magnetic resonance imaging (MRI) was performed on 24 patients (83%) and compared with preoperative MRI scans.

Results.—Preoperatively, 26 patients rated their ankles as poor and 3 as fair using the simplified symptomatology score. At last follow-up, 9 were classified as excellent, 14 as good, 5 as fair, and 1 as poor using the same score. The mean AOFAS score improved from 50.1 to 85.9 (range, 65-100). The mean Tegner activity score improved from 1.6 to 4.3 ($P < .0001$). The mean Finsen score (modified Weber score) showed significant improvement from 13.7 to 5.1 ($P < .0001$).

Conclusion.—Autologous chondrocyte implantation of the talus yields improvement in all parameters tested with enduring long-term results in patients who have failed previous surgery for OLTs (Fig 3).

▶ As the authors note, management of osteochondritis dissecans (OCD) of the talus is challenging at best. This contribution is important because it demonstrates good results with autologous chondrocyte grafting when used as a salvage for a failed previous intervention. The sample size is adequate, and the surveillance extends up to 10 years. Using several objective and subjective measurement tools, one can agree with their conclusion (Fig 3). In general, 23 of 29 (80%) benefited from the procedure. The technique itself is somewhat demanding and time-consuming, but these outcomes are encouraging.

B. F. Morrey, MD

Influence of foot ulceration on cause-specific mortality in patients with diabetes mellitus
Brownrigg JRW, Griffin M, Hughes CO, et al (St Georges Vascular Inst, London, UK; et al)
J Vasc Surg 60:982-986, 2014

Objective.—The purpose of this study was to assess the odds of all-cause mortality in individuals with diabetic foot ulceration (DFU) compared with those with diabetes and no history of DFU. In addition, we sought to determine the strength of association of DFU with cardiovascular and nonvascular mortality.

Methods.—We obtained data for a cohort of patients who attended a secondary care diabetic foot clinic or a general diabetes clinic between 2009 and 2010. A clinic cohort of patients with diabetes and no history of DFU provided a control group. Cause-specific mortality was recorded during a median follow-up duration of 3.6 years (interquartile range,

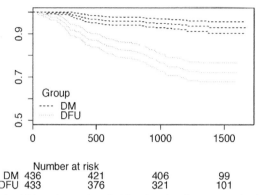

FIGURE 1.—Kaplan-Meier estimate of survival functions for all-cause mortality in diabetes mellitus (*DM*) vs diabetic foot ulceration (*DFU*). The 95% confidence intervals (CIs) are presented. All standard errors <.02 (Supplementary Table I, online only). (Reprinted from the Journal of Vascular Surgery. Brownrigg JRW, Griffin M, Hughes CO, et al. Influence of foot ulceration on cause-specific mortality in patients with diabetes mellitus. *J Vasc Surg*. 2014;60:982-986, Copyright 2014, with permission from the Society for Vascular Surgery.)

3.3-4.2 years). The association between DFU and all-cause mortality was evaluated by Cox regression. The association between DFU and cardiovascular mortality was determined by competing risk modeling.

Results.—We recorded 145 events of all-cause mortality and 27 events of cardiovascular mortality among 869 patients with diabetes. After adjustment for potential confounders, DFU was associated with both cardiovascular disease (hazard ratio, 2.53; 95% confidence interval, 0.98-6.49; $P = .05$) and all-cause mortality (hazard ratio, 3.98; 95% confidence interval, 2.55-6.21; $P < .001$). The proportion of deaths attributable to cardiovascular disease was similar between the groups (18% with diabetes only and 19% with DFU; $P = .91$).

Conclusions.—DFU is associated with premature death from vascular and nonvascular causes (Fig 1).

▶ The presence of and morbidity associated with diabetic foot ulcers (DFU) is well known by all who manage diabetes and all foot surgeons. The relationship of DFU with ultimate amputation and ultimately death is also well known. It is difficult to appreciate whether the ulcer is somehow an independent variable or is actually just a reflection of a cardiovascular comorbidity. This study does not answer that question but does reinforce the relationship with cardiovascular disease, and most importantly, it reveals the dramatic adverse effect DFU has on the survival of the patient (Fig 1).

B. F. Morrey, MD

Efficacy of topical recombinant human platelet-derived growth factor for treatment of diabetic lower-extremity ulcers: Systematic review and meta-analysis

Zhao X-H, Gu H-F, Xu Z-R, et al (Zhejiang Univ, P.R. China)
Metabolism 63:1304-1313, 2014

Objective.—Recombinant human platelet-derived growth factor (rhPDGF) is used topically in the treatment of diabetic lower-extremity ulcers. There have been few meta-analyses of the efficacy of rhPDGF in this treatment context. The aim of this study was to perform an updated systematic review and meta-analysis to assess the clinical efficacy of rhPDGF in the treatment of diabetic lower-extremity ulcers.

Methods.—We searched the MEDLINE, Cochrane Library, EMBASE and Web of Knowledge databases up to April 30, 2014. Studies were identified and selected, and data were extracted by two independent reviewers. The primary efficacy outcome was complete healing rate. Adverse events were also assessed. The studies were evaluated for quality and publication bias.

Results.—A total of 6 randomized controlled trials including 992 patients were selected from 173 identified studies. The studies compared rhPDGF treatment in the context of standard of care (SOC) to placebo or SOC alone. In the absence of study heterogeneity, a fixed-effects model was performed, and the combined odds ratio (OR) indicated a significantly greater complete healing rate in patients treated with rhPDGF compared to placebo or SOC alone. The ORs ranged from 0.58 to 2.77, with a combined OR of 1.53 (95% CI = 1.14 to 2.04, $p = 0.004$). A sensitivity analysis (leave-one-out method) indicated good study reliability, and a funnel plot with Egger test showed no publication bias.

Conclusion.—These results indicate that rhPDGF is efficacious in the treatment of diabetic lower-extremity ulcers (Table 2).

▶ This interesting meta-analysis from China selected 6 articles from which to draw a conclusion. That this represents about 3% of the literature surveyed further indicates the overall poor quality of musculoskeletal literature. The study did find that recombinant platelet-derived growth factor does improve diabetic foot ulcer treatment as defined by complete healing of the ulcer compared to the control. However, it should be noted that the healing rate is still only approximately 50% with little information about recurrence (Table 2). This does represent an advance in therapy, but it is costly. That the study was performed in China also underscores the global nature of the problem.

B. F. Morrey, MD

TABLE 2.—Summary of Participants in Included Studies

Author (Year)	Treatment Groups	Number of Patients	Mean Age (Years)	Female/Male (%)	Type 1 DM/Type 2 DM/Unspecified (%)	Duration of DM (Years), Mean	Baseline HbA1c (%), Mean (SD)	Baseline BMI, Mean (SD)	Baseline Area of Ulcer (cm^2), mean ± SD	Complete Healing Rate (%)
Blume (2011) [16]	Ad5-PDGF-B (GAM501) + SOC	72	57.9	31/69	8/88/4	15	8.06 (1.82)	33.70 (7.54)	3.1 ± 1.7	41[b]
	Formulated collagen gel + SOC[a]	33	56.2	24/76	6/88/6	14	8.07 (1.45)	33.08 (7.13)	2.9 ± 1.1	35[b]
Jaiswal (2010) [21]	SOC	19	54.8	21/79	11/84/5	13	7.85 (1.34)	34.15 (7.18)	2.8 ± 1.3	31[b]
	rhPDGF (becaplermin) 100 µg/g) + SOC	25	49.9	24/76	Type 1 or type 2	Median 5	NA	22.9	30.0 ± 3.5	60
Robson (2005) [9]	Placebo + SOC	25	56.2	8/92	Type 1 or type 2	Median 10	NA	21.8	26.5 ± 2.5	72
	rhPDGF (becaplermin) 100 µg/g) + SOC	74	NA	NA	Type 1 or type 2	17.9	NA	NA	1.5 (median)	42[c]
Wieman (1998) [22]	SOC	72	NA	NA	Type 1 or type 2	14.7	Healed: 7.2 (1.2) Not healed: 6.9 (1.7)	NA	1.6 (median)	35[c]
	rhPDGF (becaplermin) 30 µg/g) + SOC	132	58	38/62	Type 1 or type 2	NA	NA	NA	2.6 ± 2.7	36
	rhPDGF (becaplermin) 100 µg/g) + SOC	123	57	33/67	Type 1 or type 2	NA	Healed: 7.0 (1.3) Not healed: 7.1 (1.4)	NA	2.6 ± 3.4	50
	Placebo + SOC	127	58	28/72	Type 1 or type 2	NA	Healed: 6.5 (1.1) Not healed: 6.7 (1.5)	NA	2.8 ± 4.1	35

d'Hemecourt (1998) [23]	rhPDGF (becaplermin) 100 μg/g) + SOC	34	59	29/71	Type 1 or type 2	NA	NA	Height: 175.8 (9.3) cm Weight: 99.8 (20.1) kg	2.4 ± 2.0	44
	Placebo + SOC	70	57	30/70	Type 1 or type 2	NA	NA	Height: 177.6 (10.5) cm Weight: 93.0 (21.03) kg	3.2 ± 2.8	36
	SOC	68	60	21/79	Type 1 or type 2	NA	NA	Height: 176.8 (11.1) cm Weight: 97.8 (25.8) kg	3.5 ± 3.5	22
Steed (1995) [30]	rhPDGF (becaplermin) 30 μg/g) + SOC	61	63	30/70	Type 1 or type 2	NA	NA	NA	5.5 ± 8.5	48
	Placebo + SOC	57	58	19/81	Type 1 or type 2	NA	NA	NA	9.0 ± 16.0	25

Ad5-PDGF-B: E1-deleted adenovirus serotype 5 encoding human platelet-derived growth factor-B; BMI: body mass index; DM: diabetes mellitus; GAM501 Gene Activated Matrix 501, a proprietary product; HbA1c: glycated hemoglobin; NA: not available; rhPDGF: recombinant human platelet-derived growth factor; SD: standard deviation; SOC: standard of care.

Editor's Note: Please refer to original journal article for full references.

[a] The formulated collagen gel group was not included in the control group.

[b] Patient numbers for evaluating complete healing rate were 51, 17 and 13 for patients treated with rhPDGF, formulated collagen gel and SOC, respectively.

[c] The total number for evaluating efficacy was 143 patients.

Reprinted from Metabolism Clinical and Experimental. Zhao X-H, Gu H-F, Xu Z-R, et al. Efficacy of topical recombinant human platelet-derived growth factor for treatment of diabetic lower-extremity ulcers: Systematic review and meta-analysis. *Metabolism.* 2014;63:1304-1313, with permission from Elsevier.

Low Wound Complication Rates for the Lateral Extensile Approach for Calcaneal ORIF When the Lateral Calcaneal Artery Is Patent

Bibbo C, Ehrlich DA, Nguyen HML, et al (Hosp of the Univ of Pennsylvania, Philadelphia)
Foot Ankle Int 35:650-656, 2015

Background.—Historically, the lateral extensile approach for calcaneal fracture osteosynthesis has had relatively high rates of wound healing problems. The vascular territory (angiosome) of the lateral foot is now known to be dependent upon the lateral calcaneal branch of the peroneal artery (LCBP artery). We postulated that patency of the LCBP artery may have a profound positive impact on incisional wound healing for calcaneal open reduction and internal fixation (ORIF).

Methods.—Ninety consecutive calcaneal fractures that met operative criteria were preoperatively evaluated for the presence of a Doppler signal in the LCBP artery and were followed for the development of wound healing problems.

Results.—Among these 90 fractures, 85 had a positive preoperative Doppler signal along the course of the LCBP artery (94%) and 5 had no Doppler signal (6%). All patients underwent ORIF via a lateral extensile approach. Overall, incisional wound healing problems occurred in 6 of 90 calcaneal incisions (6.5%). All 5 feet that exhibited an absent Doppler signal in the LCPB artery developed an incisional wound healing

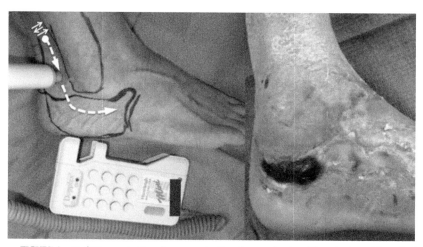

FIGURE 3.—(Left) Demonstration of preoperative Doppler examination of lateral calcaneal branch of peroneal artery. (Right) Photo of foot with displaced calcaneal fracture with a large area of progressive skin changes over several weeks; a Doppler signal was not present at initial presentation. Elevation of the flap via extensile lateral approach would have likely led to devastating wound complications. (Copyright © 2014, by the American Orthopaedic Foot and Ankle Society, Inc., originally published in Foot & Ankle International. Bibbo C, Ehrlich DA, Nguyen HML, et al. Low wound complication rates for the lateral extensile approach for calcaneal ORIF when the lateral calcaneal artery is patent. *Foot Ankle Int.* 2015;35:650-656, and reproduced here with permission.)

complication (5/6, approximately 83%): 2 large apical wounds and 3 major dehiscence/slough. However, among the 84 feet that possessed a positive preoperative Doppler signal in the LCBP artery, there was only 1 (1/84, approximately 1%) incisional wound healing problem (*P* < .0001, Fischer's exact test). Smokers with a positive Doppler signal in the LCBP artery did not develop a wound healing complication.

Conclusions.—This study suggests a strong link to low incisional wound healing complications for the lateral extensile approach to the calcaneus when a preoperative Doppler signal is present in the LCBP artery. We believe this simple examination should be routinely performed prior to calcaneal ORIF.

Level of Evidence.—Level III, comparative case series (Fig 3).

▶ I consider this to be a very helpful article, especially because we just had a grand rounds on the topic at University of Texas Health Science Center San Antonio last week. It is well known that the limiting factor in the progressive management of calcaneal fractures relates to wound complications. The trend is to use an extensile lateral exposure elevating a proximally based flap. The authors offer the useful observation that there is variation in the lateral calcaneal branch of the peroneal artery. The simple recommendation is to assess presence and patency before the incision is made. If there is no flow, avoid this incision (Fig 3).

B. F. Morrey, MD

Does the Subtalar Joint Compensate for Ankle Malalignment in End-stage Ankle Arthritis?

Wang B, Saltzman CL, Chalayon O, et al (Shanghai Inst of Traumatology and Orthopaedics, China; Univ of Utah, Salt Lake City; et al)
Clin Orthop Relat Res 473:318-325, 2015

Background.—Patients with ankle arthritis often present with concomitant hindfoot deformity, which may involve the tibiotalar and subtalar joints. However, the possible compensatory mechanisms of these two mechanically linked joints are not well known.

Questions/Purposes.—In this study we sought to (1) compare ankle and hindfoot alignment of our study cohort with endstage ankle arthritis with that of a control group (2) explore the frequency of compensated malalignment between the tibiotalar and subtalar joints in our study cohort and (3) assess the intraobserver and interobserver reliability of classification methods of hindfoot alignment used in this study.

Methods.—Between March 2006 and September 2013, we performed 419 ankle arthrodesis and ankle replacements (380 patients). In this study, we evaluated radiographs for 233 (56%) ankles (226 patients) which met the following inclusion criteria: (1) no prior subtalar arthrodesis (2) no previously failed total ankle replacement or ankle arthrodesis (3) with complete conventional radiographs (all three ankle views were required: mortise, lateral, and hindfoot alignment view). Ankle and hindfoot alignment was assessed by measurement of the medial distal tibial angle, tibial talar surface angle, talar tilting angle, tibiocalcaneal axis angle, and moment arm of calcaneus. The obtained values were compared with those observed in the control group of 60 ankles from 60 people. Only those without obvious degenerative changes of the tibiotalar and subtalar joints and without previous surgeries of the ankle or hindfoot were included in the control group. Demographic data for the patients with arthritis and the control group were comparable (sex, $p = 0.321$ age, $p = 0.087$). The frequency of compensated malalignment between the tibiotalar and subtalar joints, defined as tibiocalcaneal angle or moment arm of the calcaneus being greater or smaller than the same 95% CI statistical cutoffs from the control group, was tallied. All ankle radiographs were independently measured by two observers to determine the interobserver reliability. One of the observers evaluated all images twice to determine the intraobserver reliability.

Results.—There were differences in medial distal tibial surface angle ($86.6° \pm 7.3°$ [95% CI, $66.3°-123.7°$] versus $89.1° \pm 2.9°$ [95% CI, $83.0°-96.3°$], $p < 0.001$), tibiotalar surface angle ($84.9° \pm 14.4°$ [95% CI, $45.3°-122.7°$] versus $89.1° \pm 2.9°$ [95% CI, $83.0°-96.3°$], $p < 0.001$), talar tilting angle ($-1.7° \pm 12.5°$ [95% CI, $-41.3°-30.3°$] versus $0.0° \pm 0.0°$ [95% CI, $0.0°-0.0°$], $p = 0.003$), and tibiocalcaneal axis angle ($-7.2° \pm 13.1°$ [95% CI, $-57°-33°$] versus $-2.7° \pm 5.2°$ [95% CI, $-13.3°-9.0°$], $p < 0.001$) between patients with ankle arthritis and the control group. Using the classification system based on the tibiocalcaneal angle, there were 62 (53%) and 22 (39%) compensated ankles in the varus and valgus groups, respectively. Using the classification system based on the moment arm of the calcaneus, there were 68 (58%) and 20 (35%) compensated ankles in the varus and valgus groups, respectively. For all conditions or methods of measurement, patients with no or mild degenerative change of the subtalar joint have a greater likelihood of compensating coronal plane deformity of the ankle with arthritis ($p < 0.001 - p = 0.032$). The interobserver and intraobserver reliability for all radiographic measurements was good to excellent (the correlation coefficients range from 0.820 to 0.943).

Conclusions.—Substantial ankle malalignment, mostly varus deformity, is common in ankles with endstage osteoarthritis. The subtalar joint often compensates for the malaligned ankle in static weightbearing.

Level of Evidence.—Level III, diagnostic study.

▶ I have had a personal interest in the question of subtalar compensation for ankle malposition since we recognized that ankle fusions typically result in hind-foot stiffness with little subsequent potential for angular alignment compensation. These authors represent a truly massive practice with almost 420 ankle fusions over a 7-year period. This study is retrospective and thus suffers from the known limitations. Nonetheless, the demonstration of the common deformity of ankle arthritis as one of varus malalignment is confirmed in this study. The authors, however, document the ability of the hind foot to adapt to the varus angulation in the coronal plane in the majority of patients. This surprised me because my impression is that the subtalar joint often seems to become stiff with progressive ankle arthritis.

B. F. Morrey, MD

Comparison of Cannulated Screws Versus Compression Staples for Subtalar Arthrodesis Fixation

Herrera-Pérez M, Andarcia-Bañuelos C, Barg A, et al (Univ Hosp of Canary Islands, La Laguna, Tenerife, Spain; Univ Hosp of Basel, Switzerland; et al)
Foot Ankle Int 36:203-210, 2015

Background.—Different fixation techniques have been described in the literature for isolated subtalar arthrodesis (ISA). The purpose of this study was to compare the fusion rate and clinical outcome of ISA using cannulated compression screws or compression staples.

Methods.—Thirty-three patients (33 feet) underwent ISA using screw (17 feet) or staples (16 feet) fixation. Patients were followed for 42.7 ± 6.4 months (range, 24.5-84.3 months). The subtalar fusion was assessed radiographically and clinically. Clinical outcome measures included the visual analog scale (VAS) for pain and American Orthopaedic Foot and Ankle Society (AOFAS) hindfoot score.

Results.—The average pain score decreased significantly from 6.4 ± 1.1 (range, 5-9) to 0.8 ± 1.3 (range, 0-4) ($P < .001$). In the screws group, the average AOFAS hindfoot score increased significantly from 54.6 ± 8.8 (range, 37-67) preoperatively to 86.1 ± 7.1 (range, 71-91) postoperatively ($P < .001$). In the staples group, the average AOFAS hindfoot score increased significantly from 53.4 ± 11.1 (range, 33-69) preoperatively to 83.4 ± 6.9 (range, 71-91) postoperatively ($P < .001$). The AOFAS hindfoot score was comparable in both groups ($P = .149$). Only the AOFAS hindfoot score function subgroup in the screw fixation was significantly higher than in the staples fixation group ($P = .005$). There were 4 cases of nonunion at the site of subtalar arthrodesis (2 from screws group, 2 from staples group). The complication rate was comparable in both groups.

Conclusion.—The fusion rate was comparable in both groups, while the postoperative functional outcome was significantly better in the screw fixation group.

Level of Evidence.—Level III, retrospective comparative cohort study.

▶ As the authors describe, there is little in the literature directly comparing these 2 accepted and commonly performed techniques. The sample is relatively small, but the fact that these were all performed by the same surgeon improves the reliability of the observations. The findings are easy to summarize and are useful: no overall difference except improved function according to the American Orthopaedic Foot and Ankle Society. This is an important difference and would favor the screw fixation technique. Of concern is the nonunion rate of more than 10% in each group is a little high. Also, we have no information on the manner of patient selection or of the operative times.

B. F. Morrey, MD

Arthroscopic Treatment of Anterior Ankle Impingement: A Prospective Study of 46 Patients With 5-Year Follow-up
Walsh SJ, Twaddle BC, Rosenfeldt MP, et al (Unisports Sports Medicine, Auckland, New Zealand)
Am J Sports Med 42:2722-2726, 2014

Background.—Midterm outcomes after arthroscopic debridement in patients with anterior ankle impingement without osteoarthritis are currently unclear.

Purpose.—To assess the functional and radiological outcomes after arthroscopic treatment of anterior ankle impingement with a minimum 5-year follow-up in patients without osteoarthritis.

Study Design.—Case series; Level of evidence, 4.

Methods.—From September 1999 to March 2006, a consecutive series of eligible patients without ankle osteoarthritis and with anterior ankle impingement, who had persistent ankle pain and activity restrictions despite at least 6 months of nonoperative management, underwent standardized arthroscopic debridement and followed uniform postoperative management. Patients were assessed preoperatively and at 6 weeks, 6 months, and 12 months and then at 1-year intervals after surgery until a minimum of 5 years' follow-up had been achieved, with weight-bearing ankle dorsiflexion, Foot Functional Index (FFI), and plain radiography including Scranton and McDermott classification (SMC) grade and tibial osteophyte size.

Results.—A total of 46 patients (42 male, 4 female) were prospectively assessed, with a mean age at surgery of 29 years (range, 16-44 years) and a mean follow-up duration of 5.1 years (range, 5.0-7.5 years). Preoperative ankle radiographs demonstrated a median SMC grade of 2 and a mean tibial osteophyte size of 5.1 mm. At a minimum of 5 years postoperatively, patients demonstrated limited improvement in ankle dorsiflexion (mean, 24.7° [preoperatively] vs 27.0° [final follow-up]; $P = .049$); however, they demonstrated substantial improvement in the FFI (mean, 20.5 [preoperatively] vs 2.7 [final follow-up]; $P < .001$). Postoperatively, 84% of patients showed a recurrence of radiological osteophytes, with plain radiographs at final follow-up demonstrating no significant difference in the SMC grade ($P = .107$) or tibial osteophyte size ($P = .212$) compared with preoperative imaging. There was no significant effect of patient age, sex, body mass index, or SMC grade at the time of surgery on any of the postoperative outcome measures.

Conclusion.—In this prospective outcome study of 46 patients without osteoarthritis managed arthroscopically for anterior ankle impingement,

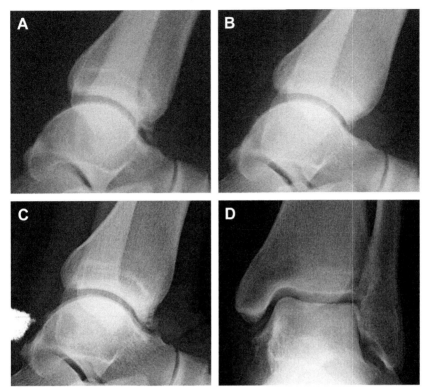

FIGURE 1.—Weightbearing lateral radiographs of the ankle in terminal dorsiflexion of a 26-year-old male patient. (A) Preoperative radiograph, demonstrating anterior ankle impingement with a prominent tibial osteophyte (Scranton and McDermott classification grade 2). (B) Radiograph taken 6 weeks after arthroscopic treatment, demonstrating satisfactory removal of an anterior tibial osteophyte. (C) Radiograph taken 5 years after arthroscopic treatment, demonstrating the recurrence of an anterior tibial osteophyte. (D) Weightbearing anteroposterior radiograph of the ankle 5 years after arthroscopic treatment, demonstrating no significant osteoarthritic change. The 5-year functional scores for this patient were excellent. (Reprinted from Walsh SJ, Twaddle BC, Rosenfeldt MP, et al. Arthroscopic treatment of anterior ankle impingement: a prospective study of 46 patients with 5-year follow-up. *Am J Sports Med.* 2014;42:2722-2726, with permission from The Author(s).)

the functional outcome scores had significantly improved at 5 years postoperatively despite a recurrence of radiographic osteophytes (Fig 1, Table 1).

▶ There are relatively few data regarding the long-term outcome of anterior osteophyte resection for anterior tibio/talar impingement. A sample of 46 patients with a minimum of 5-year surveillance with careful outcome measurements is of value. As is known, arthroscopic techniques are capable of removing the anterior osteophyte, but there is a tendency for the lesion to recur with time (Fig 1). Although improved dorsiflexion is only modest, all components of the Forefoot Index (FFI) remain improved (Table 1). Hence, this is a viable treatment option.

TABLE 1.—Results of Arthroscopic Treatment of Anterior Ankle Impingement at Minimum 5-Year Follow-up (N = 46 Patients)[a]

Variable	Preoperative	Final Follow-up	P Value
Ankle dorsiflexion, deg	24.7 ± 6.3	27.0 ± 7.5	.049
FFI score	20.5 ± 17.6	2.7 ± 4.8	<.001
Pain subscale	25.0 ± 21.0	3.1 ± 5.2	<.001
Difficulty subscale	21.6 ± 22.7	3.1 ± 6.9	<.001
Activity subscale	13.3 ± 15.5	1.2 ± 3.4	<.001
SMC grade, median ± SD	2.0 ± 0.7	2.0 ± 0.9	.107
Tibial osteophyte size, mm	5.1 ± 2.7	4.3 ± 3.1	.212

[a]Values are reported as mean ± SD unless otherwise indicated. FFI, Foot Function Index; SMC, Scranton and McDermott classification.

Reprinted from Walsh SJ, Twaddle BC, Rosenfeldt MP, et al. Arthroscopic treatment of anterior ankle impingement: a prospective study of 46 patients with 5-year follow-up. *Am J Sports Med.* 2014;42:2722-2726, with permission from The Author(s).

Unfortunately, I was unable to find a statement of the satisfaction of the patient cohort, which would be helpful, in addition to all of the objective measurements.

B. F. Morrey, MD

Cryopreserved Human Amniotic Membrane Injection for Plantar Fasciitis: A Randomized, Controlled, Double-Blind Pilot Study

Hanselman AE, Tidwell JE, Santrock RD, et al (West Virginia Univ School of Medicine, Morgantown)
Foot Ankle Int 36:151-158, 2015

Background.—Treatment options for plantar fasciitis have resulted in varied patient outcomes. The aim of this study was to compare a novel treatment, cryopreserved human amniotic membrane (c-hAM), to a traditional treatment, corticosteroid. Our hypothesis was that c-hAM would be safe and comparable to corticosteroids for plantar fasciitis in regard to patient outcomes.

Methods.—A randomized, controlled, double-blind, single-center pilot study was completed. Patients were randomized into one of 2 treatment groups: c-hAM or corticosteroid. Patients received an injection at their initial baseline visit with an option for a second injection at their first 6-week follow-up. Total follow-up was obtained for 12 weeks after the most recent injection. The primary outcome measurement was the Foot Health Status Questionnaire (FHSQ). The secondary outcome measurements were the Visual Analog Scale (VAS) and verbally reported percentage improvement. Data were analyzed between groups for the 2 different cohorts (1 injection versus 2 injections). Twenty-three patients had complete follow-up. Fourteen were randomized to receive corticosteroid and 9 were randomized to receive c-hAM.

Results.—Three patients in each group received second injections. With the numbers available, the majority of outcome measurements showed no statistical difference between groups. The corticosteroid did, however, have greater FHSQ shoe fit improvement ($P = .0244$) at 6 weeks, FHSQ general health improvement ($P = .0132$) at 6 weeks, and verbally reported improvement ($P = .041$) at 12 weeks in the one-injection cohort. Cryopreserved hAM had greater FHSQ foot pain improvement ($P = .0113$) at 18 weeks in the 2-injection cohort.

Conclusion.—Cryopreserved hAM injection may be safe and comparable to corticosteroid injection for treatment of plantar fasciitis. This is a pilot study and requires further investigation.

Level of Evidence.—Level I, prospective randomized trial.

▶ I have recently been assessing the use of human amniotic membrane (HAM) in the treatment of tendinopathy. I am very impressed by its safety and efficacy. This randomized, controlled trial pilot using HAM for the treatment of plantar fasciitis further supports the potential value of this approach. The improvement over a 12-week period is markedly better than the control steroid injection. We don't know the long-term value, but certainly in the short term the safety and efficacy is impressive. I await the cost-effectiveness data.

B. F. Morrey, MD

Effect of Pathology on Union of First Metatarsophalangeal Joint Arthrodesis
Korim MT, Allen PE (Univ Hosps Leicester, UK)
Foot Ankle Int 36:51-54, 2015

Background.—Arthrodesis is an established treatment for symptomatic degeneration of the first metatarsophalangeal (MP) joint. The published case series have often been small with different surgeons using a variety of joint preparation and fixation methods. The nonunion frequency comparing the different pathologies has not been described. We describe the senior author's results comparing the union of an MP arthrodesis in hallux valgus, hallux rigidus, inflammatory arthropathy, and salvage surgery with identical joint preparation and fixation methods.

Methods.—The logbook of the senior author was used to identify the first MP joint arthrodeses from 2003 to 2011. The radiographic data were reviewed on the Picture Archiving and Communication system to assess the severity of deformity, radiographic union, type of fixation, and need for revision surgery. If there was no definite radiographic union of the last radiograph, the medical notes were reviewed. In all, 134 MP joint arthrodeses were performed in 78 females and 38 males, with a mean age of 65 ± 12 years (range, 20-94). Fixation was achieved by crossed screws (124) and dorsal plate (10). The primary diagnoses were hallux valgus in

49 joints (36.6%), hallux rigidus in 46 joints (34%), inflammatory arthropathy in 34 joints (25.4%), and salvage surgery in 5 joints (3.7%).

Results.—The overall radiographic union rate was 91.8% (123/134). There were significantly more nonunions in the hallux valgus group (14.3% vs 0%, OR 16, $P = .05$).

Conclusion.—Biplanar cuts and crossed screw fixation gave similar union frequencies to published case series. Hallux valgus was associated with higher nonunion frequencies in this single surgeon series. It may be that the hallux valgus group needs a stronger construct to achieve comparable union frequencies to the hallux rigidus group.

Level of Evidence.—Level III, retrospective comparative study.

▶ Although this represents a single-experience case series, there is merit in the question being asked as well as the findings. As pointed out, first metatarsophalangeal fusion is a common procedure for a host of pathologies, hallux valgus being 1 of these. The preferred technique of biplanar osteotomy with cross screw fixation is successful in over 90% of patients, but those with hallux valgus have a higher rate of failure ($P < .05$) based on reoperation rate. So the question is straightforward, as are the findings.

B. F. Morrey, MD

An Anatomical Study Comparing Two Surgical Approaches for Isolated Talonavicular Arthrodesis

Higgs Z, Jamal B, Fogg QA, et al (Glasgow Royal Infirmary, Scotland, UK; Univ of Glasgow, Scotland, UK)
Foot Ankle Int 35:1063-1067, 2014

Background.—Two operative approaches are commonly used for isolated talonavicular arthrodesis: the medial and the dorsal approach. It is recognized that access to the lateral aspect of the talonavicular joint can be limited when using the medial approach, and it is our experience that using the dorsal approach addresses this issue. We performed an anatomical study using cadaver specimens, to compare the amount of articular surface that can be accessed by each operative approach.

Methods.—Medial and dorsal approaches to the talonavicular joint were performed on each of 11 cadaveric specimens (10 fresh frozen, 1 embalmed). Distraction of the joint was performed as used intraoperatively and the accessible area of articular surfaces was marked for each of the 2 approaches using a previously reported technique. Disarticulation was performed and the marked surface area was quantified using an immersion digital microscribe, allowing a 3-dimensional virtual model of the articular surfaces to be assessed.

Results.—The median percentage of total accessible talonavicular articular surface area for the medial and dorsal approaches was 71% and 92%, respectively (Wilcoxon signed-rank test, $P < .001$).

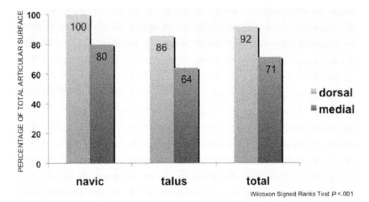

FIGURE 2.—Percentage of total articular surface area accessed by each of the dorsal (left column) and medial (right column) approaches. Statistically significant increase in area seen with the dorsal approach ($P < .001$ Wilcoxon signed-rank test). (Copyright © 2014, by the American Orthopaedic Foot and Ankle Society, Inc., originally published in Foot & Ankle International. Higgs Z, Jamal B, Fogg QA, et al. An anatomical study comparing two surgical approaches for isolated talonavicular arthrodesis. *Foot Ankle Int.* 2014;35:1063-1067, and reproduced here with permission.)

Conclusion.—This study provides quantifiable measurements of the articular surface accessible by the medial and dorsal approaches to the talonavicular joint.

Clinical Relevance.—These data support for the use of the dorsal approach for talonavicular arthrodesis, particularly in cases where access to the lateral half of the joint is necessary (Fig 2).

▶ I was attracted to this report because I thought it had direct clinical relevance. Recognizing that much of what we do is based on preference, often masked by our interpretation of the "data," studies such as this are rather refreshing. Although the technique was somewhat gross in its observations, the results do show the superiority of the dorsal approach, largely because of the nature of the medial navicular prominence with this disease (Fig 2). It would seem this is a reasonable approach for isolated fusion of the talonavicular joint for osteoarthritis.

B. F. Morrey, MD

Correction of Moderate to Severe Hallux Valgus With Isometric First Metatarsal Double Osteotomy

Siekmann W, Watson TS, Roggelin M (Argon-Orthopaedie Hamburg, Germany; Desert Orthopaedic Ctr, Las Vegas, NV)
Foot Ankle Int 35:1122-1130, 2014

Background.—The operative treatment for the moderate to severe bunion continues to present challenges. The indications for a single, double, or triple first ray osteotomy remain controversial. In addition, it is not clear whether an opening wedge osteotomy leads to clinically relevant arthritis at the first metatarsophalangeal joint. However, it is this theoretical concern that has led the authors to develop an isometric correction of the first ray.

Methods.—Thirty-two patients underwent operative correction of hallux valgus with a double osteotomy of the first metatarsal using an opening wedge proximally and a closing wedge distally. The mean follow-up period was 59.3 months with a range of 55 to 65 months.

Results.—The 1-2 intermetatarsal angle preoperatively was a mean of 18.9 degrees (range 17-23), correcting postoperatively to a mean angle of 8.6 degrees (range 5-12), for an average correction of 10.4 degrees (range 6-16). The postoperative AOFAS scores were 39.4 out of 40 points for pain, 42.4 out of 45 points for function, and 15 points for alignment. The total score was excellent with 94.2 out of 100 possible points. Radiographic union occurred in all cases. There was one case of painful edema of the foot and two cases of early avascular necrosis (AVN) diagnosed by residual pain at the hallux metatarsophalangeal joint and transient osteopenia of the metatarsal head on radiographs. No late sequelae associated with AVN such as arthritis or metatarsal head collapse were noted with long-term follow-up. These healed within months without specific treatment.

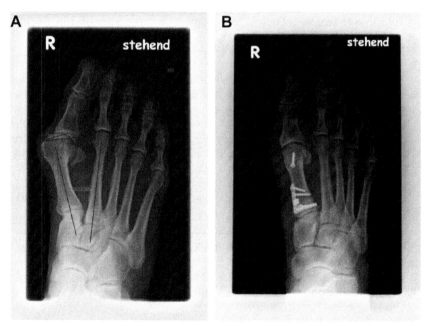

FIGURE 3.—A typical patient with a preop increased IMA and DMAA, corrected well with isometric technique at 5 years postop. (Copyright © 2014, by the American Orthopaedic Foot and Ankle Society, Inc., originally published in Foot & Ankle International. Siekmann W, Watson TS, Roggelin M. Correction of moderate to severe hallux valgus with isometric first metatarsal double osteotomy. *Foot Ankle Int.* 2014;35:1122-1130, and reproduced here with permission.)

Conclusion.—A double osteotomy of the first metatarsal with a non-locking, low-profile plate was an effective procedure for correcting severe hallux valgus that carried a low complication rate and high patient satisfaction. It has clear advantages over isolated opening wedge procedures, including potentially better correction especially in those bunions associated with an increased distal metatarsal articular angle.

Level of Evidence.—Level IV, retrospective case series (Fig 3).

▶ Severe bunion deformity remains a difficult surgical problem with several suggested corrective techniques. This case series demonstrates considerable improvement with a proximal opening and a distal closing double osteotomy (Fig 3). The overall angular improvement of 10 degrees is usually sufficient to obtain an acceptable correction. However, rather wide variation in the correction overall and at each level was documented.

The authors report no clinical sequence. Although it is a fairly complex procedure, it does appear to be a technique worth considering.

B. F. Morrey, MD

A comparison of proximal and distal Chevron osteotomy, both with lateral soft-tissue release, for moderate to severe hallux valgus in patients undergoing simultaneous bilateral correction: a prospective randomised controlled trial

Lee KB, Cho NY, Park HW, et al (Chonnam Natl Univ, Gwangju, Korea)

Bone Joint J 97-B:202-207, 2015

Moderate to severe hallux valgus is conventionally treated by proximal metatarsal osteotomy. Several recent studies have shown that the indications for distal metatarsal osteotomy with a distal soft-tissue procedure could be extended to include moderate to severe hallux valgus.

The purpose of this prospective randomised controlled trial was to compare the outcome of proximal and distal Chevron osteotomy in patients undergoing simultaneous bilateral correction of moderate to severe hallux valgus.

The original study cohort consisted of 50 female patients (100 feet). Of these, four (8 feet) were excluded for lack of adequate follow-up, leaving 46 female patients (92 feet) in the study. The mean age of the patients was 53.8 years (30.1 to 62.1) and the mean duration of follow-up 40.2 months (24.1 to 80.5). After randomisation, patients underwent a proximal Chevron osteotomy on one foot and a distal Chevron osteotomy on the other.

At follow-up, the American Orthopedic Foot and Ankle Society (AOFAS) hallux metatarsophalangeal interphalangeal (MTP-IP) score, patient satisfaction, post-operative complications, hallux valgus angle, first-second intermetatarsal angle, and tibial sesamoid position were similar in each group. Both procedures gave similar good clinical and radiological outcomes.

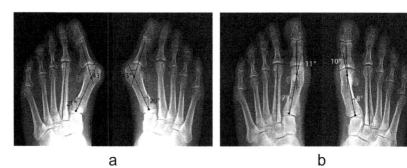

a   b

FIGURE 2.—Anteroposterior radiographs of a 57-year-old woman who underwent simultaneous correction by proximal Chevron (left) and distal Chevron (right) osteotomy for bilateral severe hallux valgus, showing the hallux valgus angle and the first-second intermetatarsal angle a) pre-operatively, and b) at final follow-up. (Reprinted from Lee KB, Cho NY, Park HW, et al. A comparison of proximal and distal chevron osteotomy, both with lateral soft-tissue release, for moderate to severe hallux valgus in patients undergoing simultaneous bilateral correction: a prospective randomised controlled trial. *Bone Joint J.* 2015;97-B:202-207, The British Editorial Society of Bone & Joint Surgery.)

This study suggests that distal Chevron osteotomy with a distal soft-tissue procedure is as effective and reliable a means of correcting moderate to severe hallux valgus as proximal Chevron osteotomy with a distal soft-tissue procedure (Fig 2).

▶ It is uncommon to have randomized controlled trials (RCTs) comparing surgical procedures for many reasons, not the least of which is the difficulty of enrollment when patient preference is a major factor. Because bunion surgery is one of the most common of all foot procedures, an RCT of 2 popular techniques is an important contribution. The answer, based on good measurement tools and assessment protocol, is that there is no difference between proximal or distal Chevron correction (Fig 2). In fact, the similarities in the results and even in the complications are striking. My personal preference has been the distal Chevron correction. However, the key appears to be that, with experience, surgeon preference is an acceptable basis of selection.

B. F. Morrey, MD

Minimally Invasive Reconstruction of the Lateral Ankle Ligaments Using Semitendinosus Autograft or Tendon Allograft

Xu X, Hu M, Liu J, et al (Shanghai Jiao Tong Univ School of Medicine, China)
Foot Ankle Int 35:1015-1021, 2014

Background.—The purpose of the study was to retrospectively compare the therapeutic effect between semitendinosus autograft and tendon allograft for lateral ankle ligaments reconstruction.

Methods.—From September 2006 to June 2011, 68 patients (41 males, 27 females) with chronic ankle instability underwent anatomical reconstruction of the lateral ligaments using semitendinosus autograft (autograft group, 32 patients) or tendon allograft (allograft group, 36 patients) via a minimally invasive approach. All patients were followed up for at least 12 months. The American Orthopaedic Foot and Ankle Society Ankle-Hindfoot Scale score (AOFAS score) and stress tests were used to evaluate the clinical outcomes. Operation time, time to heal and complications were also recorded.

Results.—Compared with allograft group, the average operation time was significantly increased (85.5 ± 11.5 minutes vs 58.1 ± 10.2 minutes, $P < .0001$), but the mean time to heal was significantly shorter (11.2 ± 4.1 months vs 13.5 ± 5.2 months, $P = .0458$) in the autograft group. Although the mean AOFAS score was significantly increased at the final follow-up in the autograft group (95.1 ± 7.5 vs 62.3 ± 8.2, $P = .0001$) and allograft group (94.8 ± 5.5 vs 60.2 ± 8.4, $P < .0001$), no significant difference in AOFAS was found between these 2 groups. Similarly, there was no significant difference in talar tilt or shift between autograft and allograft groups. In addition, no patients complained of weakness or disability at the donor site in the autograft group, while incisional swelling was observed in 4 patients in the allograft group, which was resolved via dressing change, oral use of indomethacin or dexamethasone.

Conclusion.—Reconstruction of the lateral ankle ligaments using a semitendinosus tendon autograft and a minimally invasive approach was safe and effective for ankle instability with a relatively short time for healing and minimal donor site problems.

Level of Evidence.—Level III, comparative case series.

▶ This review resulted in a bit of a surprise for me. First, I was impressed with the ability to successfully reconstruct the lateral ligament complex through a series of small puncture wounds. Furthermore, my interpretation of the findings and the authors' conclusion was somewhat different. I would conclude there is no statistical difference in the auto- or allograft tissue. The conclusion of the authors favors the autograft.

Regardless, the fact that 608 procedures were done in only a few years indicates that this is truly a referral practice with, I would suspect, a considerable learning curve.

B. F. Morrey, MD

Accelerated Versus Traditional Rehabilitation After Anterior Talofibular Ligament Reconstruction for Chronic Lateral Instability of the Ankle In Athletes

Miyamoto W, Takao M, Yamada K, et al (Teikyo Univ School of Medicine, Tokyo, Japan)
Am J Sports Med 42:1441-1447, 2014

Background.—Although several reconstruction procedures for chronic lateral ankle instability using autografts have been reported, all have recommended postoperative immobilization and a nonweightbearing period.

Hypothesis.—Reconstructive surgery with a gracilis autograft using an interference fit anchoring system for chronic lateral ankle instability enables early accelerated rehabilitation and recovery with a return to activity without requiring immobilization.

Study Design.—Cohort study; Level of evidence, 3.

Methods.—A total of 33 patients (33 feet) who underwent reconstruction of the anterior talofibular ligament with a gracilis autograft using interference screws were included; 15 were followed for 4 weeks with postoperative cast immobilization (group I), while 18 were followed with accelerated rehabilitation without immobilization (group A). Clinical and radiological results were evaluated based on the Karlsson and Peterson score, talar tilt angle, anterior displacement of the talus on stress radiography, and time between surgery and return to full athletic activity.

Results.—The mean Karlsson and Peterson scores before and 2 years after surgery were the following: for group I: 62.3 ± 4.7 (range, 54-72) and 94.4 ± 7.1 (range, 76-100), respectively (*P* < .001), and for group A: 64.1 ± 4.8 (range, 57-70) and 91.7 ± 7.7 (range, 74-100), respectively (*P* < .001). The mean difference in the talar tilt angle compared with the contralateral side and mean displacement of the talus on stress radiography before and 2 years after surgery were the following: for group I: 8.7° ± 2.6° and 7.7 ± 1.8 mm and 3.8° ± 1.5° and 4.0 ± 1.6 mm, respectively, and for group A: 10.5° ± 3.4° and 8.7 ± 2.1 mm and 4.3° ± 1.8° and 4.3 ± 1.2 mm, respectively. Radiography revealed significantly improved postoperative outcomes in both groups (*P* < .0001). No significant differences in the score and any parameters on stress radiography were evident at 2 years after surgery between the groups. The mean time between surgery and return to full athletic activity was significantly higher in group I (18.5 ± 3.5 weeks) than in group A (13.4 ± 2.2 weeks)

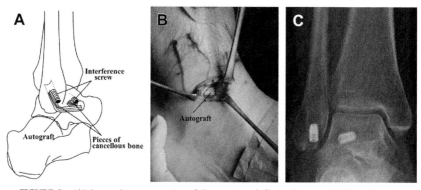

FIGURE 5.—(A) Anatomic reconstruction of the anterior talofibular ligament (ATFL) using an interference fit anchoring system with a gracilis autograft. (B) Intraoperative photograph showing the implanted autograft. (C) Postoperative radiograph showing adequate positioning of each interference screw at the fibular and talar attachments of the ATFL. (Reprinted from Miyamoto W, Takao M, Yamada K, et al. Accelerated versus traditional rehabilitation after anterior talofibular ligament reconstruction for chronic lateral instability of the ankle in athletes. *Am J Sports Med.* 2014;42:1441-1447, with permission from The Author(s).)

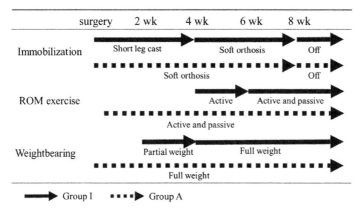

FIGURE 6.—Postoperative rehabilitation program in group I with cast immobilization and in group A with accelerated rehabilitation without cast immobilization. ROM, range of motion. (Reprinted from Miyamoto W, Takao M, Yamada K, et al. Accelerated versus traditional rehabilitation after anterior talofibular ligament reconstruction for chronic lateral instability of the ankle in athletes. *Am J Sports Med.* 2014;42:1441-1447, with permission from The Author(s).)

TABLE 1.—Treatment Outcomes[a]

	Before Surgery	2 Years After Surgery	P Value
Group I			
Karlsson and Peterson score	62.3 ± 4.7 (54-72)	94.4 ± 7.1 (76-100)	<.0001
Talar tilt angle compared with contralateral side, deg	8.7 ± 2.6 (7-16)	3.8 ± 1.5 (1-6)	<.0001
Anterior displacement of the talus, mm	7.7 ± 1.8 (6-12)	4.0 ± 1.6 (2-8)	<.0001
Group A			
Karlsson and Peterson score	64.1 ± 4.8 (57-70)	91.7 ± 7.7 (74-100)	<.0001
Talar tilt angle compared with contralateral side, deg	10.5 ± 3.4 (6-15)	4.3 ± 1.8 (2-6)	<.0001
Anterior displacement of the talus, mm	8.7 ± 2.1 (6-13)	4.3 ± 1.2 (3-7)	<.0001

[a]Values are expressed as mean ± standard deviation (range).
Reprinted from Miyamoto W, Takao M, Yamada K, et al. Accelerated versus traditional rehabilitation after anterior talofibular ligament reconstruction for chronic lateral instability of the ankle in athletes. *Am J Sports Med.* 2014;42:1441-1447, with permission from The Author(s).

($P < .0001$). No cases of reinjury were reported, and no differences in athletic performance ability were observed between the groups.

Conclusion.—Patients in group A returned to full athletic activity 5 weeks earlier than those in group I, demonstrating the advantage of accelerated rehabilitation after surgery (Figs 5 and 6, Table 1).

▶ The question of the most effective rehabilitation allowing safe return to full activity is a universal one. This is an impressive study of 33 patients rehabilitated by traditional protection, group I, and accelerated functional rehabilitation, group

A. The features of the reconstruction include an anatomic replication of the anterior talofibular ligament with a gracilis autograft secured with an interference screw (Fig 5). Patients were stratified into 1 of 2 programs as shown in Fig 6. Careful postprocedure assessment resulted in documentation of improved function and increased rotatory and translational stability in the accelerated rehabilitation Group A (Table 1). This study makes a strong case for a more aggressive and rapid rehabilitation program that might be applicable to other joint ligamentous reconstructions.

B. F. Morrey, MD

Arthrodesis After Failed Total Ankle Replacement

Deleu P-A, Bevernage BD, Maldague P, et al (Foot & Ankle Inst, Bruxelles, Belgium)
Foot Ankle Int 35:549-557, 2014

Background.—The literature on salvage procedures for failed total ankle replacement (TAR) is sparse. We report a series of 17 patients who had a failed TAR converted to a tibiotalar or a tibiotalocalcaneal arthrodesis.

Methods.—Between 2003 and 2012, a total of 17 patients with a failed TAR underwent an arthrodesis. All patients were followed on a regular basis through chart review, clinical examination and radiological evaluation. The following variables were analyzed: pre- and postoperative Meary angle, cause of failure, method of fixation, type of graft, time to union, complications, and postoperative American Orthopaedic Foot and Ankle Society (AOFAS) score. The average follow-up was 30.1 months. The average period from the original arthroplasty to the arthrodesis was 49.8 months.

Results.—Thirteen of the 17 ankles were considered radiographically healed after the first attempt in an average time of 3.7 months and 3 after repeat arthrodesis. Bone grafts were used in 16 patients. The median postoperative AOFAS score was 74.5. The mean Meary angle of the hindfoot was 5 degrees of valgus.

Conclusion.—Tibiotalar and tibiotalocalcaneal arthrodeses were effective salvage procedures for failed TAR. Massive cancellous allografts were a good alternative to compensate for the large bone defect after removal of the prosthesis and to preserve the leg length (Figs 2 and 3, Table 2).

▶ With the resurgence of ankle replacement, the need for information regarding the salvage procedure is of value. Compared with the literature, this is a typical sample size, but the follow-up is rather short at 29 months (Table 2). That both tibial-talar, (Fig 2) and tibio-talar-calcaneal (Fig 3) techniques were used renders the data a bit more heterogeneous. The success rate of approximately 75% might be considered acceptable given the considerable bone loss that is often

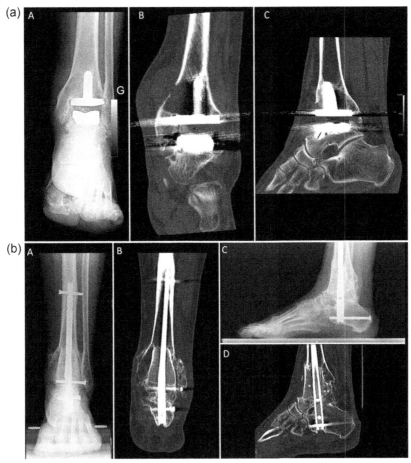

FIGURE 2.—. (a) Tibiotalocalcaneal arthrodesis after failed total ankle replacement: (A) preoperative anteroposterior (AP) view of Ankle Evolutive System prosthesis (Biomet France S.A.R.L., Valence, France); (B, C) preoperative computed tomography (CT) scan representing the frontal and sagittal view of the ankle and the hindfoot. One can observe the massive osteolysis around the tibial component, the migration of the talar component and the cystic fistula above the malleolus. (b) Postoperative AP (A) and lateral views (C) of the tibiotalocalcaneal arthrodesis (follow-up at 12 months) and the postoperative CT scan (B, D) at 12 months: *integration of the cancellous tibial allograft + **mixture of cancellous graft with demineralized bone matrix was placed posteriorly to the cancellous allograft. (Reprinted from Deleu P-A, Bevernage BD, Maldague P, et al. Arthrodesis after failed total ankle replacement. *Foot Ankle Int.* 2014;35:549-557, Copyright © 2014, by the American Orthopaedic Foot and Ankle Society, Inc., originally published in *Foot & Ankle International*, [AMA], and reproduced here with permission.)

(a)

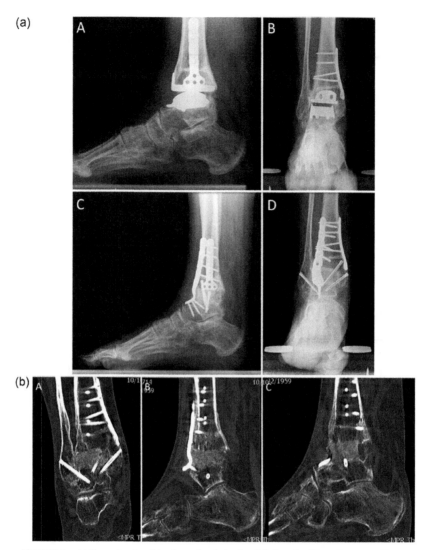

FIGURE 3.—(a) Example of a tibiotalar arthrodesis after failed total ankle replacement (TAR; case 17). The bone grafts included bone marrow from the iliac crest in association with demineralized bone matrix (DBM) and a cancellous allograft: (A, B) preoperative conventional anteroposterior and lateral weightbearing x-rays (follow-up at 3 months); (C, D) postoperative conventional anteroposterior and lateral weightbearing x-rays (follow-up at 3 months): one can observe the bone graft with the host and the additional stability procured by the screws from the medial and lateral malleoli to the talus and bone graft. (b) Example of a tibiotalar arthrodesis after failed TAR (case 17). The bone grafts were from the iliac crest in association with DBM and a cancellous allograft: (A-C) postoperative computed tomography scan: frontal and sagittal views: the bone formation made from bone marrow from the iliac crest association with DBM (B) and the cancellous femoral head allograft (C). (Reprinted from Deleu P-A, Bevernage BD, Maldague P, et al. Arthrodesis after failed total ankle replacement. *Foot Ankle Int*. 2014;35:549-557, Copyright © 2014, by the American Orthopaedic Foot and Ankle Society, Inc., originally published in Foot & Ankle International, [AMA], and reproduced here with permission.)

TABLE 2.—Review of Previous Studies Concerning "Arthrodesis After Failed Total Ankle Replacement"

Study	Year	No. of Subjects	Age, y	Time to Failure, mo	Type of Fusion	Graft, %	Time to Union, mo	Healed After First Attempt, %	Complications, %	Follow-up, mo
Kitaoka and Romness[15]	1992	38	57	42	33 TT; 5 TTC	89	NR	87	13	96
Carlsson et al[4]	1998	21	59	40	20 TT; 1 TTC	100	NR	62	38	NR
Gabrion et al[9]	2004	8	57	36	6 TT; 2 TTC	25	3.1	87	13	56
Anderson et al[1]	2005	16	55	62	16 TTC	88	43	69	31	34
Zwipp and Grass[26]	2005	4	42	45	3 TT; 1 TTC	100	3.5	75	25	37.5
Hopgood et al[13]	2006	23	62	41	16 TT; 7 TTC	61	4	74	26	29
Kotnis et al[16]	2006	16	64.7	33	10 TTC; 1 KA; 5 RTAR	100	8	94	6	12
Schill[21]	2007	15	56	115	15 TTC	100	3.9	87	13	23
Culpan et al[6]	2007	16	54	41	16 TT	100	3	94	6	44
Moor et al[19]	2008	3	NR	NR	3 TTC	100	3	100	0	32
Carlsson[5]	2008	3	49	76	3 TT	100	/	0	100	37
Thomason and Eyres[23]	2008	3	66	72	3 TTC	100	3	100	0	32
Doets and Zürcher[8]	2010	18	55	49	7 TT; 11 TTC	100	6.3	61	39	NR
Henricson and Rydholm[11]	2010	13	NR	84	13 TTC	100	NR	92	8	17
Berkovitz et al[2]	2011	12; 12	58; 65.3	41.3; 63.1	12 TT; 12 TTC	83; 100	NR; NR	92; 59	8; 41	57.9; 33.2
Jehan and Hill[14]	2012	4	66.5	20	4 TT	100	3.5	100	0	NR
McCoy et al[18]	2012	7	52	70.9	4 TT; 3 TTC	0	6.3	100	0	58
Our study	2013	17	57.3	49.8	5 TT; 12 TTC	94	3.7	76.5	23.5	29.1

KA, knee amputation; NR, not reported; RTAR, revision arthroplasty; TT, tibiotalar arthrodesis; TTC, tibiotalocalcaneal arthrodesis.

Editor's Note: Please refer to original journal article for full references.

present (Fig 2). I do have some reservations about fusing an otherwise normal subtalar joint and subsequent potential arthrosis at Chopart's joint.

B. F. Morrey, MD

10 Sports Medicine

Introduction

As most know, the sports scene is currently dominated by all aspects of the anterior cruciate ligament (ACL), including normal anatomy, pathoanatomy, implication of associated injuries, long-term outcomes, and the efforts to distinguish different technical approaches to the problem. As in the past, I have specifically attempted to limit the reviews in this section so as not to have this section become synonymous with the ACL. Hence, just over half of the articles relate in some way to the ACL, and these articles were very carefully selected to provide important insights rather than be "me too."

As in the past, issues regarding head trauma have been included, as this continues to be a much discussed and important issue both for orthopedic surgeons and for society as a whole. There are articles that relate to almost every anatomic area, and some of these studies could have been placed in the anatomic-specific area, such as the elbow, shoulder, and foot. However, they are included in this section because they helped balance the anterior cruciate ligament literature. Overall, the sports literature is very rich with a spectrum of contributions, and these do reflect overall improved management of patients.

Bernard F. Morrey, MD

Levels of Evidence in the Clinical Sports Medicine Literature: Are We Getting Better Over Time?

Grant HM, Tjoumakaris FP, Maltenfort MG, et al (Jefferson Med College, Philadelphia, PA; Thomas Jefferson Univ, Philadelphia, PA)
Am J Sports Med 42:1738-1742, 2014

Background.—There has been an increased emphasis on improving the level of evidence used as the basis for clinical treatment decisions. Several journals now require a statement of the level of evidence as a basic gauge of the study's strength.

Purpose.—To review the levels of evidence in published articles in the clinical sports medicine literature and to determine if there has been an improvement in the levels of evidence published over the past 15 years.

Study Design.—Systematic review.

Methods.—All articles from the years 1995, 2000, 2005, and 2010 in *The American Journal of Sports Medicine* (*AJSM*), *Arthroscopy*, and sports medicine–related articles from *The Journal of Bone and Joint Surgery-American* (*JBJS*–*A*) were analyzed. Articles were categorized by type and ranked for level of evidence according to guidelines from the Centre for Evidence-Based Medicine. Excluded were animal, cadaveric, and basic science articles; editorials; surveys; special topics; letters to the editor; and correspondence. Statistical analysis was performed with chi-square.

Results.—A total of 1580 articles over the 4 periods met the inclusion criteria. The percentage of level 1 and 2 studies increased from 6.8% to 12.6%, 22.9%, and 23.5%, respectively ($P < .0001$), while level 4 and 5 studies decreased from 78.9% to 72.4%, 63.9%, and 53.0% ($P < .0001$). *JBJS-A* had a significant increase in level 1 and 2 studies (4.1%, 5.1%, 28.2%, 27.8%; $P < .0001$), as did *AJSM* (9.4%, 17.1%, 36.1%, 30.1%; $P < .0001$). *Arthroscopy* showed no significant change over time. Diagnostic, therapeutic, and prognostic studies all showed significant increases in level 1 and 2 studies over time ($P < .05$).

Conclusion.—There has been a statistically significant increase in the percentage of level 1 and 2 studies published in the sports medicine literature over the past 15 years, particularly in *JBJS-A* and *AJSM*. The largest increase was seen in diagnostic studies, while therapeutic and prognostic studies demonstrated modest improvement. The emphasis on increasing

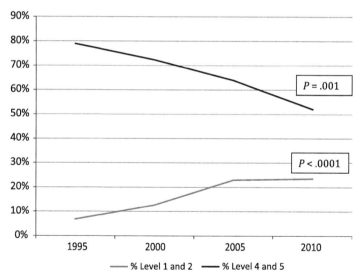

FIGURE 2.—The percentage of high (1 and 2) and low (4 and 5) levels of evidence over time. (Reprinted from Grant HM, Tjoumakaris FP, Maltenfort MG, et al. Levels of evidence in the clinical sports medicine literature: are we getting better over time? *Am J Sports Med.* 2014;42:1738-1742, with permission The Author(s).)

levels of evidence to guide treatment decisions for sports medicine patients may be taking effect (Fig 2).

▶ So there is hope! This simple analysis tallied the volume and percentage of article submission to major journals to determine the trend being investigated. Fig 2 says it all, or almost all. There is a definite increase in high-quality manuscripts in the orthopedic community, especially in the *Journal of Bone and Joint Surgery* and *American Journal of Sports Medicine*. Of interest, the *Journal of Arthroscopy* showed no change in the "quality" of manuscripts being published. As noted, this is encouraging and necessary.

B. F. Morrey, MD

Impact of a State Concussion Law on Pediatric Emergency Department Visits

Mackenzie B, Vivier P, Reinert S, et al (Alpert Med School of Brown Univ, Providence, RI; Brown Univ, Providence, RI)
Pediatr Emerg Care 31:25-30, 2015

Objective.—Many states have passed concussion laws that mandate that players undergo medical clearance before returning to play. Few data have been collected on the impact of such laws on emergency department (ED) visits. This study measures the impact of Rhode Island concussion legislation on sports-related concussion visits to a pediatric ED.

Methods.—*International Classification of Diseases, Ninth Revision, Clinical Modification* codes with injury mechanism—associated E-codes were extracted from hospital databases from 2004 to 2011 for both sports-related concussions and sports-related ankle ligamentous injuries (comparison group). Visit rates for sports-related concussions were compared before and after the passage of the state concussion law. Secondary outcome measures included rates of head imaging per ED visit for concussion before and after passage of the law. Times series analysis was used to analyze season-to-season count and rate changes.

Results.—Overall rate of sports-related concussion visits more than doubled (2.2-fold increase; 95% confidence interval, 1.3—3.6; adjusted $P = 0.01$) during the fall sports season following the implementation of legislation (2010) relative to the previous year (3.6% vs 1.4%). Rates of sports-related ankle sprain visits tended to increase during the fall sports season but did not achieve statistical significance. Rates of computed tomography scan imaging of the head did not change over time.

Conclusions.—The data from this study revealed an increase in pediatric ED visits for sports-related concussions, without a corresponding increase in head imaging, suggesting that the passage of a state concussion law has led to increased vigilance in evaluation of sports-related concussions, without an increase in diagnostic computed tomography scans.

▶ The question of sports-related concussion remains a topic in the public media and in the YEAR BOOK OF ORTHOPEDICS. This study asks an interesting question, and frankly, I was surprised by the answer. The introduction of concussion-specific legislation in the state of Rhode Island (being from Texas, I do not recognize Rhode Island as the hot bed of high school football) did result in an increased number of sports-related visits to the emergency department. Surprisingly, this did not increase the imaging surveillance for concussion. Yet this legislation seems to have had an impact on the recognition of concussion, which increased as a diagnosis from 1.4% to 3.6% of emergency department visits. For me, the key is we must be more sensitive to the features of concussion and be prepared to properly take care of not only the young, but also of the mature athlete.

B. F. Morrey, MD

Are pediatric concussion patients compliant with discharge instructions?
Hwang V, Trickey AW, Lormel C, et al (Inova Fairfax Hosp, Falls Church, VA)
J Trauma Acute Care Surg 77:117-122, 2014

Background.—Concussions are commonly diagnosed in pediatric patients presenting to the emergency department (ED). The primary objective of this study was to evaluate compliance with ED discharge instructions for concussion management.

Methods.—A prospective cohort study was conducted from November 2011 to November 2012 in a pediatric ED at a regional Level 1 trauma center, serving 35,000 pediatric patients per year. Subjects were aged 8 years to 17 years and were discharged from the ED with a diagnosis of concussion. Exclusion criteria included recent (past 3 months) diagnosis of head injury, hospital admission, intracranial injury, skull fracture, suspected nonaccidental trauma, or preexisting neurologic condition. Subjects were administered a baseline survey in the ED and were given standardized discharge instructions for concussion by the treating physician. Telephone follow-up surveys were conducted at 2 weeks and 4 weeks after ED visit.

Results.—A total of 150 patients were enrolled. The majority (67%) of concussions were sports related. Among sports-related concussions, soccer (30%), football (11%), lacrosse (8%), and basketball (8%) injuries were most common. More than one third (39%) reported return to play (RTP) on the day of the injury. Physician follow-up was equivalent for sport and nonsport concussions (2 weeks, 58%; 4 weeks, 64%). Sports-related concussion patients were more likely to follow up with a trainer (2 weeks, 25% vs. 10%, $p = 0.06$; 4 weeks, 29% vs. 8%, $p < 0.01$). Of the patients who did RTP or normal activities at 2 weeks (44%), more than one third (35%) were symptomatic, and most (58%) did not receive

TABLE 5.—Compliance Among Patients With Sports Versus Non—Sports-Related Concussions

	Sports Concussions		Nonsports Concussions		
	Available Data, n	n (%)	Available Data, n	n (%)	p*
2-wk follow-up					
Completed follow-up	100	85 (85)	50	40 (80)	0.439
Symptomatic	85	51 (60)	40	21 (53)	0.445
RTP or normal activities	85	35 (41)	40	20 (50)	0.354
RTP with symptoms	35	14 (40)	20	5 (25)	0.760
Received medical clearance if RTP	35	19 (54)	20	4 (20)	0.013
No stages skipped	81	71 (88)	39	34 (87)	0.999
4-wk follow-up					
Completed follow-up	100	77 (77)	50	39 (78)	0.999
Symptomatic	77	32 (42)	39	19 (49)	0.553
RTP or normal activities	77	46 (60)	39	28 (72)	0.202
RTP with symptoms	46	8 (17)	28	10 (36)	0.075
Received medical clearance if RTP	46	28 (61)	28	12 (43)	0.132
No stages skipped	72	63 (88)	36	31 (86)	0.999

*p values were calculated using W2 tests or Fisher's exact tests when assumptions for W2 tests were not met.
Reprinted from Hwang V, Trickey AW, Lormel C, et al. Are pediatric concussion patients compliant with discharge instructions? *J Trauma Acute Care Surg.* 2014;77:117-122.

medical clearance. Of the patients who had returned to activities at 4 weeks (64%), less than one quarter (23%) were symptomatic, and most (54%) received medical clearance.

Conclusion.—Pediatric patients discharged from the ED are mostly compliant with concussion instructions. However, a significant number of patients RTP on the day of injury, while experiencing symptoms or without medical clearance.

Level of Evidence.—Care management, level IV. Epidemiologic study, level III. (Table 5).

▶ With the ever-growing awareness of the long-term implications of concussion, a study of this nature in the adolescent age group is particularly relevant. I was struck by the high percentage of individuals who returned to play on the day of injury—40%. The full article should be read because there is much useful information contained therein. As a team doctor for a local high school, I have recently cared for 3 such injuries. It is interesting that more than 2 weeks are required for symptoms to resolve in approximately 35%, and symptoms persist after 4 weeks in 23%. Overall, I was favorably impressed with the general compliance of both the sports- and non-sports-related injury (Table 5). Finally, I was reminded of the high risk of soccer: There is a 3 times greater chance in soccer than football to sustain a concussion in this age group. Some of this is, of course, due to the number of participants, but this is still an impressive statistic.

B. F. Morrey, MD

Functional Outcomes and Return to Sports After Acute Repair, Chronic Repair, and Allograft Reconstruction for Proximal Hamstring Ruptures

Rust DA, Giveans MR, Stone RM, et al (Minnesota Orthopedic Sports Medicine Inst at Twin Cities Orthopedics, Edina)
Am J Sports Med 42:1377-1383, 2014

Background.—There are limited data regarding outcomes and return to sports after surgery for acute versus chronic proximal hamstring ruptures.

Hypothesis.—Surgery for chronic proximal hamstring ruptures leads to improved outcomes and return to sports but at a lower level than with acute repair. Proximal hamstring reconstruction with an Achilles allograft for chronic ruptures is successful when direct repair is not possible.

Study Design.—Cohort study; Level of evidence, 3.

Methods.—Between 2002 and 2012, a total of 72 patients with a traumatic proximal hamstring rupture (51 acute, 21 chronic) underwent either direct tendon repair with suture anchors (n = 58) or Achilles allograft tendon reconstruction (n = 14). Results from the Single Assessment Numeric Evaluation (SANE) for activities of daily living (ADL) and sports-related activities, Short Form−12 (SF-12), visual analog scale (VAS), and a patient satisfaction questionnaire were obtained.

Results.—The mean time to surgery in the chronic group was 441.4 days versus 17.8 days in the acute group. At a mean follow-up of 45 months, patients with chronic tears had inferior sports activity scores (70.2% vs 80.3%, respectively; $P = .026$) and a trend for decreased ADL scores (86.5% vs 93.3%, respectively; $P = .085$) compared with those with acute tears. Patients with chronic tears, however, reported significant improvements postoperatively for both sports activity scores (30.3% to 70.2%; $P < .01$) and ADL scores (56.1% to 86.5%; $P < .01$). Greater than 5 to 6 cm of retraction in the chronic group was predictive of the need for allograft reconstruction ($P = .015$) and resulted in ADL and sports activity scores equal to those of chronic repair ($P = .507$ and $P = .904$, respectively). There were no significant differences between groups in SF-12, VAS, or patient satisfaction outcomes (mean, 85.2% satisfaction overall).

Conclusion.—Acute repair was superior to chronic surgery with regard to return to sports. Acute and chronic proximal hamstring repair and allograft reconstruction had favorable results for ADL. For low-demand patients or those with medical comorbidities, delayed repair or reconstruction might be considered with an expected 87% return to normal ADL. For patients who desire to return to sports, acute repair is recommended.

▶ This study provides useful information. There is relatively little information regarding the outcome to be expected from repair or reconstruction of the proximal hamstring ruptures. The clear definition of acute and chronic lesions allows confidence in the findings, because expected acute ruptures do better than reconstructions, especially if retraction is greater than 5 cm. The outcomes are relevant for return to sport, but the reconstruction is useful even for the less active patient because of improvements in the ability to perform activities of daily living. This experience can aid in clinical decision making.

B. F. Morrey, MD

Chronic Complaints After Ankle Sprains: A Systematic Review on Effectiveness of Treatments

van Ochten JM, van Middelkoop M, Meuffels D, et al (Erasmus Univ Med Ctr, Rotterdam, the Netherlands)

J Orthop Sports Phys Ther 44:862-871, 2014

Study Design.—Systematic review.

Objective.—To determine the effectiveness of treatments for patients with chronic complaints after ankle sprain.

Background.—Though most people recover completely after a lateral inversion ankle injury, a considerable percentage have persistent complaints. Currently, it is still unclear which treatment options are best for these patients.

Methods.—Major databases, including PubMed, Embase, CINAHL, and PEDro, were searched for randomized controlled trials and controlled clinical trials conducted from 1966 to October 2012. Due to clinical heterogeneity, the data were analyzed using a best-evidence synthesis.

Results.—A total of 20 randomized controlled trials and 1 controlled clinical trial were included in the analysis. The included studies compared different treatments (training programs, physiotherapy, chiropractic/manual therapy, surgery, postoperative training, and functional treatment). For pain and function outcomes, limited to moderate evidence was found for effectiveness of a training program compared to conservative treatment. Two studies found a decrease of recurrences after a proprioceptive training program. Four studies showed good results for different surgical methods but did not include a nonsurgical control group for comparison. Limited evidence was found for the effectiveness of an early mobilization program after surgery.

Conclusion.—In chronic ankle complaints after an ankle sprain, a training program gives better results for pain and function, and a decrease of recurrent ankle sprains, than a wait-and-see policy. There was insufficient evidence to determine the most effective surgical treatment, but limited evidence suggests that postoperative, early mobilization was more effective than a plaster cast.

Level of Evidence.—Therapy, level 1a−.

▶ Yet another systemic review of the literature regarding a common and relevant question. With the methodology employed, these investigators demonstrated the value of proprioceptive rehabilitation in contrast to doing nothing. They considered but were unable to comment on the optimal postoperative rehabilitation program. The important message is a simple one: There is merit to a focused and well-constructed rehabilitation program for ankle injuries, even chronic recurrent injuries.

B. F. Morrey, MD

Achilles Tendon Injury Risk Factors Associated with Running
Lorimer AV, Hume PA (Auckland Univ of Technology, New Zealand)
Sports Med 44:1459-1472, 2014

Background.—Research into the nature of overuse Achilles tendon injuries is extensive, yet uncertainty remains around how to identify athletes susceptible to Achilles tendon injury.

Objective.—To identify the strength of evidence for biomechanical risk factors associated with Achilles tendon injuries.

Research Methods.—SPORTDiscus, CINAHL, Web of Science and PubMed were searched for Achilles tendon injury risk factors and biomechanical measures which are altered in runners with Achilles tendon injuries, excluding ruptures. Fifteen articles were included in the analysis.

Results.—Two variables, high vertical forces and high arch, showed strong evidence for reduced injury risk. High propulsive forces and running on stiffer surfaces may also be protective. Only one biomechanical variable, high braking force, showed clear evidence for increasing Achilles injury risk.

Discussion.—Gait retraining to direct the centre of mass further forward to reduce high braking force could be useful in decreasing the risk of Achilles injury. The majority of biomechanical risk factors examined showed unclear results, which is likely due to the multifactorial nature of Achilles overuse injuries. Many risk factors are related to how the athlete's body interacts with the environment during gait, including ground reaction forces, muscle activity both prior to landing and immediately post ground contact, and joint motion throughout stance.

Conclusion.—Multiple risk factors have been associated with the development of Achilles tendon injuries in running athletes but most effects remain unclear. Advice for athletes recovering from Achilles tendon injuries could include avoiding soft surfaces and reducing the pace of recovery runs. Orthotic intervention could assist athletes with low arches but modification of pronation should be viewed with caution. Strength training and gait retraining could be beneficial for reducing injury risk.

▶ This is an excellent study. Of almost 3000 articles dealing with Achilles' tendon injury in runners, only 15 were selected to provide input to the study and conclusions. After a detailed analysis, only 2 variables were identified to protect against injury: high peak ground reaction force and a high arch. One variable was identified to be causative: running on soft surfaces. The discussion is excellent and points out the multifactorial nature of the problem. From a practical perspective, there are 2 recommendations that can be made to a patient: use of arch supports for those with flat feet or low arches and avoidance of excessive running on soft, synthetic surfaces.

B. F. Morrey, MD

Acromial Apophysiolysis: Superior Shoulder Pain and Acromial Nonfusion in the Young Throwing Athlete
Roedl JB, Morrison WB, Ciccotti MG, et al (Thomas Jefferson Univ Hosp, Philadelphia, PA)
Radiology 274:201-209, 2015

Purpose.—To describe the frequency of acromial apophysiolysis and its association with incomplete fusion and superior shoulder pain, to determine risk factors of acromial apophysiolysis, and to assess whether acromial apophysiolysis is associated with the development of an os acromiale and rotator cuff tears.

Materials and Methods.—Institutional review board approval was obtained for this HIPAA-compliant study; requirement for informed consent was waived. A retrospective report review of 2372 consecutive patients between 15 and 25 years of age who underwent shoulder magnetic resonance (MR) imaging for shoulder pain was performed. Individuals with edema at the acromial apophyses and no other abnormalities on MR images were included in the study group. Association of acromial edema with incomplete fusion, pitching, and clinical findings was determined in the study group and in an age- and sex-matched control group, with both univariate and multivariate binary logistic regression analyses. Association with the development of an os acromiale and rotator cuff tears later in life was assessed with follow-up imaging after age 25 years.

Results.—Edema at the acromial apophyses was found in 2.6% (61 of 2372) of patients and was associated with incomplete fusion of the acromial apophyses (χ^2, $P < .001$) and superior shoulder tenderness ($P < .001$). The entity was named acromial apophysiolysis. A pitch count of more than 100 pitches per week was shown to be a risk factor for acromial apophysiolysis (odds ratio [OR] = 6.5, $P = .017$). Follow-up imaging showed that acromial apophysiolysis was significantly associated with the development of an os acromiale (OR = 138, $P < .001$) and rotator cuff tears (OR = 5.4, $P = .015$) after age 25 years.

Conclusion.—Acromial apophysiolysis is characterized by incomplete fusion and edema at the acromial apophyses. It is associated with superior shoulder pain in young patients (<25 years old), and pitching is a risk factor. It predisposes the patient to the development of an os acromiale and rotator cuff tears after age 25 years.

▶ This is a very good study from a reputable institution. The methodology is sound, the question being addressed is relevant, and the conclusions are credible. The summary says it all. Approximately 2.5% of young pitchers with shoulder pain will have this condition. It is associated with more than 100 pitches per week in the young pitcher. The finding of edema is the key to the MRI diagnosis (Fig 2 in the original article). Importantly, the investigators go on to demonstrate late effects of an increased frequency of os acromiale as well as with rotator cuff problems in those older than 25 years. Overall, a very important study.

B. F. Morrey, MD

A Systematic Review of Ulnar Collateral Ligament Reconstruction Techniques

Watson JN, McQueen P, Hutchinson MR (Univ of Illinois at Chicago)
Am J Sports Med 42:2510-2516, 2014

Background.—Ulnar collateral ligament (UCL) reconstruction of the elbow has become increasingly more frequent among elite overhead athletes. The purpose of this study was to conduct a systematic review comparing the clinical outcomes and biomechanical results of the Jobe, modified Jobe, docking, modified docking, Endobutton, and interference screw techniques for UCL reconstruction.

Hypothesis.—The docking technique will have significantly fewer complications and improved return-to-play rate.

Study Design.—Systematic review; Level of evidence, 4.

Methods.—Using the Medline PubMed, Cochrane, and EMBASE databases, a search was performed of all published articles, including randomized controlled trials, cohort studies, and case series, examining UCL reconstructions performed using one of the above noted techniques and excluding case reports and hybrid techniques. Statistical analysis was performed using a χ^2 test of independence and 2-proportion Z test.

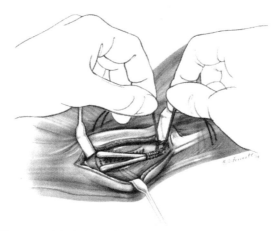

FIGURE 1.—Illustration of the docking technique. The anterior limb was passed into the humeral tunnel, and the sutures from both limbs were tied over the bone bridge to secure the graft. (Reprinted with permission from David W. Altchek.)

Results.—A total of 21 studies, 7 biomechanical and 14 clinical, met the inclusion criteria. There were 1368 patients. The overall complication rate was 18.6% (255/1368), further subdivided into 21 for the Jobe technique (29.2%), 203 for the modified Jobe technique (19.1%), 2 for the interference screw technique (10.0%), 2 (4.3%) for the modified docking technique, and 10 for the docking technique (6.0%). The most common complication across all studies was ulnar nerve neurapraxia in 176 patients (12.9%). The overall rate of return to play was 78.9%.

Conclusion.—Ulnar collateral ligament reconstruction utilizing the docking technique results in a significantly higher rate of return to play and a lower complication rate when compared with the Jobe and modified Jobe techniques.

Clinical Relevance.—A lower complication rate can lead to increased rates of return to play and better outcomes postoperatively (Fig 1).

▶ I was a bit surprised by the findings of this study. As is emerging as a standard, a systematic review attempting to identify and interpret quality articles were reviewed to glean insight into this question. The study has easy end points: success of the stabilization and incidence of complication. As might have been anticipated, the docking procedure or a modification of the technique emerged as effective, with a lower complication rate. It should be noted that the most frequent complication was that of ulnar nerve irritation. Dr Jobe was aware of this problem and modified his original technique to address the issue. To be honest, one reason to include this article was not just that it demonstrated the value of the docking technique but to give credit to Dr Jobe for his courage and innovation, which truly changed 1 aspect of "America's pastime." Dr Jobe died earlier this year; he is and will be missed.

B. F. Morrey, MD

Factors Related to the Need for Surgical Reconstruction After Anterior Cruciate Ligament Rupture: A Systematic Review of the Literature
Eggerding V, Meuffels DE, Bierma-Zeinstra SMA, et al (Erasmus Univ Med Ctr, Rotterdam, the Netherlands)
J Orthop Sports Phys Ther 45:37-44, 2015

Study Design.—Systematic literature review.

Objectives.—To summarize and evaluate research on factors predictive of progression to surgery after nonoperative treatment for an anterior cruciate ligament (ACL) rupture.

Background.—Anterior cruciate ligament rupture is a common injury among young, active individuals. Surgical reconstruction is often required for patients who do not regain satisfactory knee function following nonsurgical rehabilitation. Knowledge of factors that predict the need for surgical reconstruction of the ACL would be helpful to guide the decision-making process in this population.

Methods.—A search was performed for studies predicting the need for surgery after nonoperative treatment for ACL rupture in the Embase, MEDLINE (OvidSP), Web of Science, CINAHL, Cochrane Central Register of Controlled Trials, PubMed, and Google Scholar digital databases from inception to October 2013. Two reviewers independently selected the studies and performed a quality assessment. Best-evidence synthesis was used to summarize the evidence of factors predicting the need for surgical reconstruction after nonoperative treatment for an ACL rupture.

Results.—Seven studies were included, 3 of which were of high quality. Based on these studies, neither sex (strong evidence) nor the severity of knee joint laxity (moderate evidence) can predict whether, soon after ACL injury, a patient will need ACL reconstruction following nonoperative treatment. All other factors identified in this review either had conflicting or only minimal evidence as to their level of association with the need for surgical reconstruction. Noteworthy is that 1 high-quality study reported that the spherical shape of the femoral condyle was predictive of the need for ACL reconstruction.

Conclusion.—Sex and knee joint laxity tests do not predict the need for ACL reconstruction soon after an ACL rupture. Independent validation in future research will be necessary to establish whether knee shape is a predictive factor.

▶ I am not sure how to interpret this study. Obviously a rigorous process was employed to review almost 4000 citations and select only 7 for study, only 3 of which were considered of "high quality." I was sure the finding of meniscal pathology would be a factor in determining to stabilize after a period of observation. This was not the case. In addition, the study specifically noted that neither gender nor laxity predicted those undergoing stabilization procedures after a period of nonoperative management. My conclusion is that our literature is simply not adequate to address this question, or that although the process is rigorous, it does not accurately capture the clinical reality. For me, and based on numerous articles in the literature, a positive pivot shift is a clinical finding that requires surgery.

B. F. Morrey, MD

Incidence and Trends of Anterior Cruciate Ligament Reconstruction in the United States

Mall NA, Chalmers PN, Moric M, et al (Regeneration Orthopedics, St Louis, MO; Rush Univ Med Ctr, Chicago, IL)
Am J Sports Med 42:2363-2370, 2014

Background.—Anterior cruciate ligament (ACL) injury is among the most commonly studied injuries in orthopaedics. The previously reported incidence of ACL injury in the United States has varied considerably and is often based on expert opinion or single insurance databases.

Purpose.—To determine the incidence of ACL reconstruction (ACLR) in the United States; to identify changes in this incidence between 1994 and 2006; to identify changes in the demographics of ACLR over the same time period with respect to location (inpatient vs outpatient), sex, and age; and to determine the most frequent concomitant procedures performed at the time of ACLR.

Study Design.—Descriptive epidemiological study.

Methods.—*International Classification of Diseases, 9th Revision* (ICD-9) codes 844.2 and 717.83 were used to search the National Hospital Discharge Survey (NHDS) and the National Survey of Ambulatory Surgery (NSAS) for the diagnosis of ACL tear, and the procedure code 81.45 was used to search for ACLR. The incidence of ACLR in 1994 and 2006 was determined by use of US Census Data, and the results were then stratified based on patient age, sex, facility, concomitant diagnoses, and concomitant procedures.

Results.—The incidence of ACLR in the United States rose from 86,687 (95% CI, 51,844-121,530; 32.9 per 100,000 person-years) in 1994 to 129,836 (95% CI, 94,993-164,679; 43.5 per 100,000 person-years) in 2006 (*P* = .015). The number of ACLRs increased in patients younger

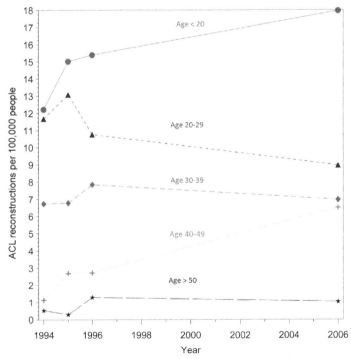

FIGURE 2.—Number of ACL reconstructions performed in the United States based on age. (Reprinted Mall NA, Chalmers PN, Moric M, et al. Incidence and trends of anterior cruciate ligament reconstruction in the United States. *Am J Sports Med.* 2014;42:2363-2370, with permission The Author(s).)

than 20 years and those who were 40 years or older over this 12-year period. The incidence of ACLR in females significantly increased from 10.36 to 18.06 per 100,000 person-years between 1994 and 2006 ($P =.0003$), while that in males rose at a slower rate, with an incidence of 22.58 per 100,000 person-years in 1994 and 25.42 per 100,000 person-years in 2006. In 2006, 95% of ACLRs were performed in an outpatient setting, while in 1994 only 43% of ACLRs were performed in an outpatient setting. The most common concomitant procedures were partial meniscectomy and chondroplasty.

Conclusion.—The incidence of ACLR increased between 1994 and 2006, particularly in females as well as those younger than 20 years and those 40 years or older. Research efforts as well as cost-saving measures may be best served by targeting prevention and outcomes measures in these groups. Surgeons should be aware that concomitant injury is common (Fig 2).

▶ As stated in previous editions, I make a real effort to avoid this section being synonymous with "anterior cruciate ligament (ACL) issues." I was interested to see the objective data of what is known to be occurring. There are more and more ACL reconstructions being done from 33 in 100 000 in 1994 to 43 in 100 000 in 2006; $P < .015$. The issue is then, why? The answer is provided: There are more procedures being done on those aged under 20 and over 40 years (Fig 2). Documentation of the accepted standard of this as an outpatient procedure is reflected by 95% being outpatient procedures in 2006. Today it must be close to 100%. What I would like to know is the motivation or basis for the dramatic increase in this procedure. One can only speculate; I would hope it is based on data demonstrating the ACL reconstruction is protective against future pathology, as opposed to some other less scientific motivation.

B. F. Morrey, MD

Anterior Cruciate Ligament Tears in Children and Adolescents: A Meta-analysis of Nonoperative Versus Operative Treatment

Ramski DE, Kanj WW, Franklin CC, et al (St Luke's Univ Health Network Orthopaedic Residency Program, Bethlehem, PA; Harvard Combined Orthopaedic Residency Program, Boston, MA; Shriners Hosp for Children, Philadelphia, PA; et al)
Am J Sports Med 42:2769-2776, 2014

Background.—Debate regarding the optimal initial treatment for anterior cruciate ligament (ACL) injuries in children and adolescents has not resulted in a clear consensus for initial nonoperative treatment or operative reconstruction.

Hypothesis/Purpose.—The purpose of this meta-analysis was to systematically analyze aggregated data from the literature to determine if a benefit exists for either nonoperative or early operative treatment for ACL injuries in the pediatric patient. The hypothesis was that combined results would favor early operative reconstruction with respect to posttreatment episodes of instability/pathological laxity, symptomatic meniscal tears, clinical outcome scores, and return to activity.

Study Design.—Meta-analysis.

Methods.—A literature selection process included the extraction of data on the following clinical variables: symptomatic meniscal tears, return to activities, clinical outcome scores, return to the operating room, and posttreatment instability/pathological laxity. A symptomatic meniscal tear was defined as occurring after the initial presentation, limiting activity, and requiring further treatment. Instability/pathological laxity was defined for the sake of this study as having an episode of giving way, a grade ≥ 2 Lachman/pivot-shift test result, or a side-to-side difference of >4 mm as measured by the KT-1000 arthrometer. All studies were evaluated using a formal study quality analysis. Meta-analysis was conducted for aggregated data in each category.

Results.—Six studies (217 patients) comparing operative to nonoperative treatment and 5 studies (353 patients) comparing early to delayed reconstruction were identified. Three studies reported posttreatment instability/pathological laxity; 13.6% of patients after operative treatment experienced instability/pathological laxity compared with 75% of patients after nonoperative treatment ($P < .01$). Two studies reported symptomatic meniscal tears; patients were over 12 times more likely to have a medial meniscal tear after nonoperative treatment than after operative treatment (35.4% vs 3.9%, respectively; $P = .02$). A significant difference in scores between groups was noted in 1 of 2 studies reporting International Knee Documentation Committee (IKDC) scores ($P = .002$) and in 1 of 2 studies reporting Tegner scores ($P = .007$). Two studies reported return to activity; none of the patients in the nonoperative groups returned to their previous level of play compared with 85.7% of patients in the operative groups ($P < .01$). Study quality analysis revealed that the majority of the studies were inconsistent in reporting outcomes.

Conclusion.—Meta-analysis revealed multiple trends that favor early surgical stabilization over nonoperative or delayed treatment. Patients after nonoperative and delayed treatment experienced more instability/pathological laxity and inability to return to previous activity levels than did patients treated with early surgical stabilization (Fig 2).

▶ With most, if not all, such studies, we anticipate the final conclusion that more data from better constructed studies are needed, and this report is no exception. Yet, despite using only 11 of 3324 published reports, it does provide some useful information. Even in the adolescent athlete, reconstructing the anterior cruciate ligament is of value. The limited data do show greater stability after reconstruction, *P* < .01 (Fig 2). The data also show fewer subsequent meniscal injuries and a greater likelihood of returning to sport. So, while we

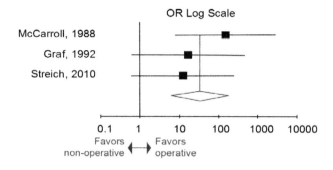

Study	Patients with instability/pathologic laxity		Weight of study (based on number of patients)	Odds Ratio (95% CI)
	Non-op	Op		
McCarroll (1988)	16/16	4/24	36%	150.3 (7.5-2997.8)
Graf (1992)	8/8	2/4	29%	17 (0.6-483.5)
Streich (2010)	3.5/12.5	0.5/16.5	35%	12.44 (0.6-269.1)
Totals	27.5/36.5	6.5/44.5	100%	33.75 (5.6-205.33)

FIGURE 2.—Results of aggregate analysis for comparison of instability/pathological laxity. (Reprinted from Ramski DE, Kanj WW, Franklin CC, et al. Anterior cruciate ligament tears in children and adolescents: a meta-analysis of nonoperative versus operative treatment. *Am J Sports Med.* 2014;42:2769-2776, with permission from The Author(s).)

await multicenter randomized studies, we do have some information to guide our way forward.

B. F. Morrey, MD

Are Magnetic Resonance Imaging Recovery and Laxity Improvement Possible After Anterior Cruciate Ligament Rupture in Nonoperative Treatment?

van Meer BL, Oei EH, Bierma-Zeinstra SM, et al (Univ Med Ctr Rotterdam, The Netherlands; et al)
Arthroscopy 30:1092-1099, 2014

Purpose.—This study aimed to determine whether anterior cruciate ligament (ACL) features on magnetic resonance imaging (MRI) and knee laxity are improved 2 years after ACL rupture treated nonoperatively and to analyze the relation between changes in scores of ACL features and changes in laxity.

Methods.—One hundred fifty-four eligible patients were included in a prospective multicenter cohort study with 2-year follow-up. Inclusion criteria were (1) ACL rupture diagnosed by physical examination and MRI, (2) MRI within 6 months after trauma, and (3) age 18 to 45 years. Laxity tests and MRI were performed at baseline and at 2-year follow-up. Fifty of 143 patients, for whom all MRI data was available, were treated nonoperatively and were included for this study. Nine ACL features were scored using MRI: fiber continuity, signal intensity, slope of ACL with respect to the Blumensaat line, distance between the Blumensaat line and the ACL, tension, thickness, clear boundaries, assessment of original insertions, and assessment of the intercondylar notch. A total score was determined by summing scores for each feature.

Results.—Fiber continuity improved in 30 patients (60%), and the empty intercondylar notch resolved for 22 patients (44%). Improvement in other ACL features ranged from 4% to 28%. Sixteen patients (32%) improved on the Lachman test (change from soft to firm end points [n = 14]; decreased anterior translation [n = 2]), one patient (2%) showed improvement with the KT-1000 arthrometer (MEDmetric, San Diego, CA) and 4 patients (8%) improved on the pivot shift test. Improvement on the Lachman test was moderately negatively associated with the total score of ACL features at follow-up. Analyzing ACL features separately showed that only signal intensity improvement, clear boundaries, and intercondylar notch assessment were positively associated with improvement on the Lachman test.

Conclusions.—Two years after ACL rupture and nonoperative management, patients experienced partial recovery on MRI, and some knee laxity improvement was present. Improvement of ACL features on MRI correlates moderately with improved laxity.

Level of Evidence.—Level II, Prospective comparative study (Fig 1).

▶ As we increasingly rely on imaging to make our clinical diagnosis and even substitute the findings for clinical judgment, this is a useful assessment. The methodology would seem legitimate to answer the question: Can we rely on

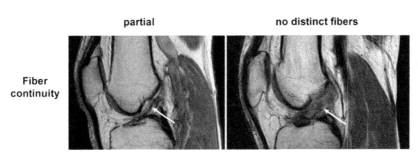

FIGURE 1.—Fiber continuity (arrows: partially visible; no distinct fibers visible). MRI sequence: sagittal proton density weighted turbo spin echo (TSE); slice thickness, 3 mm; repetition time (TR)/time echo (TE), 2700/27 ms. (Reprinted from Arthroscopy: The Journal of Arthroscopic and Related Surgery. van Meer BL, Oei EH, Bierma-Zeinstra SM, et al. Are magnetic resonance imaging recovery and laxity improvement possible after anterior cruciate ligament rupture in nonoperative treatment? *Arthroscopy.* 2014;30:1092-1099, Copyright 2014, with permission from the Arthroscopy Association of North America.)

magnetic resonance imaging (MRI) to assess status of a nonoperated anterior cruciate ligament (ACL) tear? This particular study reveals that not all features of MRI correlate with the clinical findings. This includes the most important finding, fiber continuity (Fig 1). The authors' conclusion of a moderate correlation seems generous. I would conclude that MRI is not a reliable substitute for clinical assessment in the determination of ACL function after a nontreated ACL tear.

B. F. Morrey, MD

Cost-Effectiveness Analysis of Early Reconstruction Versus Rehabilitation and Delayed Reconstruction for Anterior Cruciate Ligament Tears
Mather RC III, Hettrich CM, Dunn WR, et al (Duke Univ School of Medicine, Durham, NC; Univ of Iowa School of Medicine; Univ of Wisconsin Med Ctr, Madison; et al)
Am J Sports Med 42:1583-1591, 2014

Background.—An initial anterior cruciate ligament (ACL) tear can be treated with surgical reconstruction or focused rehabilitation. The KANON (Knee Anterior cruciate ligament, NON-surgical versus surgical treatment) randomized controlled trial compared rehabilitation plus early ACL reconstruction (ACLR) to rehabilitation plus optional delayed ACLR and found no difference at 2 years by an intention-to-treat analysis of total Knee injury and Osteoarthritis Outcome Score (KOOS) results.

Purpose.—To compare the cost-effectiveness of early versus delayed ACLR.

Study Design.—Economic and decision analysis; Level of evidence, 2.

Methods.—A Markov decision model was constructed for a cost-utility analysis of early reconstruction (ER) versus rehabilitation plus optional delayed reconstruction (DR). Outcome probabilities and effectiveness were derived from 2 sources: the KANON study and the Multicenter Orthopaedic Outcomes Network (MOON) database. Collectively, these 2 sources provided data from 928 ACL-injured patients. Utilities were measured by the Short Form—6 dimensions (SF-6D). Costs were estimated from a societal perspective in 2012 US dollars. Costs and utilities were discounted in accordance with the United States Panel on Cost-Effectiveness in Health and Medicine. Effectiveness was expressed in quality-adjusted life-years (QALYs) gained. Principal outcome measures were average incremental costs, incremental effectiveness (as measured by QALYs), and net health benefits. Willingness to pay was set at $50,000, which is the currently accepted standard in the United States.

Results.—In the base case, the ER group resulted in an incremental gain of 0.28 QALYs over the DR group, with a corresponding lower overall cost to society of $1572. Effectiveness gains were driven by the low utility of an unstable knee and the lower utility for the DR group. The cost of rehabilitation and the rate of additional surgery drove the increased cost of the DR group. The most sensitive variable was the rate of knee

TABLE 2.—Results of Analysis for Base Case[a]

	Average Cost	Average QALYs Gained	Average Cost Difference	Average Difference in QALYs Gained	Cost-Effectiveness Ratio	Incremental Cost-Effectiveness Ratio
ER group	$19,883	5.12	—	+0.28	$3881/QALY	—
DR group	$21,454	4.84	$1572	—	$4434/QALY	Dominated[b]

[a]Costs are in US dollars. DR, delayed reconstruction; ER, early reconstruction; QALY, quality-adjusted life-year.

[b]The DR group resulted in a lower number of average QALYs gained while also at a higher average cost to the payer and is therefore "dominated" by the early anterior cruciate ligament (ACL) reconstruction strategy for the treatment of an ACL tear in the base case.

Reprinted from Mather RC III, Hettrich CM, Dunn WR, et al. Cost-Effectiveness Analysis of Early Reconstruction Versus Rehabilitation and Delayed Reconstruction for Anterior Cruciate Ligament Tears. *Am J Sports Med.* 2014;42:1583-1591.

instability after initial rehabilitation. When the rate of instability falls to 51.5%, DR is less costly, and when the rate of instability falls below 18.0%, DR becomes the preferred cost-effective strategy.

Conclusion.—An economic analysis of the timing of ACLR using data exclusively from the KANON trial, MOON cohort, and national average reimbursement revealed that early ACLR was more effective (improved QALYs) at a lower cost than rehabilitation plus optional delayed ACLR. Therefore, early ACLR should be the preferred treatment strategy from a societal health system perspective (Table 2).

▶ This is an excellent and very useful study. The question of the value of early vs late reconstruction is straightforward. The analysis to answer the question is surprisingly complex. A large, detailed database is necessary to address such a question. This is another example of the value of the MOON collaborative database. As a result of this analysis, the conclusion is cleanly documented in Table 2 and stated in the abstract. Early reconstruction is less costly by about $1570, primarily because of savings from less therapy utilization. This represents an approximately 7% lower cost. The impact of quality of life also favors early reconstruction (Table 2). However, it should be noted that this does not mean all patients should have an early reconstruction. The threshold analysis also demonstrated the potential value of initial trial of therapy in those with a lower-demand lifestyle. Overall, this is an excellent contribution.

B. F. Morrey, MD

Femoral Nerve Block Is Associated With Persistent Strength Deficits at 6 months After Anterior Cruciate Ligament Reconstruction in Pediatric and Adolescent Patients

Luo TD, Ashraf A, Dahm DL, et al (Mayo Clinic, Rochester, MN; Texas Tech Univ Health Sciences, Lubbock; et al)
Am J Sports Med 43:331-336, 2015

Background.—Femoral nerve block (FNB) has become a popular method of postoperative analgesia for anterior cruciate ligament (ACL) reconstruction in pediatric and adolescent patients. Successful rehabilitation after surgery involves return of quadriceps and hamstring strength.

Purpose.—To compare knee strength and function 6 months after ACL reconstruction in pediatric and adolescent patients who received FNB versus patients with no nerve block.

Study Design.—Cohort study; Level of evidence, 3.

Methods.—Patients 18 years or younger who underwent primary ACL reconstruction between 2000 and 2010 at a single institution were identified. If the patient was skeletally immature, a transphyseal ACL reconstruction was performed. Of these patients, 68% underwent reconstruction with a patellar tendon autograft, and in 32% of patients a hamstring autograft was utilized. There were 124 patients who met the study inclusion criteria, including 62 in the FNB group (31 males, 31 females) and 62 patients in the control group (25 males, 37 females). All study patients participated in a comprehensive rehabilitation program that included isokinetic strength and functional testing at 6 months postoperatively.

Results.—Univariate analysis showed a significantly higher deficit at 6 months in the FNB group with respect to fast isokinetic extension strength (17.6% vs 11.2%; $P = .01$) as well as fast (9.9% vs 5.7%; $P = .04$) and slow (13.0% vs 8.5%; $P = .03$) isokinetic flexion strength. There was no difference in slow isokinetic extension strength deficit between the 2 groups (FNB, 22.3% vs control, 18.7%; $P = .20$). With respect to function, there were no differences in deficit for vertical jump (FNB, 9.4% vs control, 11.3%; $P = .30$), single hop (7.6% vs 7.5%; $P = .96$), or triple hop (8.0% vs 6.6%; $P = .34$) between the 2 groups. A significantly higher percentage of patients in the control group met functional and isokinetic criteria for return to sports at 6 months (90.2% vs 67.7%; odds ratio, 4.37; $P = .002$).

Conclusion.—Pediatric and adolescent patients treated with FNB for postoperative analgesia after ACL reconstruction had significant isokinetic deficits in knee extension and flexion strength at 6 months when compared with patients who did not receive a nerve block. Patients without a block were 4 times more likely to meet criteria for clearance to return to sports at 6 months.

▶ The title of this study is enough to warrant its review. The authors enrolled more than 120 patients into the 1 arms of the study. The finding of delayed strength recovery is notable and relevant in the rehabilitative period to allow return to sport. I was especially impressed to note that the difference was a factor of 4 times the control—quite a difference. Interpretation and implication is obvious: Avoid a femoral nerve block in the adolescent. But what about the mature adult?

B. F. Morrey, MD

Anterior Cruciate Ligament Injury and Radiologic Progression of Knee Osteoarthritis: A Systematic Review and Meta-analysis

Ajuied A, Wong F, Smith C, et al (Guy's & St Thomas' NHS Foundation Trust, London, UK)
Am J Sports Med 42:2242-2252, 2014

Background.—Knee osteoarthritis after anterior cruciate ligament (ACL) injury has previously been reported. However, there has been no meta-analysis reporting the development and progression of osteoarthritis.

Purpose.—We present the first meta-analysis reporting on the development and progression of osteoarthritis after ACL injury at a minimum mean follow-up of 10 years, using a single and widely accepted radiologic classification, the Kellgren & Lawrence classification.

Study Design.—Meta-analysis.

Method.—Articles were included for systematic review if they reported radiologic findings of ACL-injured knees and controls using the Kellgren & Lawrence classification at a minimum mean follow-up period of 10 years. Appropriate studies were then included for meta-analysis.

Results.—Nine studies were included for systematic review, of which 6 studies were further included for meta-analysis. One hundred twenty-one of 596 (20.3%) ACL-injured knees had moderate or severe radiologic changes (Kellgren & Lawrence grade III or IV) compared with 23 of 465 (4.9%) uninjured ACL-intact contralateral knees. After ACL injury, irrespective of whether the patients were treated operatively or nonoperatively, the relative risk (RR) of developing even minimal osteoarthritis was 3.89 ($P < .00001$), while the RR of developing moderate to severe osteoarthritis (grade III and IV) was 3.84 ($P < .0004$). Nonoperatively treated ACL-injured knees had significantly higher RR (RR, 4.98; $P < .00001$) of developing any grade of osteoarthritis compared with those treated with reconstructive surgery (RR, 3.62; $P < .00001$). Investigation of progression to moderate or severe osteoarthritis (grade III or IV only) after 10 years showed that ACL-reconstructed knees had a significantly higher RR (RR, 4.71; $P < .00001$) compared with nonoperative management (RR, 2.41; $P = .54$). It was not possible to stratify for return to sports among the patients undergoing ACL reconstruction.

Conclusion.—Results support the proposition that ACL injury predisposes knees to osteoarthritis, while ACL reconstruction surgery has a role in reducing the risk of developing degenerative changes at 10 years. However, returning to sports activities after ligament reconstruction may exacerbate the development of arthritis (Figs 5 and 6).

▶ Once again, we turn to a meta-analysis to better understand an important issue within the discipline of sports medicine: What are the long-term implications of anterior cruciate ligament (ACL) injury and subsequent arthritis, with or without reconstruction? The research included almost 600 knees with a mean of 10 years' surveillance. The analysis revealed the anticipated correlation of ACL tear and subsequent arthrosis. It is noteworthy that this occurred in knees that

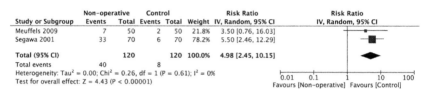

| Study or Subgroup | ACL Reconstruction | | Control | | Weight | Risk Ratio IV, Random, 95% CI | Risk Ratio IV, Random, 95% CI |
	Events	Total	Events	Total			
Hoffelner 2012	1	28	0	28	1.7%	3.00 [0.13, 70.64]	
Meuffels 2009	12	50	2	50	7.5%	6.00 [1.41, 25.44]	
Oiestad 2011	149	210	53	210	66.7%	2.81 [2.19, 3.60]	
Sutherland 2010	36	79	6	79	20.2%	6.00 [2.68, 13.43]	
van der Hart 2008	8	28	1	28	4.0%	8.00 [1.07, 59.81]	
Total (95% CI)		**395**		**395**	**100.0%**	**3.62 [2.40, 5.47]**	
Total events	206		62				

Heterogeneity: Tau² = 0.05; Chi² = 4.83, df = 4 (P = 0.31); I² = 17%
Test for overall effect: Z = 6.11 (P < 0.00001)

0.01 0.1 1 10 100
Favours [Reconstruction] Favours [Control]

FIGURE 5.—Forest plot of anterior cruciate ligament—reconstructed knees versus contralateral knees (control) in developing osteoarthritis. Relative risk = 3.62 ($P < .00001$), with heterogeneity of 17% ($P = .31$). (Reprinted from Ajuied A, Wong F, Smith C, et al. Anterior cruciate ligament injury and radiologic progression of knee osteoarthritis: a systematic review and meta-analysis. *Am J Sports Med.* 2014;42:2242-2252, with permission from The Author(s).)

| Study or Subgroup | Non-operative | | Control | | Weight | Risk Ratio IV, Random, 95% CI | Risk Ratio IV, Random, 95% CI |
	Events	Total	Events	Total			
Meuffels 2009	7	50	2	50	21.8%	3.50 [0.76, 16.03]	
Segawa 2001	33	70	6	70	78.2%	5.50 [2.46, 12.29]	
Total (95% CI)		**120**		**120**	**100.0%**	**4.98 [2.45, 10.15]**	
Total events	40		8				

Heterogeneity: Tau² = 0.00; Chi² = 0.26, df = 1 (P = 0.61); I² = 0%
Test for overall effect: Z = 4.43 (P < 0.00001)

0.01 0.1 1 10 100
Favours [Non-operative] Favours [Control]

FIGURE 6.—Forest plot of nonoperatively managed anterior cruciate ligament—injured knees versus contralateral knees (control) in developing osteoarthritis. Relative risk = 4.98 ($P < .00001$), with heterogeneity of 0% ($P = .61$). (Reprinted from Ajuied A, Wong F, Smith C, et al. Anterior cruciate ligament injury and radiologic progression of knee osteoarthritis: a systematic review and meta-analysis. *Am J Sports Med.* 2014;42:2242-2252, with permission from The Author(s).)

underwent reconstruction (Fig 5) as well as those treated without surgery (Fig 6). It is encouraging that those with reconstruction did have significantly less tendency to develop arthrosis. This supports the trend to offer reconstruction to both return the athlete to sport but also protect against the development of arthritis later in life.

B. F. Morrey, MD

Anterior Cruciate Ligament Injury, Return to Play, and Reinjury in the Elite Collegiate Athlete: Analysis of an NCAA Division I Cohort

Kamath GV, Murphy T, Creighton RA, et al (Univ of North Carolina at Chapel Hill)
Am J Sports Med 42:1638-1643, 2014

Background.—Graft survivorship, reinjury rates, and career length are poorly understood after anterior cruciate ligament (ACL) reconstruction in the elite collegiate athlete. The purpose of this study was to examine the outcomes of ACL reconstruction in a National Collegiate Athletic Association (NCAA) Division I athlete cohort.

Study Design.—Case series; Level of evidence, 4.

Methods.—A retrospective chart review was performed of all Division I athletes at a single public university from 2000 to 2009 until completion of

TABLE 2.—Incidence of ACL Reinjuries: Graft Failure or Contralateral Knee[a]

	Intracollegiate ACL Reconstruction (n = 54)	Precollegiate ACL Reconstruction (n = 35)
ACL reinjuries, n	7	14
Contralateral	6	7
Ispilateral	1	7[b]
Incidence, %	12.9	40.0

[a]ACL, anterior cruciate ligament.
[b]One athlete sustained a reinjury to the ACL revision.
Reprinted from Kamath GV, Murphy T, Creighton RA, et al. Anterior Cruciate Ligament Injury, Return to Play, and Reinjury in the Elite Collegiate Athlete: Analysis of an NCAA Division I Cohort. *Am J Sports Med.* 2014;42:1638-1643.

TABLE 4.—Total Years Played After Surgery and Percentage of Eligibility Used[a]

	During High School (n = 35 Athletes)	Freshman (n = 15 Athletes)	Sophomore (n = 15 Athletes)	Junior (n = 13 Athletes)	Senior (n = 11 Athletes)
Average years played after injury	3.11	2.00	1.73	0.77	0
Percentage of eligibility used	77.9	66.7	86.7		N/A
No. of patients with subsequent surgery	18	5	6	4	1
No. of revision ACL reconstructions	7	0	1	0	0
No. of contralateral ACL reconstructions	7	3	1	2	N/A

[a]All collegiate injuries/eligibility used = 76.7%. Return-to-play rate after primary ACL injury for intracollegiate group = 88.3%. Utilization of 100% eligibility = 60.0% (precollegiate group) and 65.1% (intracollegiate group). ACL, anterior cruciate ligament; N/A, not applicable.
Reprinted from Kamath GV, Murphy T, Creighton RA, et al. Anterior Cruciate Ligament Injury, Return to Play, and Reinjury in the Elite Collegiate Athlete: Analysis of an NCAA Division I Cohort. *Am J Sports Med.* 2014;42:1638-1643.

eligibility. Athletes were separated into 2 cohorts: those who underwent precollegiate ACL reconstruction (PC group) and those who underwent intracollegiate reconstruction (IC group). Graft survivorship, reoperation rates, and career length information were collected.

Results.—Thirty-five athletes were identified with precollegiate reconstruction and 54 with intracollegiate reconstruction. The PC group had a 17.1% injury rate with the original graft, with a 20.0% rate of a contralateral ACL injury. For the IC group, the reinjury rates were 1.9% with an ACL graft, with an 11.1% rate of a contralateral ACL injury after intracollegiate ACL reconstruction. The athletes in the PC group used 78% of their total eligibility (average, 3.11 years). The athletes in the IC group used an average of 77% of their remaining NCAA eligibility; 88.3% of those in the IC group played an additional non-redshirt year after their injury. The reoperation rate for the PC group was 51.4% and was 20.4% for the IC group.

Conclusion.—Reoperation and reinjury rates are high after ACL reconstruction in the Division I athlete. Precollegiate ACL reconstruction is associated with a very high (37.1%) rate of repeat ACL reinjuries to the graft or opposite knee. The majority of athletes are able to return to play after successful reconstruction (Tables 2 and 4).

▶ This study addresses 2 relevant issues. What is the likelihood of reinjury after anterior cruciate ligament reconstruction? This question is further stratified into those reconstructed before and during their college athletic career. In this sample, the risk of reinjury to the knee is placed at 40% of those entering college with a reconstructed knee; the incidence is only 13% of reinjury if this occurs during collegiate play (Table 2). Of interest, the majority, up to 80%, of injuries are to the contralateral knee. The additional question addresses the ability to effectively return to competition. This cohort exhibited 68% to 87% completion of eligibility, depending on the year injured (Table 4). The results are clean and of prognostic use to the surgeon caring for the collegiate athlete.

B. F. Morrey, MD

A Radiographic Assessment of Failed Anterior Cruciate Ligament Reconstruction: Can Magnetic Resonance Imaging Predict Graft Integrity?

Waltz RA, Solomon DJ, Provencher MT (Naval Health Clinic New England, Newport, RI; Marin Orthopedics and Sports Medicine, Novato, CA; Massachusetts General Hosp, Boston)
Am J Sports Med 42:1652-1660, 2014

Background.—Magnetic resonance imaging (MRI) showing an "intact" anterior cruciate ligament (ACL) graft may not correlate well with examination findings. Reasons for an ACL graft dysfunction may be from malpositioned tunnels, deficiency of secondary stabilizers, repeat injuries, or a combination of factors.

Purpose.—To evaluate the concordance/discordance of an ACL graft assessment between an arthroscopic evaluation, physical examination, and MRI and secondarily to evaluate the contributing variables to discordance.

Study Design.—Case series; Level of evidence, 4.

Methods.—A total of 50 ACL revisions in 48 patients were retrospectively reviewed. The ACL graft status was recorded separately based on Lachman and pivot-shift test data, arthroscopic findings from operative reports, and MRI evaluation and was categorized into 3 groups: intact, partial tear, or complete tear. Two independent evaluators reviewed all of the preoperative radiographs and MRI scans, and interrater and intrarater reliability were evaluated. Concordance and discordance between a physical examination, arthroscopic evaluation, and MRI evaluation of the ACL graft were calculated. Graft position and type, mechanical axis, collateral ligament injuries, chondral and meniscal injuries, and

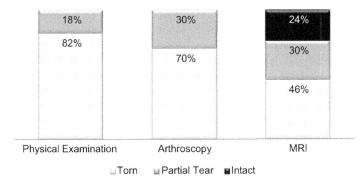

FIGURE 5.—This chart compares anterior cruciate ligament graft integrity on the 3 assessment modalities. No grafts were found to be intact on physical examination or arthroscopic evaluation; however, 24% of grafts were read as intact on magnetic resonance imaging. (Reprinted from Waltz RA, Solomon DJ, Provencher MT. A radiographic assessment of failed anterior cruciate ligament reconstruction: Can magnetic resonance imaging predict graft integrity? *Am J Sports Med.* 2014;42:1652-1660, with permission from The Author(s).)

mechanism of injury were evaluated as possible contributing factors using univariate and multivariate analyses. Sensitivity and specificity of MRI to detect a torn ACL graft and meniscal and chondral injuries on arthroscopic evaluation were calculated.

Results.—The interobserver and intraobserver reliability for the MRI evaluation of the ACL graft were moderate, with combined κ values of .41 and .49, respectively. The femoral tunnel position was vertical in 88% and anterior in 46%. On MRI, the ACL graft was read as intact in 24%; however, no graft was intact on arthroscopic evaluation or physical examination. The greatest discordance was between the physical examination and MRI, with a rate of 52%. An insidious-onset mechanism of injury was significantly associated with discordance between MRI and arthroscopic evaluation of the ACL ($P =.0003$) and specifically with an intact ACL graft on MRI ($P =.0014$). The sensitivity and specificity of MRI to detect an ACL graft tear were 60% and 87%, respectively.

Conclusion.—Caution should be used when evaluating a failed ACL graft with MRI, especially in the absence of an acute mechanism of injury, as it may be unreliable and inconsistent (Fig 5).

▶ This study had to be included in my selections because it emphasizes one of my major themes in diagnosis: examination must not be abandoned in favor of elaborate imaging. The study is quite relevant as we consistently rely on the magnetic resonance imaging (MRI) scan to determine the intactness of the reconstruction. This may be a mistake. The nicely designed evaluation employs a simple end point of arthroscopic demonstration of the presence or absence of the cruciate graft. Given this, the examination was markedly superior to MRI in determining the integrity of the anterior cruciate ligament reconstruction. The sensitivity of 60% is not only very useful, it would prompt me not to rely on an imaging modality to understand what is happening. The examination is more accurate, and because it measures instability, and not a shadow, it is more relevant.

B. F. Morrey, MD

11 Trauma and Amputation

Pelvic and Acetabular Fracture

Treatment of Acetabulum Fractures Through the Modified Stoppa Approach: Strategies and Outcomes
Isaacson MJ, Taylor BC, French BG, et al (Doctors' Hosp, Columbus, OH; Grant Med Ctr, Columbus, OH)
Clin Orthop Relat Res 472:3345-3352, 2014

Background.—Since the original description by Letournel in 1961, the ilioinguinal approach has remained the predominant approach for anterior acetabular fixation. However, modifications of the original abdominal approach described by Stoppa have made another option available for reduction and fixation of pelvic and acetabular fractures.

Questions/Purposes.—We evaluated our results in patients with acetabulum fractures with the modified Stoppa approach in terms of (1) hip function as measured by the Merle d'Aubigne hip score (2) complications and (3) quality of fracture reduction and percentage of fractures that united.

Methods.—Between September 2008 and August 2012, 289 patients with acetabular fractures were treated at our Level I trauma center. Twelve percent (36 of 289) of patients were treated operatively using the modified Stoppa approach. Ninety-seven percent (35 of 36) of our patients had fracture patterns involving displacement of the posterior column. Six (17%) were converted early to a total hip arthroplasty, and 14 (39%) were lost to final followup, leaving 22 of 36 for subjective clinical outcome analysis at a mean of 32 months (range, 9—59 months). Our general indications for this approach during the period in question were fractures of the anterior column and anterior wall, anterior column with posterior hemitransverse fractures, both column fractures, transverse fractures, and T-type fractures. Followup included regularly scheduled office visits with radiographs (AP pelvis, Judet views) that were graded by the treating surgeon and by the authors of this study (MJI, BCT) and patient outcome surveys.

Results.—Merle d'Aubigne hip scores were very good in 55% (12 of 22), good in 9% (two of 22), medium in 18% (four of 22), fair in 5% (one of 22), and poor in 14% (three of 22), and 70% (23 of 33) of patients were able to ambulate without any assistive devices. Complications included one superficial infection and three deep infections, two patients with temporary lateral thigh numbness, no obturator nerve palsies, and one inguinal hernia. Three deaths in the cohort were seen in followup as a result of unrelated causes. Radiographic grading of fracture reductions after surgery revealed that 27 (75%) were anatomic, six (17%) were satisfactory, and three (8%) were unsatisfactory. A total of 94% of the fractures united.

Conclusions.—In agreement with prior published data, our results show good functional outcomes with minimal complications using the modified Stoppa approach for a variety of acetabular fractures. Our results highlight the difficulty but feasibility in treating posterior column displacement through an anterior approach. Consideration for dual approaches with posterior column involvement may be warranted to optimize fracture reduction and functional outcomes.

Level of Evidence.—Level IV, therapeutic study. See Guidelines for Authors for a complete description of levels of evidence.

▶ The use of the modified Stoppa approach in the treatment of acetabular fractures has gained popularity recently. This approach provides access to parts of the anterior and posterior column as well as the quadrilateral surface. Its usefulness is most evident in the treatment of the anterior column posterior hemitransverse fracture pattern, a pattern commonly encountered in geriatric acetabular fractures. These fractures demonstrate the medialization of the femoral head as the entire quadrilateral surface is displaced medially. Controlling these fractures through a standard ilioinguinal approach relied on "drop-down" screws placed through an anterior column plate into the quadrilateral surface and posterior column. These screws were susceptible to toggling and subsequent displacement of the fracture. The modified Stoppa approach allows direct fixation of the quadrilateral surface with a buttress plate for increased resistance to displacement.

The complication rate in this study demonstrates that this approach is safe and can be performed with lower risks compared with historic controls using the ilioinguinal approach. This approach should be considered an option when the acetabular surgeon encounters fractures with significant quadrilateral surface involvement.

S. A. Sems, MD

Acetabular fractures with marginal impaction: mid-term results
Giannoudis PV, Kanakaris NK, Delli Sante E, et al (Leeds Teaching Hosps NHS Trust, UK; et al)
Bone Joint J 95-B:230-238, 2013

Over a five-year period, adult patients with marginal impaction of acetabular fractures were identified from a registry of patients who underwent acetabular reconstruction in two tertiary referral centres. Fractures were classified according to the system of Judet and Letournel. A topographic classification to describe the extent of articular impaction was used, dividing the joint surface into superior, middle and inferior thirds. Demographic information, hospitalisation and surgery-related complications, functional (EuroQol 5-D) and radiological outcome according to Matta's criteria were recorded and analysed. In all, 60 patients (57 men, three women) with a mean age of 41 years (18 to 72) were available at a mean follow-up of 48 months (24 to 206). The quality of the reduction was 'anatomical' in 44 hips (73.3%) and 'imperfect' in 16 (26.7%). The originally achieved anatomical reduction was lost in 12 patients (25.8%). Radiologically, 33 hips (55%) were graded as 'excellent', 11 (18.3%) as 'good', one (1.7%) as 'fair' and 15 (25%) as 'poor'. A total of 11 further operations were required in 11 cases, of which six were total hip replacements.

Univariate linear regression analysis of the functional outcome showed that factors associated with worse pain were increasing age and an inferior location of the impaction. Elevation of the articular impaction leads to joint preservation with satisfactory overall medium-term functional results, but secondary collapse is likely to occur in some patients.

▶ Marginal impaction occurs during acetabular fractures when the femoral head is driven into the acetabular cartilage and it flattens the contour of the acetabulum as the femoral head is displacing. Previous studies have shown that this is an independent predictor of poor outcome and subsequent need for further surgery and hip arthroplasty. This study presents midterm results of acetabular fractures with marginal impaction. The ultimate outcomes in this cohort, which had a mean follow-up of 48 months, are comparable with the results of previous studies, with 10% requiring total hip arthroplasty. In this study, better reductions were associated with better outcomes, and the development of less heterotopic bone was also associated with better outcomes.

When marginally impacted segments are mobilized and reduced into their anatomic locations, a defect is left. In this study, graft substitutes were used to fill this defect almost 60% of the time with autologous bone graft being used 20% of the time. In more than 20% of cases in this study, no graft was used to support the marginally impacted segments. The authors did note that better outcomes were associated with the use of bone graft, particularly the graft substitutes. Given this finding and the understanding that large defects occur following elevation of marginally impacted segments, the use of bone grafts or bone grafts substitutes is highly recommended.

Postoperative CT scans are helpful to assess the quality of the postoperative reduction, particularly for posterior wall fractures. This study just used plain radiographs to evaluate the subsequent reductions, but the CT scans give much more information in detail regarding the quality of the reduction of the marginally impacted segments. Surgeons may find the information they get from postoperative CT scans helpful to objectively evaluate their performance in reducing the fracture.

S. A. Sems, MD

Open Reduction and Internal Fixation of Acetabulum Fractures: Does Timing of Surgery Affect Blood Loss and OR Time?

Dailey SK, Archdeacon MT (Univ of Cincinnati, OH)
J Orthop Trauma 28:497-501, 2014

Objectives.—The purpose of this study was to investigate the timing of surgical intervention for fractures of the acetabulum and its influence on perioperative factors.

Design.—Retrospective review.

Setting.—Level I trauma center.

Patients.—Two hundred eighty-eight consecutive patients who sustained either posterior wall (*PW*), associated both column (*ABC*), or anterior column posterior hemitransverse (*ACPHT*) acetabulum fractures were included in the study.

Intervention.—One hundred seventy-six PW fractures were treated through a Kocher—Langenbeck approach, and 112 ABC/ACPHT fractures were treated through an anterior intrapelvic approach.

Main Outcome Measurements.—Estimated blood loss (EBL), operative time.

Results.—EBL (800 vs. 400 mL), operative time (270 vs.154 minutes), and hospital stay (11 vs. 7 days) were greater for the ABC/ACPHT fractures compared with the PW fractures. When comparing early (≤48 hours) versus late (>48 hours) treatment of PW fractures, there was no difference in EBL (400 vs. 400 mL, $P = 0.37$) or operative time (150 vs. 156 minutes, $P = 0.50$). In comparison of early versus late treatment of ABC/ACPHT fractures, no significant difference was noted in EBL (725 vs. 800 mL, $P = 0.30$) or operative time (258.5 vs. 272 minutes, $P = 0.21$).

Conclusions.—We found no advantage or disadvantage in terms of EBL or operative time for early (≤48 hours) versus late (>48 hours) fixation for either PW or ABC/ACPHT acetabular fractures.

Level of Evidence.—Therapeutic Level III. See Instructions for Authors for a complete description of levels of evidence.

▶ Open reduction and internal fixation of acetabular fractures is a challenging and time-consuming endeavor. The most reliable predictor of outcomes after the surgical treatment of these fractures is the quality of the reduction, so surgeons treating these fractures should be patient, focused, and willing to spend as much time as necessary performing the surgery to get the best outcome possible.

The decision on when to operate on these fractures is influenced by many factors, including the associated injuries and the status of the patient's resuscitation. In this retrospective study, the patients who underwent fixation less than 48 hours from injury had the same amount of blood loss as patients whose surgery was delayed past 48 hours. Unsurprisingly, the Injury Severity Scores in the delayed group were higher than the early group, yet these more severely injured patients did not experience more blood loss.

This article reinforces that early fixation of acetabular fractures in certain patients, particularly those with isolated injuries, can be considered without concern for increased blood loss. Although the patients who were treated with early fixation also experienced shorter lengths of stay, these authors were unable to conclude that early fixation caused the shorter length of stay, just that they were associated. Without controlling for the associated injuries and reason the surgery occurred at the time that it did, this relationship is unclear.

The equal blood loss between the groups indicates that the method the authors use to determine the timing of fixation of acetabular fractures is practical and effective at not exposing their patients to increased risks of bleeding, either early or late. Unfortunately, this article does not describe an algorithm that the authors used to determine when to operate.

Surgeons treating acetabular fractures should not feel that they must wait more than 48 hours to perform internal fixation on a stable and resuscitated patient. Early internal fixation is a reasonable option.

S. A. Sems, MD

Indomethacin Prophylaxis for Heterotopic Ossification after Acetabular Fracture Surgery Increases the Risk for Nonunion of the Posterior Wall
Sagi HC, Jordan CJ, Barei DP, et al (Florida Orthopaedic Inst, Tampa; Harborview Med Ctr, Seattle, WA)
J Orthop Trauma 28:377-383, 2014

Objectives.—To determine if indomethacin has a positive clinical effect for the prophylaxis of heterotopic ossification (HO) after acetabular fracture surgery. To determine whether indomethacin affects the union rate of acetabular fractures.

Design.—Prospective randomized double-blinded trial.

Setting.—Level 1 regional trauma center.

Patients.—Skeletally mature patients treated operatively for an acute acetabular fracture through a Kocher-Langenbeck approach.

Intervention.—Patients were randomly allocated to 1 of 4 groups comparing placebo (group 1) to 3 days (group 2), 1 week (group 3), and 6 weeks (group 4) of indomethacin treatment.

Main Outcome Measurements.—Factors analyzed included the overall incidence, Brooker class and volume of HO, radiographic union of the acetabular fracture, and pain. Patients were followed clinically and radiographically at 6 weeks, 3 months, 6 months, and 1 year. Serum levels of indomethacin were drawn at 1 month to assess compliance. Computed tomographic scans were performed at 6 months to assess healing and volume of HO.

Results.—Ninety-eight patients were enrolled into this study, 68 completed the follow-up and had the 6-month computed tomographic scan, and there was a 63% compliance rate with the treatment regimen. Overall incidence of HO was 67% for group 1, 29% for group 2 ($P = 0.04$), 29% for group 3 ($P = 0.019$), and 67% for group 4. The volume of HO formation was 17,900 mm^3 for group 1, 33,800 mm^3 for group 2, 6300 mm^3 for group 3 ($P = 0.005$), and 11,100 mm^3 for group 4. The incidence of radiographic nonunion was 19% for group 1, 35% for group 2, 24% for group 3, and 62% for group 4 ($P = 0.012$). Seventy-seven percent of the nonunions involved the posterior wall segment. Pain visual analog scores (VASs) were significantly higher for patients with radiographic nonunion (VAS 4 vs. VAS 1, $P = 0.002$).

Conclusions.—Treatment with 6 weeks of indomethacin does not appear to have a therapeutic effect for decreasing HO formation after acetabular fracture surgery and appears to increase the incidence of nonunion. Treatment with 1 week of indomethacin may be beneficial for decreasing the volume of HO formation without increasing the incidence of nonunion.

Level of Evidence.—Therapeutic Level II. See Instructions for Authors for a complete description of levels of evidence.

▶ Heterotopic ossification after open reduction and internal fixation of acetabular fractures through the Kocher–Langenbeck approach can result in significant dysfunction and limited range of motion. Strategies to decrease the formation of heterotopic ossification after this approach have included medical treatment with indomethacin, local radiation, and thorough debridement of devitalized and traumatized musculature in the zone of injury. In this prospective, double-blinded, placebo-controlled trial, patients who sustained acetabular fractures treated through a Kocher–Langenbeck approach were randomized to receive either a placebo or differing lengths or administrations of indomethacin treatment. The patients treated for the longest time interval with indomethacin had a much higher rate of radiographic nonunion of the posterior wall. The group that received indomethacin for 1 week had a lower incidence of heterotopic ossification compared with the placebo group, yet it did not experience the high rate of nonunion seen in the group treated for 6 weeks. This study also highlights the relative poor compliance rate for patients taking indomethacin for 6 weeks (63%). The authors appropriately conclude that prolonged (6 weeks) use of indomethacin is not indicated after acetabular surgery and is associated with increased risk of acetabular nonunion. Further study is required to confirm that a 75-mg daily dose of indomethacin for 1 week results in the desired heterotopic ossification prevention without increasing nonunion rates.

S. A. Sems, MD

Femur Fractures

An anatomical study of the entry point in the greater trochanter for intramedullary nailing

Farhang K, Desai R, Wilber JH, et al (Case Western Reserve Univ, Cleveland, OH)
Bone Joint J 96-B:1274-1281, 2014

Malpositioning of the trochanteric entry point during the introduction of an intramedullary nail may cause iatrogenic fracture or malreduction.

Although the optimal point of insertion in the coronal plane has been well described, positioning in the sagittal plane is poorly defined.

The paired femora from 374 cadavers were placed both in the anatomical position and in internal rotation to neutralise femoral anteversion. A marker was placed at the apparent apex of the greater trochanter, and the lateral and anterior offsets from the axis of the femoral shaft were measured on anteroposterior and lateral photographs. Greater trochanteric morphology and trochanteric overhang were graded.

The mean anterior offset of the apex of the trochanter relative to the axis of the femoral shaft was 5.1 mm (SD 4.0) and 4.6 mm (SD 4.2) for the anatomical and neutralised positions, respectively. The mean lateral offset of the apex was 7.1 mm (SD 4.6) and 6.4 mm (SD 4.6), respectively.

Placement of the entry position at the apex of the greater trochanter in the anteroposterior view does not reliably centre an intramedullary nail in the sagittal plane. Based on our findings, the site of insertion should be about 5 mm posterior to the apex of the trochanter to allow for its anterior offset.

▶ Varus malreduction with apex anterior angulation of subtrochanteric femoral fractures during intramedullary nail fixation occurs in part due to the surgeon choosing a poor starting point for nail insertion. Lateral starting points result in varus malreduction, whereas anterior starting points contribute to flexion deformities at the fracture site. This article reviews the osseous anatomy of the proximal femur as it relates to intramedullary nail starting points in the greater trochanter. Starting the intramedullary nail slightly posterior to the apex of the greater trochanter allows the intramedullary nail to be centered in the sagittal plane. The apex of the greater trochanter on the anteroposterior view is similar in anatomic and neutralized positions and is lateral to the axis of the femoral shaft. This offset must be accounted for when placing intramedullary nails through the trochanteric entry point, and the particular geometry of each nail should be considered as the starting point is selected. Perfect intraoperative imaging is required to obtain the specific starting point that will prevent contributing to deformity. Intraoperative lateral imaging requires matching the image intensifier with the femoral neck anteversion, thus aligning the femoral head, neck, trochanter, and femoral canal. Once this view is obtained, the starting point just posterior to the apex of the greater trochanter can be identified, and an in-line starting point can be obtained.

S. A. Sems, MD

Ipsilateral Proximal Femur and Shaft Fractures Treated With Hip Screws and a Reamed Retrograde Intramedullary Nail

Ostrum RF, Tornetta P III, Watson JT, et al (Univ of North Carolina, Chapel Hill; Boston Univ Med Ctr, MA; St. Louis Univ Hosp, MO; et al)
Clin Orthop Relat Res 472:2751-2758, 2014

Background.—Although not common, proximal femoral fractures associated with ipsilateral shaft fractures present a difficult management problem. A variety of surgical options have been employed with varying results.

Questions/Purposes.—We investigated the use of hip screws and a reamed retrograde intramedullary (IM) nail for the treatment of this combined fracture pattern in terms of postoperative alignment (malunion), nonunion, and complications.

Methods.—Between May 2002 and October 2011, a total of 95 proximal femoral fractures with associated shaft fractures were treated at three participating Level 1 trauma centers; all were treated with hip screw fixation (cannulated screws or sliding hip screws) and retrograde reamed IM nails. The medical records of these patients were reviewed retrospectively for alignment, malunion, nonunion, and complications. Followup was available on 92 of 95 (97%) of the patients treated with hip screws and a retrograde nail. Forty were treated with a sliding hip screw, and 52 were treated with cannulated screws.

Results.—There were five proximal malunions in this series (5%). The union rate was 98% (90 of 92) for the femoral neck fractures and 91.3% (84 of 92) for the femoral shaft fractures after the initial surgery. There were two nonunions of comminuted femoral neck fractures after cannulated screw fixation. There was no difference in femoral neck union or alignment when comparing cannulated screws to a sliding hip screw. Four open comminuted femoral shaft fractures went on to nonunion and required secondary surgery to obtain union, and one patient developed symptomatic avascular necrosis.

Conclusions.—The treatment of ipsilateral proximal femoral neck and shaft fractures with hip screw fixation and a reamed retrograde nail demonstrated a high likelihood of union for the femoral neck fractures and a low risk of malunion. Comminution and initial displacement of the proximal femoral fracture may still lead to a small incidence of malunion or nonunion, and open comminuted femoral shaft fractures still may progress to nonunion despite appropriate surgical management.

Level of Evidence.—Level IV, therapeutic study. See Instructions for Authors for a complete description of levels of evidence.

▶ Combined injuries to the femoral shaft and femoral neck occur about 5% of the time the femoral shaft is fractured. Obtaining accurate reduction and stabilization of the femoral neck fracture may require approaches and implants that compromise antegrade nail placement for the femoral shaft fracture. This study described the technique and results of retrograde nail fixation after fixation or stabilization of the femoral neck fracture.

The described surgical technique discusses using a Shanz pin in the middle floating shaft fragment to manipulate and reduce the femoral neck fracture. Unlike femoral neck fractures with an intact femoral shaft, applying traction through a traction pin or traction boot will not allow the surgeon to control the shaft and distal aspect of the femoral neck, and reduction of the femoral neck is nearly impossible if the distal piece of the femoral neck is not controlled.

Using a Shanz pin in the femoral shaft to control this fragment will greatly improve the surgeon's chances of obtaining an anatomic reduction.

The results of this study compare favorably to studies that have used a single cephalomedullary implant. The technique of initial reduction and stabilization of the femoral neck followed by retrograde nail fixation for combined femoral neck and femoral shaft fractures appears to result in low rates of complications and high rates of union.

S. A. Sems, MD

Assessing Leg Length After Fixation of Comminuted Femur Fractures
Herscovici D Jr, Scaduto JM (Florida Orthopaedic Inst, Temple Terrace)
Clin Orthop Relat Res 472:2745-2750, 2014

Background.—Nailing comminuted femur fractures may result in leg shortening, producing significant complications including pelvic tilt, narrowing of the hip joint space, mechanical and functional changes in gait, an increase in energy expenditures, and strains on spinal ligaments, leading to spinal deformities. The frequency of this complication in patients managed with an intramedullary (IM) nail for comminuted diaphyseal fractures is unknown.

Questions/Purposes.—We therefore determined (1) the frequency of LLDs, (2) whether a specific fracture pattern was associated with LLDs, (3) the frequency of reoperation, and (4) whether revision fixation ultimately corrected the LLD.

Methods.—We studied 83 patients with 91 AO/OTA Type B or Type C fractures fixed with either an antegrade or retrograde IM nail from July 2002 through December 2005. There were 60 males and 23 females, with a mean age of 30 years (range, 15–79 years). All underwent a digitized CT scan in the immediate postoperative period. Measurements of both legs were performed. Any fixation producing a discrepancy and requiring a return to surgery was identified.

Results.—A mean LLD of 0.58 cm was found in 98% of the patients, but only six (7%) patients had an LLD of greater than 1.25 cm. No fracture pattern or the presentation of bilateral injuries demonstrated a greater incidence of LLD. Of the patients with LLD, two patients refused further surgery while the remaining four patients, two Type B and two Type C fractures, ultimately underwent revision fixation. Repeat CT scans after revision surgery of all four patients demonstrated a residual LLD of only 0.2 cm.

Conclusions.—Postoperative CT scans appear to be an efficient method to measure femoral length after IM nailing. Although residual LLDs may be common in comminuted femurs treated with IM nails, most LLDs do not appear to be functionally relevant. When an LLD of greater than 1.5 cm is identified, it should be discussed with the patient, who should be told that potential complications may occur with larger LLDs and that sometimes patients may benefit from repeat surgery.

Level of Evidence.—Level IV, therapeutic study. See Instructions for Authors for a complete description of levels of evidence.

▶ Intramedullary locked nail fixation of comminuted femoral shaft fractures may result in leg length discrepancies and rotational deformities if the nail is not locked with the limb at the proper length and alignment. This study performed computed tomography scans in the postoperative period to allow for evaluation of the femoral lengths. The majority of patients had a small discrepancy (less than a centimeter) between the femoral lengths, and no revision surgery was performed. The discussion also nicely covers the issues related to limb length discrepancy in the uninjured population and highlights the fact that many completely asymptomatic people may have measurable leg length differences.

Evaluating the femoral length after intramedullary nail fixation can be difficult for many reasons. The procedures are commonly performed on a fracture table, and the uninjured limb is not accessible in the operative field to compare the length. Surgeons can use an intraoperative ruler to measure the contralateral femur from the tip of the greater trochanter to the center of the intercondylar notch before positioning the patient on the fracture table. Then, when the injured femur is stabilized, the traction control on the table can be adjusted until the appropriate length is restored. This technique may be used in c-type fractures, which do not allow the direct assessment of length due to comminution.

S. A. Sems, MD

Hip Fracture

Predictors of failure for cephalomedullary nailing of proximal femoral fractures
Kashigar A, Vincent A, Gunton MJ, et al (Mount Sinai Hosp, Toronto, Ontario, Canada; Univ of Toronto, Ontario, Canada)
Bone Joint J 96-B:1029-1034, 2014

The purpose of this study was to identify factors that predict implant cut-out after cephalomedullary nailing of intertrochanteric and subtrochanteric hip fractures, and to test the significance of calcar referenced tip-apex distance (CalTAD) as a predictor for cut-out.

We retrospectively reviewed 170 consecutive fractures that had undergone cephalomedullary nailing. Of these, 77 met the inclusion criteria of a non-pathological fracture with a minimum of 80 days radiological follow-up (mean 408 days; 81 days to 4.9 years). The overall cut-out rate was 13% (10/77).

The significant parameters in the univariate analysis were tip-apex distance (TAD) ($p < 0.001$), CalTAD ($p = 0.001$), cervical angle difference ($p = 0.004$), and lag screw placement in the anteroposterior (AP) view (Parker's ratio index) ($p = 0.003$). Non-significant parameters were age ($p = 0.325$), gender ($p = 1.000$), fracture side ($p = 0.507$), fracture type (AO classification) ($p = 0.381$), Singh Osteoporosis Index ($p = 0.575$), lag screw placement in the lateral view ($p = 0.123$), and reduction quality (modified Baumgaertner's method) ($p = 0.575$). In the multivariate analysis, CalTAD was the only significant measurement ($p = 0.001$). CalTAD had almost perfect inter-observer reliability (interclass correlation coefficient (ICC) 0.901).

Our data provide the first reported clinical evidence that CalTAD is a predictor of cut-out. The finding of CalTAD as the only significant parameter in the multivariate analysis, along with the univariate significance of Parker's ratio index in the AP view, suggest that inferior placement of the lag screw is preferable to reduce the rate of cut-out.

▶ Cephalomedullary nail use in the treatment of proximal femoral fractures has surpassed the sliding hip screw in the past decade. Although multiple reports show varying amounts of differences between the 2 techniques, nail fixation appears to be superior for the most unstable patterns, with minimally improved results in the more stable patterns. In either technique, cutout of the screw through the femoral head is the most common method of fixation failure. Placement of the screw close to the center of the femoral head has been shown to decrease cutout of the constructs.

Varus malreductions are poorly tolerated when fixing proximal femoral fractures, and this was confirmed in this study. Techniques to avoid varus malreductions during nailing include liberal use of traction, direct reduction of the femoral neck and head segment with pins or bone hooks, obtaining the proper starting point for the femoral nail, and aggressive reaming and preparation of the entry portal for the nail through the trochanter.

When the nail is inserted through the fracture site, failure to ream the proximal femur adequately will result in the nail separating the intertrochanteric fracture and displacing the fracture into varus.

Poor positioning of the screw in the femoral head and varus malreduction are often related, and surgeons should not accept guide pin placement with an increased tip-apex distance or when the fracture remains in varus. These features should be recognized before the lag screw reaming occurs because they can still be easily corrected up until that point.

S. A. Sems, MD

Peri-operative mortality after hemiarthroplasty for fracture of the hip: does cement make a difference?
Middleton RG, Uzoigwe CE, Young PS, et al (Royal Cornwall Hosp, Truro, UK; Leicester Royal Infirmary, Leicestershire, UK; Southern General Hosp, Glasgow, Lanarkshire, UK; et al)
Bone Joint J 96-B:1185-1191, 2014

We aimed to determine whether cemented hemiarthroplasty is associated with a higher post-operative mortality and rate of re-operation when compared with uncemented hemiarthroplasty. Data on 19 669 patients, who were treated with a hemiarthroplasty following a fracture of the hip in a nine-year period from 2002 to 2011, were extracted from NHS Scotland's acute admission database (Scottish Morbidity Record, SMR01). We investigated the rate of mortality at day 0, 1, 7, 30, 120 and one-year post-operatively using 12 case-mix variables to determine the independent effect of the method of fixation. At day 0, those with a cemented hemiarthroplasty had a higher rate of mortality ($p < 0.001$) compared with those with an uncemented hemiarthroplasty, equivalent to one extra death per 424 procedures. By day one this had become one extra death per 338 procedures. Increasing age and the five-year co-morbidity score were noted as independent risk factors. By day seven, the cumulative rate of mortality was less for cemented hemiarthroplasty though this did not reach significance until day 120. The rate of re-operation was significantly higher for uncemented hemiarthroplasty. Despite adjusting for 12 confounding variables, these only accounted for 15% of the observed variability.

The debate about the choice of the method of fixation for a hemiarthroplasty with respect to the rate of mortality or the risk of re-operation may be largely superfluous. Our results suggest that uncemented hemiarthroplasties may have a role to play in elderly patients with significant co-morbid disease.

▶ Cemented hemiarthroplasty has been recommended as the treatment of choice for the geriatric patient with a displaced femoral neck fracture. This recommendation has been made based on literature that showed no increased risk of mortality when cement is used. Additionally, the subsequent risk of need for reoperation in the uncemented implants has favored the use of cemented implants in this patient population.

Reports of increased mortality in the immediate postoperative period following cemented hemiarthroplasty have caused some surgeons to choose uncemented techniques for the patient with significant comorbid disease.

This study evaluated data from a national registry to evaluate the risks of mortality when a cemented hemiarthroplasty was used in the treatment of a hip fracture. The authors report an increase in the mortality early in the perioperative period in the cemented group, and this difference dissipated within a week. When the authors evaluated the most susceptible group of patients (aged > 90) the risk of mortality on day 0 was greatly increased when cemented technique was used. Beyond day 7, the mortality rates favored the cemented group. Subsequent reoperations were more frequent in the uncemented group, consistent with previously published literature.

This study highlights the need for surgeons to consider the comorbidities of their hip fracture patients when deciding between a cemented and uncemented technique. Although a cemented hemiarthroplasty remains the preferred choice as the treatment for the geriatric hip fracture, it is reasonable to consider an uncemented implant in the patient with significant comorbidities.

S. A. Sems, MD

Knee

Plating of Patella Fractures: Techniques and Outcomes
Taylor BC, Mehta S, Castaneda J, et al (Grant Med Ctr, Columbus, OH)
J Orthop Trauma 28:e231-e235, 2014

Operative treatment of displaced patella fractures with tension band fixation remains the gold standard, but is associated with a significant rate of complications and symptomatic implants. Despite the evolution of tension band fixation to include cannulated screws, surprisingly little other development has been made to improve overall patient outcomes. In this article, we present the techniques and outcomes of patella plating for displaced patella fractures and patella nonunions.

▶ Compression plating represents the most common method of treatment for most fractures. This technique has not been widely described in the treatment of patella fractures. The most common methods of fixation of patella fractures is tension band fixation, which can be augmented with the use of interfragmentary screws and cannulated screws through which tension bands can be placed. Historically, tension band fixation has had significant rates of hardware failure, loosening, and prominence that requires subsequent hardware removal. Chronic knee dysfunction can also occur after surgical treatment of patella fractures.

This article describes the technique for compression plate fixation of patella fractures using a plate that has capabilities for locked screw fixation. The technique is described for both simple and comminuted fractures. The authors presented a small series of 8 patients who underwent treatement of their patella fracture with this technique, and all of the fractures united.

Placing a plate directly on the anterior surface of the patella would cause concern for problems with hardware prominence and difficulty in kneeling. Surprisingly, none of the patients experienced hardware prominence that required hardware removal at a mean of 13.6 months, although longer follow-up could change this result.

This article presents an alternative technique that effectively treats patella fractures and holds promise to lessen the need for hardware removal due to prominence. Larger studies with longer follow-up will be needed to confirm this preliminary finding.

S. A. Sems, MD

The outcome following fixation of bicondylar tibial plateau fractures
Ahearn N, Oppy A, Halliday R, et al (Univ Hosps Bristol NHS Foundation Trust, UK)
Bone Joint J 96-B:956-962, 2014

Unstable bicondylar tibial plateau fractures are rare and there is little guidance in the literature as to the best form of treatment. We examined the short- to medium-term outcome of this injury in a consecutive series of patients presenting to two trauma centres. Between December 2005 and May 2010, a total of 55 fractures in 54 patients were treated by fixation, 34 with peri-articular locking plates and 21 with limited access direct internal fixation in combination with circular external fixation using a Taylor Spatial Frame (TSF). At a minimum of one year post-operatively, patient-reported outcome measures including the WOMAC index and SF-36 scores showed functional deficits, although there was no significant difference between the two forms of treatment. Despite low outcome scores, patients were generally satisfied with the outcome. We achieved good clinical and radiological outcomes, with low rates of complication. In total, only three patients (5%) had collapse of the joint of > 4 mm, and metaphysis to diaphysis angulation of greater than 5°, and five patients (9%) with displacement of > 4 mm. All patients in our study went on to achieve full union.

This study highlights the serious nature of this injury and generally poor patient-reported outcome measures following surgery, despite treatment by experienced surgeons using modern surgical techniques. Our findings suggest that treatment of complex bicondylar tibial plateau fractures with either a locking plate or a TSF gives similar clinical and radiological outcomes.

▶ Bicondylar tibia plateau fractures are frequently high-energy injuries that result in significant joint dysfunction and disability. Treatment methods include internal fixation with plates and screws and limited internal fixation with screws only and the addition of an external fixator to maintain the limb alignment.

This study documents the 1-year Western Ontario and McMaster Universities Arthritis Index (WOMAC) and Short-Form Health Survey (SF-36) scores, demonstrating the poor functional scores associated with this injury. This study also evaluated the relationship of articular reduction and joint alignment to the outcome scores. Despite high rates of satisfactory reduction and restoration of limb alignment, the poor outcome scores were still encountered. This highlights the likelihood that the poor outcomes associated with bicondylar tibial plateau fractures occur despite surgical treatment performed in a technically correct manner.

The root cause of the poor outcomes associated with bicondylar tibial plateau fractures is not fully understood, and this study contributes to the understanding by demonstrating these poor outcomes despite the restoration of the articular surface and joint alignment. Other factors including soft-tissue injury, length of immobilization, restrictions of weight bearing, and variations in postoperative rehabilitation are likely to contribute to the end result.

Regardless of the method of treatment of bicondylar tibial plateau fractures, poor outcomes on the WOMAC and SF-36 scores may be expected. Fortunately, the patients were generally satisfied with their outcomes and treatment in this study. This result may represent the skill of the authors as physicians who effectively manage their patient's injuries in the operating room and their patient's expectations in the perioperative period.

S. A. Sems, MD

The usefulness of MRI and arthroscopy in the diagnosis and treatment of soft-tissue injuries associated with split-depression fractures of the lateral tibial condyle
Parkkinen M, Madanat R, Mäkinen TJ, et al (Helsinki Univ Central Hosp, Finland; Harvard Med School, Boston, MA; Univ of Toronto, Ontario, Canada; et al)
Bone Joint J 96-B:1631-1636, 2014

The role of arthroscopy in the treatment of soft-tissue injuries associated with proximal tibial fractures remains debatable. Our hypothesis was that MRI over-diagnoses clinically relevant associated soft-tissue injuries. This prospective study involved 50 consecutive patients who underwent surgical treatment for a split-depression fracture of the lateral tibial condyle (AO/OTA type B3.1). The mean age of patients was 50 years (23 to 86) and 27 (54%) were female. All patients had MRI and arthroscopy. Arthroscopy identified 12 tears of the lateral meniscus, including eight bucket-handle tears that were sutured and four that were resected, as well as six tears of the medial meniscus, of which five were resected. Lateral meniscal injuries were diagnosed on MRI in four of 12 patients, yielding an overall sensitivity of 33% (95% confidence interval (CI) 11 to 65). Specificity was 76% (95% CI 59 to 88), with nine tears diagnosed among 38 menisci that did not contain a tear. MRI identified medial meniscal injuries in four of six patients, yielding an overall sensitivity of 67% (95% CI 24 to 94). Specificity was 66% (95% CI 50 to 79), with 15 tears diagnosed in 44 menisci that did not contain tears.

MRI appears to offer only a marginal benefit as the specificity and sensitivity for diagnosing meniscal injuries are poor in patients with a fracture. There were fewer arthroscopically-confirmed associated lesions than reported previously in MRI studies.

▶ This prospective study enrolled 50 patients with split depression fractures of the tibial plateau. All fractures underwent arthroscopy before internal fixation. MRI was found to be 33% sensitive in finding lateral meniscal injuries.

The poor sensitivity of MRI in detecting lateral meniscal tears in this series is likely related to the distortion of the anatomy due to the split and depressed lateral tibial plateau fracture. This low sensitivity brings into question whether there is a role to routinely obtain an MRI before fixation of split depressed lateral tibial plateau fractures. Another consideration should be that the majority of lateral split depression tibial plateau fractures that are treated operatively will undergo arthrotomy and direct visualization of the meniscus as well as the articular surface. In all cases, surgeons should be prepared for the need to perform either partial meniscectomy or meniscal repair at the time of internal fixation of split depression lateral tibial plateau fractures. This study showed that 28% of patients who sustained split depression tibial plateau fractures also sustained lateral meniscal tears. An effective surgical strategy involves performing an anterolateral approach followed by careful submeniscal arthrotomy. The surgeon should obtain good control of the capsule and identify the periphery of the meniscus. The meniscus is often displaced into the depressed area, and it can be mobilized with a nerve hook or other instrument back into its position. Multiple sutures should be passed into the periphery of the bucket handle tears, and they can be passed through the capsule and tied down for repair. The capsule can be reapproximated back to a proximal tibial plate through small holes in the plate to prevent the meniscus from displacing medially again. This surgical approach minimizes the benefit that an MRI could provide in the diagnosis of lateral meniscal injuries in the split depressed tibial plateau fracture.

Interestingly, there were several medial meniscal injuries in this study that would not be identified from a direct approach laterally. However, the authors do note that it is possible that some of medial meniscal tears occurred before the fracture and were degenerative asymptomatic medial meniscal tears. It is unknown whether these medial meniscal tears were identified by the MRI in this study would have been symptomatic had they been left alone.

The routine use of preoperative arthroscopy is also not recommended by the authors. The low incidence of clinically relevant lesions does not justify the routine use of arthroscopy. MRI is not routinely necessary in the management of split depressed tibial plateau fractures.

S. A. Sems, MD

Early Fracture Fixation

The Cost of After-Hours Operative Debridement of Open Tibia Fractures

Schenker ML, Ahn J, Donegan D, et al (Univ of Pennsylvania, Philadelphia; The Children's Hosp of Philadelphia, PA)
J Orthop Trauma 28:626-631, 2014

Objectives.—The aim of this study was to evaluate the additional cost associated with performing after-hours operative debridement of open fractures within 6 hours of injury.

Data Sources.—The economic model is based on population estimates obtained from the National Trauma Database and the National Inpatient Sample on the number of open tibia fractures that occur annually in the United States and the number that present after-hours (between 6 PM and 2 AM) that undergo operative debridement within 6 hours. This model estimates incremental cost for after-hours surgery based on overtime wages for on-call personnel (nurses and surgical technicians) required to staff after-hours cases as published by the US Department of Labor and data from our own institution. As many level 1 hospitals are capable of performing after-hours cases without additional cost, a sensitivity analysis was performed to determine the effect of designated level of care of the trauma hospital.

Data Extraction and Synthesis.—A total of 17,414 open tibia fractures were recorded in the National Inpatient Sample for 2009, and an estimated 7485 open tibia fractures presented after-hours, 4242 of which underwent operative debridement within 6 hours of presentation. Based on wage statistics from the US Department of Labor and our own institution, the estimated total additional cost for after-hours operative debridement of open tibia fractures within 6 hours is from $2,210,895 to $4,046,648 annually, respectively. For level 2 hospitals and below, the cost of performing after-hours operative debridement of open tibia fractures is calculated as from $1,532,980 to $2,805,846 annually.

Conclusions.—The data indicated an increased overall financial cost of performing after-hours operative debridement of open tibia fractures. Given that there is minimal documented benefit to this practice, and with increased pressure to practice cost containment, elective delay of operative debridement of open fractures and/or transfer to a higher level of care trauma hospital may be an acceptable way to address these issues.

Level of Evidence.—Economic Analysis Level III. See Instructions for Authors for a complete description of levels of evidence.

▶ Historically, open fractures have been an indication for emergent operative treatment of fractures, with the concern that delaying the time to the debridement would result in increased infection rates. More recent literature has failed to confirm this previously held belief, and the time from the injury to debridement has repeatedly been shown to not affect the rate of subsequent infection.

Other time-dependent variables, such as time from injury to the administration of antibiotics and time from injury to soft tissue coverage, have been shown to have an impact on the rate of late infection in open fractures.

This study modeled the national cost of treating open fractures with urgent, after-hours debridement using 2 methods. Although the validity of each method can be debated, both found significant costs associated with this practice. Given that the risk of delaying the debridement of open fractures appears quite small, if it even exists, the total cost of continuing to routinely take open fractures to the operating room after hours is difficult to justify.

S. A. Sems, MD

Intramedullary Nailing of Tibial Diaphyseal Fractures

Insertion of distal locking screws of tibial intramedullary nails: A comparison between the free-hand technique and the SURESHOT™ Distal Targeting System

Moreschini O, Petrucci V, Cannata R (Univ of Rome "Sapienza", Italy)
Injury 45:405-407, 2014

Introduction.—Positioning of the distal locking screws of an intramedullary nail is often challenging and time consuming because of difficult localisation of the distal locking holes, potential screw malalignment and nail deformation during insertion. The standard free-hand technique under fluoroscopic control involves considerable radiation exposure of both the patient and the surgical team. In this study, we aimed to compare the free-hand technique with a new system that utilises electromagnetic (EM) tracking data (SURESHOT^{TM} Distal Targeting System) to localise distal locking holes.

Material and Methods.—Patients admitted from March 2010 to January 2013 for tibial fracture that required intramedullary nailing were analysed retrospectively. We compared intraoperative radiation exposure time and distal locking time in patients treated with the standard free-hand technique and distal locking using the EM field-generating device. Intraoperative radiation exposure time and distal locking time were used for comparison.

Results.—Data from a total of 50 patients were analysed. The standard free-hand technique and the EM field-generating device were used in 25 (group 1) and 25 (group 2) patients, respectively. Mean distal locking time was 1258.6 (450–2289) s in group 1 and 603.5 (360–1140) s in group 2. Mean radiation exposure time was 19.4 (6–33) s in group 1 and 4.6 (1–10) s in group 2.

Conclusion.—The EM field-generating device significantly reduces distal locking time and, more importantly, significantly decreases duration of exposure to ionising radiation.

▶ Placement of interlocking screws in the distal tibia is typically done using a free-hand technique by obtaining perfect circles with a fluoroscopy machine. This process can be time-consuming and expose the surgeon and patient to radiation. New technology using an electromagnetic field generator assists with targeting of these distal locking screws. This study compares the retrospective results of 1 center's experience using a Sureshot electromagnetic field generator, comparing cases in which the device was used to the traditional method. This article showed a greater than 10-minute time savings when the Sureshot device was used. It also showed significant decreases in fluoroscopy exposure during the use of the Sureshot technique.

This technique and the technology certainly hold promise for improving operating room efficiency as well as opening up the world of free-hand distal interlocking to facilities that do not have fluoroscopy. However, in this study, fluoroscopy was still used in conjunction with the Sureshot. Additionally, the equipment malfunctioned in 8% of the cases in which it was used. Unfortunately, this technology may not be ready for use completely free of fluoroscopy.

To determine whether the benefits of this technology outweigh the costs, a thorough analysis would need to be done at each individual institution considering its use. The cost of operating room time, cost of fluoroscopy, and value of decreased radiation exposure must be considered, along with the basic cost of the technology and nonreusable parts of the technique. (The Sureshot requires a piece of hardware that is used for each procedure and is generally not recommended to be reused.) These variables differ from institution to institution, so each individual surgeon must determine whether this technology is worthwhile for their practice.

This study confirms previous studies showing that this is an effective method of placing distal interlocking screws. It is an exciting new technology that holds great promise.

S. A. Sems, MD

Tibia Fractures

Definitive Plates Overlapping Provisional External Fixator Pin Sites: Is the Infection Risk Increased?
Shah CM, Babb PE, McAndrew CM, et al (Washington Univ School of Medicine, St Louis, MO; et al)
J Orthop Trauma 28:518-522, 2014

Objectives.—The purpose of this study was to compare the infection risk when internal fixation plates either overlap or did not overlap previous external fixator pin sites in patients with bicondylar tibial plateau fractures and pilon fractures treated with a 2-staged protocol of acute spanning external fixation and later definitive internal fixation.

Design.—Retrospective comparison study.

Setting.—Two level I trauma centers.

Patients/Participants.—A total of 85 OTA 41C bicondylar tibial plateau fractures and 97 OTA 43C pilon fractures treated between 2005 and 2010. Radiographs were evaluated to determine the positions of definitive plates in relation to external fixator pin sites and patients were grouped into an "overlapping" group and a "nonoverlapping" group.

Intervention.—Fifty patients had overlapping pin sites and 132 did not.

Main Outcome Measure.—Presence of a deep wound infection.

Results.—Overall, 25 patients developed a deep wound infection. Of the 50 patients in the "overlapping" group, 12 (24%) developed a deep infection compared with 13 (10%) of the 132 patients in the "nonoverlapping" group ($P = 0.033$).

Conclusions.—Placement of definitive plate fixation overlapping previous external fixator pin sites significantly increases the risk of deep infection in the 2-staged treatment of bicondylar tibial plateau and pilon fractures. Surgeons must make a conscious effort to place external fixator pins outside of future definitive fixation sites to reduce the overall incidence of deep wound infections. Additionally, consideration must be given to the relative benefit of a spanning external fixator in light of the potential for infection associated with their use.

Level of Evidence.—Therapeutic Level III. See Instructions for Authors for a complete description of levels of evidence.

▶ A staged approach to the definitive fixation of tibial pilon and plateau fractures consists of the initial application of a joint spanning external fixator followed by definitive open reduction and internal fixation once the soft-tissue envelope allows. Choosing the proper location of the initial external fixator pins can be difficult without knowing which approach or approaches will be used for the final fixation. Surgeons can minimize the risk of pin-to-plate over-lap by drawing out the surgical incisions that are likely to be used for final fix-ation before placement of the external fixator pins. Adding a cushion of a few centimeters from the predicted incision to the pin site can also minimize the risks of pin-to-plate overlap. Temporizing external fixators are used to provide initial skeletal stability and maintain the soft tissues at their anatomic length. Because these fixators are placed with these goals, and not the goals of provid-ing definitive stabilization and maximal stability, increasing the pin spacing away from the fracture is well tolerated and recommended to avoid pin-to-plate overlap and to decrease later risk of infection following final internal fix-ation. This study nicely documents the increased risk of infection when the pin sites overlap the plate position and encourages the surgeon to consider whether initial external fixation is truly necessary and where pin placement can occur without overlapping the location of the definitive fixation.

S. A. Sems, MD

Micromotion in the fracture healing of closed distal metaphyseal tibial fractures: A multicentre prospective study

Vicenti G, Pesce V, Tartaglia N, et al (Univ of Bari, Italy; Hosp Miulli, Bari, Italy)
Injury 45S:S27-S35, 2014

The dynamic locking screw (DLS) in association with minimally inva-sive plate osteosynthesis (MIPO) in a bridging construct for simple meta-diaphyseal long bone fractures enables modulation of the rigidity of the system and facilitates the development of early and triplanar bone callus.

Twenty patients affected by distal tibial fracture were treated with MIPO bridging technique and DLS at the proximal side of the fracture. Time of consolidation, quality of the reduction, complications and American Ortho-paedic Foot and Ankle Society (AOFAS) score were monitored and the results compared with those from a control group treated with only standard screws on both fracture sides. Student t-test for independent samples was used for the comparison of means between the two groups. Chi-square test was used for the comparison of proportions. A multiple logistic regres-sion model was constructed to assess the possible confounding effects. Per-formance was considered significant for $p < 0.05$. The mean healing time was 17.6 ± 2.8 weeks in the group treated with standard screws and 13.5 ± 1.8 weeks in the group treated with DLS ($t = 5.5$, $p < 0.0001$). The DLS was associated with early healing and triplanar bone callus.

▶ This study reports the results of a randomized trial of minimally invasive plate osteosynthesis of distal tibia fractures by comparing the use of dynamic locking screw with standard locking screws. The results showed that the dynamic lock-ing screw constructs were associated with early healing and more bone callus formation.

Internal fixation of fractures result in the formation of constructs that expose the fracture to certain amount of strain. The strain is defined as the change in length over the overall length of the fracture site. Strain can be modified in many ways by using plates with different materials and different geometric properties by placing screws at varying lengths from the fracture site and by using different diameter screws. This article introduces yet another variable, the dynamic locking screw. The dynamic locking screw allows motion at the near cortex while providing a more secure fixation on the far cortex. This theoretically results in more micromotion and more strain along the fracture site.

This study compared the dynamic locking screw to standard locking screws in the diaphyseal location. The role of the use of routine locking screws in the diaphysis is not fully understood, but in general, nonlocking screws are much less expensive and much more commonly used in this location without expected increased failure rates. Rather than comparing the dynamic locking screw to a standard nonlocked screw construct, the authors compared the dynamic locking screw to the more rigid locked screw construct. This leaves the reader wondering whether the increased callus and earlier healing observed in the dynamic locking screw group was a result of being compared with a very rigid fully locked construct, rather than a more standard nonlocked diaphyseal construct. This study had only 1 nonunion out of 40 cases, and the complication rates were relatively low with a few angular malalignments and superficial infections.

Although the dynamic locking screw is an exciting new innovation in the field of internal fixation, it is unknown at this time whether its use can be replaced or simulated with other techniques, such as increasing the working length of the plate, using nonlocking screws, or using smaller standard locking screws closer to the fracture site. This study did show that dynamic locking screws are a relatively safe implant that can be considered to promote early healing and callus formation.

S. A. Sems, MD

Type III Open Tibia Fractures: Immediate Antibiotic Prophylaxis Minimizes Infection

Lack WD, Karunakar MA, Angerame MR, et al (Loyola Univ Med Ctr, Chicago, IL; Carolinas Med Ctr, Charlotte, NC)
J Orthop Trauma 29:1-6, 2015

Objective.—To examine the association between antibiotic timing and deep infection of type III open tibia fractures.

Design.—Retrospective prognostic study.

Setting.—Level 1 Trauma Center.

Patients.—The study population included 137 patients after exclusions for missing data (13), nonreconstructible limbs (9), and/or absence of 90-day outcome data (3).

Intervention.—An observational study of antibiotic timing.

Main Outcome Measurement.—Deep infection within 90 days.

Results.—Age, smoking, diabetes, injury severity score, type IIIA versus 3B/C injury, and time to surgical debridement were not associated with infection on univariate analysis. Greater than 5 days to wound coverage

($P < 0.001$) and greater than 66 minutes to antibiotics ($P < 0.01$) were univariate predictors of infection. Multivariate analysis found wound coverage beyond 5 days [odds ratio, 7.39; 95% confidence interval (CI), 2.33–23.45; $P < 0.001$] and antibiotics beyond 66 minutes (odds ratio, 3.78; 95% CI, 1.16–12.31; $P = 0.03$) independently predicted infection. Immediate antibiotics and early coverage limited the infection rate (1 of 36, 2.8%) relative to delay in either factor (6 of 59, 10.2%) or delay in both factors (17 of 42, 40.5%).

Conclusions.—Time from injury to antibiotics and to wound coverage independently predict infection of type III open tibia fractures. Both should be achieved as early as possible, with coverage being dependent on the condition of the wound. Given the relatively short therapeutic window for antibiotic prophylaxis (within an hour of injury), prehospital antibiotics may substantially improve outcomes for severe open fractures.

Level of Evidence.—Prognostic Level II. See Instructions for Authors for a complete description of levels of evidence.

▶ This retrospective prognostic study evaluated 137 patients with open tibia fractures and observed the relationship of antibiotic timing with subsequent infection. A delay of more than 66 minutes from injury to antibiotic administration independently predicted infection.

This study also observed the time to debridement as well as smoking and diabetes history and did not find a relationship of these variables with infection.

Open tibia fractures that underwent soft tissue coverage more than 5 days from the injury had higher infection rates. This variable is difficult to control for in a retrospective study but is consistent with the previous literature that associated delays in coverage with infection. Surgeons should proceed with soft tissue coverage of open tibia fractures as soon as the condition of the soft tissues allow.

Surgeons should consider protocols that promote early antibiotic administration in the setting of open tibial fractures. Prehospital administration of antibiotics should be considered in the setting of open tibia fractures. To implement the routine administration of antibiotics in the prehospital setting, surgeons must work closely with first responders to develop antibiotic administration protocols.

S. A. Sems, MD

Evaluation of the Effectiveness of the Angular Stable Locking System in Patients with Distal Tibial Fractures Treated with Intramedullary Nailing: A Multicenter Randomized Controlled Trial

Höntzsch D, Schaser K-D, Hofmann GO, et al (Berufsgenossenschaftliche Unfallklinik Tübingen, Germany; Charité-Universitätsmedizin Berlin, Germany; Friedrich-Schiller-Universität Jena, Germany; et al)
J Bone Joint Surg Am 96:1889-1897, 2014

Background.—Angular stable locking of intramedullary nails has been shown to enhance fixation stability of tibial fractures in biomechanical and animal studies. The aim of our study was to assess whether use of the angular stable locking system or conventional locking resulted in earlier full weight-bearing with minimum pain for patients with a distal tibial fracture treated with an intramedullary nail.

Methods.—A prospective multicenter, randomized, patient-blinded trial was conducted with adults who had a distal tibial fracture. Patients' fractures were managed with an intramedullary nail locked with either an angular stable locking system or conventional locking screws. Outcomes were evaluated at six weeks, twelve weeks, six months, and one year after surgery. Time to full weight-bearing with minimum pain was calculated with use of daily entries from patient diaries. Secondary outcomes included pain at the fracture site under load, quality of life, gait analysis, mobility, radiographic findings, and adverse events.

Results.—One hundred and forty-two patients were randomly allocated to two treatment groups: seventy-five to the group receiving intramedullary nailing with the angular stable locking system and sixty-seven to the group receiving conventional intramedullary nailing. No clinically important differences were found for either the primary or secondary outcome parameters between the groups during the entire follow-up period.

Conclusions.—Use of an angular stable locking system with intramedullary nailing did not improve the outcome compared with conventional locking screws in the treatment of distal tibial fractures.

Level of Evidence.—Therapeutic Level I. See Instructions for Authors for a complete description of levels of evidence.

▶ Angular stable locking screws used in the distal tibia during intramedullary nail fixation provide the surgeon with an accessory method of increasing the stability of the nailing construct. This option is promoted in conjunction with nail fixation of distal tibia fractures, with the hope of promoting earlier weight bearing through increased stability.

Because fracture healing is affected by the amount of strain experienced at the fracture site, the use of angular stable locking screws introduces yet another variable that changes the amount of strain that is experienced. Other factors that affect the strain include the fracture geometry; the size, shape, and material of the nail; the diameter of the intramedullary canal; and the location, number, orientation, and size of the interlocking screws. With this many variables, the role of angular stable locking screws in contributing to healing is unknown.

However, previous animal studies have suggested that the use of angular stable locking screws would allow earlier weight bearing. This study was a well-designed, prospective, randomized, blinded trial that evaluated the role of angular stable locking screws on time to weight bearing, and it refuted the hypothesis that earlier weight bearing would occur with the use of angular stable locking screw.

Given the increased costs associated with angular stable locking screws, this technique should not be routinely used with the expectation that earlier weight bearing will occur. Patients who undergo intramedullary nail fixation of distal tibial fractures with or without angular stable locking screws should be permitted weight bearing as tolerated.

S. A. Sems, MD

Foot and Ankle Fractures

Early Ankle Movement Versus Immobilization in the Postoperative Management of Ankle Fracture in Adults: A Systematic Review and Meta-analysis

Keene DJ, Williamson E, Bruce J, et al (Univ of Oxford, UK; Univ of Warwick, Coventry, UK)
J Orthop Sports Phys Ther 44:690-701, 2014

Study Design.—Systematic review and meta-analysis.

Objectives.—To compare early ankle movement versus ankle immobilization after surgery for ankle fracture on clinical and patient-reported outcomes.

Background.—A significant proportion of patients undergoing surgery for ankle fracture experience postoperative complications and delayed return to function. The risks and benefits of movement of the ankle in the first 6 weeks after surgery are not known, and clinical practice varies widely.

Methods.—We searched bibliographic databases and reference lists to identify eligible trials. Two independent reviewers conducted data extraction and risk-of-bias assessments.

Results.—Fourteen trials (705 participants) were included in the review, 11 of which were included in the meta-analysis. The quality of the trials was universally poor. The pooled effect of early ankle movement on function at 9 to 12 weeks after surgery compared to immobilization was inconclusive (standardized mean difference, 0.46; 95% confidence interval: -0.02, 0.93; $P = .06$; $I^2 = 72\%$), and no differences were observed between groups at 1 year. The odds of venous thromboembolism were significantly lower with early ankle movement compared to immobilization (Peto odds ratio $= 0.12$; 95% confidence interval: 0.02, 0.71; $P = .02$; $I^2 = 0\%$). Deep surgical site infection (Peto odds ratio $= 7.08$; 95% confidence interval: 1.39, 35.99; $P = .02$; $I^2 = 0\%$), superficial surgical site infection, fixation failure, and reoperation to remove metalwork were more common after early ankle movement compared to immobilization.

Conclusion.—The quality of evidence is poor. The effects of early movement after ankle surgery on short-term functional outcomes are unclear, but there is no observable difference in the longer term. There is a small reduction in risk of postoperative thromboembolism with early ankle movement. Current evidence suggests that deep and superficial surgical site infections, fixation failure, and the need to remove metalwork are more common after early ankle movement.

Level of Evidence.—Therapy, level 1a—.

▶ Ankle fractures are common injuries that may require open reduction and internal stabilization depending on the fracture pattern. Stiffness is a common complaint among patients suffering ankle fractures, and a complaint that can persist over the long term. This systematic review and meta-analysis reviewed 11 trials that compared early movement to immobilization and concluded that while the short-term differences in outcome are unclear, there are no long-term differences. This finding, combined with the findings that the complications are higher with early movement, is generally discouraging to the concept of early movement. This study did find that there was a reduced risk of thrombosis/thromboembolism with early motion.

Internal fixation of ankle fractures relies on fixation of small bony fragments of the medial malleolus, and fixation with thin or low-profile hardware on the fibula because of a limited soft-tissue envelope. Because of this, immobilization with a boot or cast is commonly used in the postoperative period to protect the reconstruction and fixation. Therefore, it is not surprising that there was an increased risk of hardware failure with early motion.

The potential for decreased thrombotic events must be weighed against the increased risk for complications when the decision regarding immobilization is made. Patients should be counseled that there is unlikely to be a long-term difference in function regardless of which method is chosen.

S. A. Sems, MD

Comparison of Lag Screw Versus Buttress Plate Fixation of Posterior Malleolar Fractures

Erdem MN, Erken HY, Burc H, et al (International Kolan Hosp, Istanbul, Turkey; Anadolu Med Ctr, Istanbul, Turkey; Suleyman Demirel Univ School of Medicine, Isparta, Turkey; et al)

Foot Ankle Int 35:1022-1030, 2014

Background.—The goal of this study was to report the results of selective open reduction and internal fixation of fractures of the posterior malleolus with a posterolateral approach and to compare the results of the 2 techniques.

Methods.—We prospectively evaluated 40 patients who underwent posterior malleolar fracture fixation between 2008 and 2012. The patients were treated with a posterolateral approach. We assigned alternating patients to receive plate fixation and the next screw fixation, consecutively, based on the order in which they presented to our institution. Fixation of the posterior malleolus was made with lag screws in 20 patients and a buttress plate in 20 patients. We used American Orthopaedic Foot and Ankle Society (AOFAS) scores, range of motion (ROM) of the ankle, and radiographic evaluations as the main outcome measurements. The mean follow-up was 38.2 (range, 24-51) months.

Results.—Full union without any loss of reduction was obtained in 38 of the 40 patients. We detected a union with a stepoff of 3 mm in 1 patient in the screw group and a step-off of 2 mm in 1 patient in the plate group. At the final follow-up, the mean AOFAS score of the patients regardless of fixation type was 94.1 (range, 85-100). The statistical results showed no significant difference between the patients regardless of the fixation type of the posterior malleolus in terms of AOFAS scores and ROM of the ankle ($P > .05$).

Conclusions.—Good (AOFAS score of 94/100) and equivalent (within 3 points) results were obtained using the 2 techniques (screws or plate) for fixation after open reduction of posterior malleolar fragments.

Level of Evidence.—Level II, prospective case series.

▶ The posterolateral approach is incredibly powerful to treat fibular fractures and associated posterior malleolar fractures. It allows access by working on either side of the peroneal tendons and musculature to access both the fibula and the posterior aspect of the tibia. The posterior malleolus is easily identified and mobilized through this posterolateral approach, and an anatomic reduction can be confirmed by using cortical reads along the posterior malleolar area. It is difficult to visualize the joint through that approach, and the articular reduction must be confirmed using intraoperative fluoroscopy. This study randomly allocated 40 patients to fixation of posterior malleolar fractures using either lag screws or plate fixation. All procedures were performed through a posterolateral approach.

The authors showed no difference between plate or screw fixation of posterior malleolar fractures. Alternative methods of securing fixation of the posterior malleolar fractures include anterior to posteriorly directed screws. It is an important distinction that screws using this study were placed posterior to anterior but through a direct approach, which is likely why the excellent results were obtained. Surgeons should not interpret this study to indicate that screw-alone fixation from an anterior to posterior direction without direct reduction is equivalent to the results obtained through a posterior approach with a direct reduction.

The posterolateral approach is typically performed either in a lateral or prone position. Although it can be done supine, this often requires the surgeon to significantly internally rotate and mobilize the leg in an odd position to access the posterior malleolus. The prone position also allows a small bump to be placed under the anterior tibia so that the foot can translate forward. Often in fractures with the posterior malleolar fracture, the deformity force of the injury and the direction of instability is posterior, so placing the patient prone allows gravity to assist in the reduction rather than to deform the fracture. When performing the posterolateral approach and fixation of posterior malleolar fractures, surgeons should feel confident using either lag screws or buttress plate fixation to stabilize the fragment, knowing either technique will work.

S. A. Sems, MD

Fragility fractures of the ankle in the frail elderly patient: treatment with a long calcaneotalotibial nail

Al-Nammari SS, Dawson-Bowling S, Amin A, et al (St George's Hosp, Tooting, London, UK)
Bone Joint J 96-B:817-822, 2014

Conventional methods of treating ankle fractures in the elderly are associated with high rates of complication. We describe the results of treating these injuries in 48 frail elderly patients with a long calcaneotalotibial nail.

The mean age of the group was 82 years (61 to 96) and 41 (85%) were women. All were frail, with multiple medical comorbidities and their mean American Society of Anaesthesiologists score was 3 (3 to 4). None could walk independently before their operation. All the fractures were displaced and unstable; the majority (94%, 45 of 48) were low-energy injuries and 40% (19 of 48) were open.

The overall mortality at six months was 35%. Of the surviving patients, 90% returned to their pre-injury level of function. The mean pre- and post-operative Olerud and Molander questionnaire scores were 62 and 57 respectively. Complications included superficial infection (4%, two of 48); deep infection (2%, one of 48); a broken or loose distal locking screw (6%, three of 48); valgus malunion (4%, two of 48); and one below-knee amputation following an unsuccessful vascular operation. There were no cases of nonunion, nail breakage or peri-prosthetic fracture.

A calcaneotalotibial nail is an excellent device for treating an unstable fracture of the ankle in the frail elderly patient. It allows the patient to mobilise immediately and minimises the risk of bone or wound problems. A long nail which crosses the isthmus of the tibia avoids the risk of peri-prosthetic fracture associated with shorter devices.

▶ Treatment of fragility fractures of the ankle is fraught with challenges and complications. Standard methods of internal fixation with fibular plating and screw fixation of the medial malleolus frequently fail. The subcutaneous nature of the fibula and need to place hardware immediately beneath the skin also contribute to the development of devastating soft-tissue complications in this patient group.

This article describes the use of a retrograde calcaneotibial nail to maintain the talus in a centered position beneath the tibia to allow the fractures to stabilize with a low risk of complications. A concern with this technique is the violation of both the ankle and subtalar joints with a large intramedullary rod. This concern did not translate to functional outcomes because the Olerud and Molander scores were returned to near baseline levels.

This technique should be reserved for elderly patients with significant comorbidities who have a fragility fracture of the ankle at this point. Satisfactory outcomes with more standard internal fixation of ankle fractures in younger, healthier populations should be expected, and calcaneotibial nail fixation is not indicated in those patients. Careful patient selection is important when considering this technique to treat ankle fractures.

S. A. Sems, MD

The Effect of Syndesmosis Screw Removal on the Reduction of the Distal Tibiofibular Joint: A Prospective Radiographic Study
Song DJ, Lanzi JT, Groth AT, et al (Landstuhl Regional Med Ctr, Germany; Tripler Army Med Ctr, Honolulu, HI; et al)
Foot Ankle Int 35:543-548, 2014

Background.—Injury to the tibiofibular syndesmosis is frequent with rotational ankle injuries. Multiple studies have shown a high rate of syndesmotic malreduction with the placement of syndesmotic screws. There are no studies evaluating the reduction or malreduction of the syndesmosis after syndesmotic screw removal. The purpose of this study was to prospectively evaluate syndesmotic reduction with CT scans and to determine the effect of screw removal on the malreduced syndesmosis.

Methods.—This was an IRB-approved prospective radiographic study. Patients over 18 years of age treated at 1 institution between August 2008 and December 2011 with intraoperative evidence of syndesmotic disruption were enrolled. Postoperative CT scans were obtained of bilateral ankles within 2 weeks of operative fixation. Syndesmotic screws were removed after 3 months, and a second CT scan was then obtained 30 days after screw removal. Using axial CT images, syndesmotic reduction was evaluated compared to the contralateral uninjured ankle. Twenty-five patients were enrolled in this prospective study. The average age was 25.7 (range, 19 to 35), with 3 females and 22 males.

Results.—Nine patients (36%) had evidence of tibiofibular syndesmosis malreduction on their initial postoperative axial CT scans. In the postsyndesmosis screw removal CT scan, 8 of 9 or 89% of malreductions showed adequate reduction of the tibiofibular syndesmosis. There was a statistically significant reduction in syndesmotic malreductions ($t = 3.333$, $P < .001$) between the initial rate of malreduction after screw placement of 36% (9/25) and the rate of malreduction after all screws were removed of 4% (1/25).

Conclusions.—Despite a high rate of initial malreduction (36%) after syndesmosis screw placement, 89% of the malreduced syndesmoses spontaneously reduced after screw removal. Syndesmotic screw removal may be advantageous to achieve final anatomic reduction of the distal tibiofibular joint, and we recommend it for the malreduced syndesmosis.

Level of Evidence.—Level IV, prognostic case series.

▶ Obtaining accurate reductions of syndesmotic disruptions can be challenging. The anatomy does not lend to easy interpretation of reduction via plain radiographs. Methods to assess reduction at the time of fixation include comparison to the contralateral side, making specific measurements on the lateral radiographs, and obtaining intraoperative computed tomography (CT) or intra-operative fluoroscopic reconstruction images. Many studies have looked at postoperative CT scans to assess malreductions and have permitted subsequent revision surgery.

This study looked at a small number of patients who had syndesmotic screw placement for syndesmotic injury associated with ankle fractures. Of the 9 patients who had syndesmotic malreductions with the screws in place, 8 of the malreductions resolved after the syndesmotic screws were removed.

The optimal timing of syndesmotic screw removal is not well established. It is possible that malreduced syndesmoses may not return to the proper alignment if the screw is left in place for a prolonged period of time. This study removed the screws at an average of 107 days, which is relatively early in the postoperative period. The reader may wish to consider removal of syndesmotic screws in this time period in cases of misaligned reduction.

S. A. Sems, MD

Upper Extremity

Natural History of Anterior Chest Wall Numbness After Plating of Clavicle Fractures: Educating Patients

Christensen TJ, Horwitz DS, Kubiak EN (Univ of Utah, Salt Lake City; Geisinger Med Ctr, Dansville, PA)
J Orthop Trauma 28:642-647, 2014

Objectives.—Improved patient outcomes after plating of displaced clavicle fractures have been demonstrated by recent clinical studies. Many of these patients, however, complain of anterior chest wall numbness after this procedure; we hypothesize that numbness likely persists long term for many patients, but without effect on shoulder function.

Design.—Prospective observational cohort.

Setting.—Level 1 trauma center.

Patients/Participants.—Adult patients undergoing plating of a displaced middle third diaphyseal clavicle fracture.

Intervention.—Open reduction and internal fixation with superior clavicle plating.

Main Outcome Measurements.—The primary outcome is anterior chest wall numbness size (in square centimeters) and location as measured with a numbness transparency grid. Secondary outcomes include Visual Analog scale, Disabilities of the Arm, Shoulder, and Hand, and Constant scores 1 year postoperatively.

Results.—Twenty-five of 27 consecutive patients met inclusion/exclusion criteria, with 92% 1-year follow-up. Numbness at 2 weeks is very common, involving 83% of patients, with a mean area of 44 cm^2. Numbness at 1 year remains relatively common, involving 52% of patients, with a mean area of 15 cm^2 (66% decrease in area from 2 weeks, $P = 0.009$). Numbness at 2 weeks predicted a 63% chance of continued 1-year numbness (37% resolved); Constant, Disabilities of the Arm,

Shoulder, and Hand, and Visual Analog scale pain scores remained excellent in all patients at final follow-up, without correlation between numbness and outcome measures ($r^2 < 0.170$).

Conclusions.—Anterior chest wall numbness after open reduction internal fixation of displaced clavicle fractures is very common in the early postoperative period and may remain high 1 year postoperatively. Numbness 1 year after surgery is not associated with poor clinical outcome measures.

Level of Evidence.—Prognostic Level IV. See Instructions for Authors for a complete description of levels of evidence.

▶ Supraclavicular nerves are variable in location and size. They cross the clavicle directly and orthogonally to surgical approaches that are used to perform internal fixation of clavicle fractures. Whether clavicle plates are applied anteroinferiorly or superiorly, the supraclavicular nerves pass through the operative field. Some branches are small and readily sacrificed when some large branches that are identified during these approaches can be preserved. This study looked at 25 patients who were treated consecutively with open reduction internal fixation of clavicle fractures. They found that 52% of patients had numbness at 1 year, but this was not associated with poor clinical outcomes, measured with Disabilities of the Arm, Shoulder, and Hand and Constant scores. The average area of numbness did decrease over time, with the initial area of numbness averaging 44 cm^2, decreasing to 15 cm^2 at 1 year follow-up.

Preoperative counseling of patients who are planned to undergo internal fixation of clavicle fractures should include discussion about the likelihood that patients will experience permanent or long-standing postoperative numbness in the anterior chest wall. Surgeons should educate patients that although they will do everything possible to preserve large supraclavicular nerves, this numbness may be unavoidable and patients should expect it in about half of cases. Patients should be counseled that although this numbness will persist, it will not have any effect on shoulder function. As clavicle fracture fixation is increasing in popularity for various reasons, this discussion will need to be a more common occurrence in fracture clinics.

S. A. Sems, MD

Factors Predicting Complication and Reoperation Rates Following Surgical Fixation of Proximal Humeral Fractures

Petrigliano FA, Bezrukov N, Gamradt SC, et al (David Geffen School of Medicine at the Univ of California at Los Angeles; Univ of Southern California)
J Bone Joint Surg Am 96:1544-1551, 2014

Background.—The purpose of this study was to report complication and reoperation rates following non-arthroplasty fixation of shoulder fractures determined on the basis of observational, population-based data from all inpatient admissions in California over an eleven-year period.

Methods.—Records from all inpatient hospital discharges and subsequent readmissions related to operative non-arthroplasty treatment of proximal humeral fractures were obtained for patients in California from December 1994 through December 2005. These admissions were evaluated to identify patient and hospital characteristics associated with short and intermediateterm complications (within and after ninety days, respectively) as well as reoperation rates. Procedures performed included open reduction and internal fixation in 9254 patients, closed reduction and internal fixation in 1903 patients, and internal fixation without reduction in 302 patients.

Results.—The short-term complications included mortality in 401 patients (3.5%), which was associated with a higher Charlson comorbidity index (odds ratio [OR] = 1.5, $p < 0.001$) and male sex (OR = 1.7, $p < 0.001$); and pulmonary embolism in sixty patients (0.5%), which was associated with male sex (OR = 2.2, $p = 0.007$) and patient age of seventyfive years or older (OR = 3.6, $p = 0.001$). Intermediate-term reoperations included conversion to hemiarthroplasty in 174 patients (1.5%); and conversion to total shoulder arthroplasty in eight patients (0.07%), which was associated with an age of fifty to sixty-four years (hazard ratio = 2.8, $p = 0.007$). Overall, an age of sixty-five years or older, male sex, residence in an area with an income in the lowest two quintiles, and the presence of preexisting comorbidities were associated with elevated risks of short-term complications but not of intermediate-term conversion to arthroplasty. The ninety-day revision rate was 5.3%.

Conclusions.—Surgical fixation of proximal humeral fractures has a low complication and mortality profile. The data provided in this study can serve in counseling patients about risks associated with operative fixation of displaced proximal humeral fractures.

▶ Deciding when and when not to operate on geriatric proximal humerus fractures can be a difficult thing. Although most proximal humerus fractures in the geriatric population can be treated without surgical intervention, certain fracture patterns may benefit from internal fixation. Complications are poorly tolerated in this patient population, and this study will assist the reader in determining risks of patients developing these complications postoperatively.

Access to health care varies by location and socioeconomic standing of the patient. This study confirmed that surgery was chosen as a treatment method most often in patients from the higher income areas. This finding should encourage the reader to stop and consider their biases (recognized or unrecognized) toward their patient's socioeconomic status that affects their decisions to perform surgery.

Overall, the complication and reoperation rates were low. This study also highlights the higher complication rate of closed reduction and internal fixation compared with open reduction and internal fixation. Surgeons should consider the indications for closed reduction and internal fixation in the geriatric population and consider the risks associated with that method of treatment.

S. A. Sems, MD

Lack of Benefit of Physical Therapy on Function Following Supracondylar Humeral Fracture: A Randomized Controlled Trial

Schmale GA, Mazor S, Mercer LD, et al (Seattle Children's Hosp, WA)
J Bone Joint Surg Am 96:944-950, 2014

Background.—The goal of the study was to evaluate the efficacy of physical therapy in restoring function and mobility after a pediatric supracondylar humeral fracture.

Methods.—The study included sixty-one patients from five to twelve years of age with a supracondylar humeral fracture that was treated with casting or with closed reduction and pinning followed by casting. Patients were randomized to receive either no further treatment (no-PT group) or six sessions of a standardized hospital-based physical therapy program (PT group). The ASK-p (Activities Scale for Kids-performance version) and self-assessments of activity were used to assess function at one, nine, fifteen, and twenty-seven weeks after injury. Motion was measured at nine and fifteen weeks after injury by a blinded therapist. Anxiety was measured at one and nine weeks after injury with a self-assessment. Differences in ASK-p scores and anxiety level were analyzed with use of multivariate generalized estimating equations.

Results.—ASK-p scores were significantly better in the no-PT group at nine and fifteen weeks after injury ($p = 0.02$ and 0.01, respectively) but the difference at twenty-seven weeks was not significant. There were no differences between groups with respect to performance of activities of daily living or time to return to sports. Anxiety at nine weeks was associated with worse ASK-p scores at nine and fifteen weeks in the PT group and with better ASK-p scores in the no-PT group at these time points ($p = 0.01$ and 0.02, respectively). There were no differences between the groups with respect to elbow motion in the injured arm at any time. Severity of injury had no impact on function or elbow motion in either the PT or the no-PT group.

Conclusions.—Children undergoing closed treatment of a supracondylar humeral fracture that was limited to approximately three weeks of cast immobilization received no benefit involving either return of function or elbow motion from a short course of physical therapy.

Level of Evidence.—Therapeutic Level I. See Instructions for Authors for a complete description of levels of evidence.

▶ Pediatric supracondylar humerus fractures are common injuries requiring surgical stabilization, but with restoration of alignment and internal fixation, excellent outcomes can be expected. Nondisplaced injuries can be treated with initial cast immobilization. The subsequent rehabilitation focuses on regaining range of motion followed by functional exercises and then strengthening. This study randomized 61 patients to either hospital-based physical therapy or no physical therapy. The results showed that 3 weeks of immobilization followed by initiation of motion will have similar results whether physical therapy is used or not.

Surgeons who treat pediatric supracondylar humerus fractures also interface with the parents and families of the injured child. These usually well-meaning families are looking for every option available to allow their child to make a full recovery from their injury. Surgeons are often asked to initiate physical therapy at the request of these families. This excellent study provides the surgeon with quality information to provide to families and parents when the decision is made not to use physical therapy. Surgeons can reassure parents that the range of motion and overall function of the arm will not be impaired if physical therapy is not initiated. The cost-saving implications of this study are great given the frequency with which this injury occurs. Surgeons should feel comfortable recommending that physical therapy not be initiated after closed treatment of pediatric supracondylar humerus fractures.

S. A. Sems, MD

Treatment of Olecranon Fractures With 2.4- and 2.7-mm Plating Techniques
Wellman DS, Lazaro LE, Cymerman RM, et al (Hosp for Special Surgery, NY; New York Presbyterian Hosp)
J Orthop Trauma 29:36-43, 2015

Objectives.—To evaluate the outcomes of olecranon fractures treated with 2.4- and 2.7-mm plate constructs.

Design.—Retrospective Case Series.

Setting.—One-level 1 trauma center and 1 tertiary care hospital.

Patients.—Thirty-five consecutive patients meeting inclusion criteria.

Intervention.—A 2.7- or 2.4-mm reconstruction plate was placed on the dorsal ulnar cortex and contoured to allow passage of either a 2.7- or 3.5-mm intramedullary screw. In 9 patients, additional plates were required to control comminution. Available computed tomographic (CT) scans were evaluated for the presence of comminution.

Main Outcome Measurements.—Average Disabilities of the Arm, Shoulder, and Hand (DASH) and Mayo Elbow Performance Score (MEPS).

Results.—All fractures were united. Average extension deficit was 4.2 degrees, and average flexion angle was 137.4 degrees. Outcome scores were completed by 94% (33/35) of study patients. Average DASH score was 6.6, and average MEPS score was 94.5. Implants were removed in 18 patients. In the cohort of patients with CT scans, 6 of the 7 fractures thought to be simple on plain film analysis were found to have occult comminution on CT scan.

Conclusions.—Comminution should be considered in all olecranon fractures, even when plain films display simple patterns; although this did not affect treatment in this series of plated patients, it may be important if selecting tension band wiring. Fixation with 2.4- and 2.7-mm plates addresses comminution in olecranon fractures, avoiding the pitfalls of tension band wiring. In patients with completed outcome scores, 97% (32/33) reported their outcomes as good or excellent according to the MEPS.

Level of Evidence.—Therapeutic Level IV. See Instructions for Authors for a complete description of levels of evidence.

▶ Fixation of olecranon fractures can be accomplished with many techniques, including plate and screw, tension band, and intramedullary screw fixation. Each technique has specific advantages.

Plate and screw fixation is generally preferred in the setting of comminuted olecranon fractures because it allows more points of fixation of the fragments and does not necessarily rely on interfragmentary compression for stability. Intramedullary screws and tension band wiring may not support smaller fragments encountered in the setting of comminution, and the comminuted areas may not be bridged, resulting in shortening and malreduction of the articular surface.

Plate fixation relies on the placement of a plate along the subcutaneous border of the olecranon, and this plate can be prominent, resulting in soft tissue irritation and subsequent plate removal. The fixation is typically performed using a 3.5-mm plate, but this study presents the results of the plating of olecranon fractures using smaller 2.4- and 2.7-mm plates.

These smaller plates sacrifice some strength compared with the larger 3.5-mm plate, but they may be less prominent and better tolerated than 3.5-mm plates. The concern with the smaller plates is whether they will be strong enough to hold the fixation and whether increased rates of hardware failure and reoperation would be encountered. This study has shown that these plates have adequate strength to be used for the treatment of olecranon fractures because they were able to get all 35 fractures to unite.

Interestingly, 22 of the 35 patients underwent hardware removal, with 14 removals due to prominent hardware. This is consistent with previously published results, despite the use of the smaller plates.

In cases in which the patient's anatomy or smaller stature makes the use of a 3.5-mm plate undesirable, a smaller-sized plate can be substituted, and similar results should be expected.

S. A. Sems, MD

The Effect of C-Arm Position on Radiation Exposure During Fixation of Pediatric Supracondylar Fractures of the Humerus

Hsu RY, Lareau CR, Kim JS, et al (The Warren Alpert Med School of Brown Univ, Providence, RI)
J Bone Joint Surg Am 96:e129(1-6), 2014

Background.—Closed reduction and percutaneous pinning of a pediatric supracondylar fracture of the humerus requires operating directly next to the C-arm to hold reduction and perform fixation under direct imaging. This study was designed to compare radiation exposure from two C-arm configurations: with the image intensifier serving as the operating surface, and with a radiolucent hand table serving as the operating surface and the image intensifier positioned above the table.

Methods.—We used a cadaveric specimen in this study to determine radiation exposure to the operative elbow and to the surgeon at the waist and neck levels during simulated closed reduction and percutaneous pinning of a pediatric supracondylar fracture of the humerus. Radiation exposure measurements were made (1) with the C-arm image intensifier serving as the operating surface, with the emitter positioned above the operative elbow; and (2) with the image intensifier positioned above a hand table, with the emitter below the table.

Results.—When the image intensifier was used as the operating surface, we noted 16% less scatter radiation at the waist level of the surgeon but 53% more neck-level scatter radiation compared with when the hand table was used as the operating surface and the image intensifier was positioned above the table. In terms of direct radiation exposure to the operative elbow, use of the image intensifier as the operating surface resulted in 21% more radiation exposure than from use of the other configuration. The direct radiation exposure was also more than two orders of magnitude greater than the neck and waist-level scatter radiation exposure.

Conclusions.—Traditionally, there has been concern over increased radiation exposure when the C-arm image intensifier is used as an operating surface, with the emitter above, compared with when the image intensifier is positioned above the operating surface, with the emitter below. We determined that, although there was a statistically significant difference in radiation exposure between the two configurations, neither was safer than the other at all tested levels.

Clinical Relevance.—In contrast to traditional teaching regarding radiation exposure, neither C-arm configuration—with the image intensifier serving as the operating surface or with the image intensifier positioned above a radiolucent hand table—was shown to be clearly safer for pediatric supracondylar humeral fracture fixation.

▶ Orthopedic surgeons frequently use intraoperative fluoroscopy, and the procedures being performed require the surgeon to be close to the image intensifier and source of radiation. Despite the familiarity with the use of the intraoperative C-arm, many orthopedic surgeons do not understand the manner in which the radiation is dispersed and reflected from the structures in the operative field. This article studied the amount of radiation exposure that occurs at the different anatomic areas of the surgeon when the C-arm was used in 2 common configurations used to treat supracondylar humerus fractures.

The authors used cadaveric specimen to simulate closed reduction and percutaneous pinning of a supracondylar humerus fracture. Two configurations of C-arm were tested: 1 with the receiver used as the operating surface, and 1 with the receiver above the table and the emitter below the table. Scatter radiation bouncing off the receiver and patient resulted in increased exposure to the neck area of the surgeon when the receiver was used as the operating table. However, there was less scatter radiation at the surgeon's waist level when this arrangement was used. The direct exposure to the patient was more when the intensifier was used as the operating table.

The use of protective lead is commonplace among orthopedic surgeons using intraoperative fluoroscopy. However, the use of thyroid shields and leaded eyewear is likely not as common. This study highlights the importance of understanding the role that backscatter plays in exposing surgeons to radiation during C-arm use. When using the image intensifier as a table during percutaneous pinning of supracondylar humerus fractures, the use of leaded eyewear and thyroid shields should be given serious consideration in the event that the surgeon does not typically use these protective devices.

S. A. Sems, MD

12 Orthopedic Oncology

Introduction

Thank you for your interest in the Orthopedic Oncology section of the YEAR BOOK OF ORTHOPEDICS 2015. As in previous years, I have sought to bring together a collection of articles that includes those of interest to practicing tumor surgeons, as well as more general articles that will have immediate clinical use to surgeons who do not directly practice in this field.

As always, metastatic disease treatment and tumor resection and reconstruction papers figure prominently. This year I have included a pair of papers that rigorously evaluate surgical site infection in tumor surgery, a topic relevant to all surgeons in this field. Also, a number of studies are included that document patient outcomes and even look into new technologies to evaluate patient function after tumor resection. Several papers on rare reconstructions are included; while these are small series, they inform surgeons of options and techniques as they confront unique clinical scenarios. I hope this collection is useful to surgeons as they encounter patients in clinical practice.

Peter S. Rose, MD

General Tumor

Prognostic Effect of Erroneous Surgical Procedures in Patients with Osteosarcoma: Evaluation Using Propensity Score Matching

Chung SW, Han I, Oh JH, et al (Konkuk Univ Hosp, Seoul, Republic of Korea; Seoul Natl Univ Hosp, Republic of Korea; Seoul Natl Univ Bundang Hosp, Republic of Korea; et al)
J Bone Joint Surg Am 96:e60(1-8), 2014

Background.—Little is known concerning erroneous surgical procedures of malignant bone tumors, and the prognostic effect of erroneous surgical procedures in osteosarcoma has not been determined.

Methods.—We retrospectively reviewed 240 patients with initially non-metastatic high-grade osteosarcoma of the pelvis and extremities and, of these, identified twenty-six who had undergone previous less appropriate surgical procedures due to misdiagnosis followed by adequate treatment at our institution. We evaluated the clinicopathologic characteristics of these twenty-six patients compared with the remaining 214 patients treated with regular protocol. Subsequently, thirtyeight patients (nineteen in the matched case group and nineteen in the matched control group) were matched for multiple different variables using propensity score matching, and the oncologic results in terms of event-free survival and overall survival were analyzed.

Results.—The patients undergoing erroneous surgical procedures were typically older, with small, non-osteoblastic-type tumors that were in an unusual location, showed an osteolytic pattern on radiographs, had a tendency toward marginal or intralesional excision with positive histologic margin, and had not been treated with neoadjuvant chemotherapy (all $p < 0.05$). After adjustment of confounding variables by propensity score matching, there was no significant difference between matched groups with regard to event-free survival ($p = 0.46$) and overall survival ($p = 0.99$).

Conclusions.—Distinct differences existed in the clinicopathologic characteristics of the patients who underwent erroneous surgical procedures due to misdiagnosis. We failed to detect a prognostic relevance of the presence of previous erroneous procedures followed by adequate treatment.

▶ This group from Korea sought to characterize patients who underwent non-oncologic surgical procedures erroneously for osteosarcoma and to evaluate their outcome with a matched cohort. They identified 26 patients of 240 with localized high-grade osteosarcoma who initially underwent inappropriate surgical procedures in their tumor experience.

The patients who underwent erroneous procedures were older and had small nonosteoblastic sarcomas, often in an atypical location. None were treated with preoperative chemotherapy before manipulation. Using propensity matching, the authors assembled a cohort for comparison and found no significant difference between the patients who underwent erroneous operations and those who had conventional treatment with respect to event-free and overall survival. Although the amputation rate was not statistically different given the numbers involved, at least 2 patients in the erroneous surgical group underwent amputations as a direct consequence of their operations.

It is worth noting that the authors make some rather strong conclusions regarding their propensity score matching, claiming that it can take advantage of the randomization effect even in a retrospective study (they qualify this statement later in a more rigorous fashion). Readers should not confuse this with a truly prospective randomized study, despite the verbiage the authors have used in their article. It is also worth noting that other studies examining the outcome of patients undergoing unplanned manipulations of osteosarcoma have reached different conclusions.

This article is useful to the practicing clinician in identifying patients who are at risk of being misdiagnosed and undergoing surgical misadventure for osteosarcoma. It also brings forth the hope that their oncologic outcome can be salvaged similar to the experience with unplanned excisions of soft-tissue sarcomas. Certainly, the best outcome is to recognize these patients properly at presentation.

P. S. Rose, MD

Sarcoma Chemotherapy

Walczak BE, Irwin RB (Mayo Clinic, Rochester, MN; McLaren Cancer Inst, Mount Clemens, MI)
J Am Acad Orthop Surg 21:480-491, 2013

Sarcomas are a rare, heterogeneous group of malignant tumors of the bone or soft tissue. Although historically intended for the pharmaceutical treatment of microbes, today chemotherapy is used in orthopaedic oncology and is arguably the primary reason for improved survivorship. Agents such as anthracyclines (eg, doxorubicin), alkylating agents (eg, cyclophosphamide, ifosfamide), antimetabolites (eg, methotrexate), topoisomerase inhibitors (eg, etoposide [VP-16]), vinca alkaloids (eg, vincristine), and cytotoxic antibiotics (eg, actinomycin D) are used in various combinations to manage different types of tumors. Side effects are common and range from mild to severe. The effectiveness of the chemotherapy regimen correlates with the extent of tumor necrosis.

▶ I have included this article in the YEAR BOOK as a nice review of sarcoma chemotherapy. It can serve as a refresher for active clinicians and a nice teaching tool for residents, fellows, or colleagues who may interact with these patients. The article briefly reviews the history and rationale for sarcoma chemotherapy and gives data on specific agents and regimens used in the treatment of osteosarcoma, Ewing sarcoma, and soft-tissue sarcoma (including the adverse effects of chemotherapy agents that surgical oncologists are likely to encounter in the care of patients). As such, this is a useful reference article on this topic for orthopedic oncologists.

P. S. Rose, MD

Surgical Site Infection in Orthopaedic Oncology

Gradl G, de Witte PB, Evans BT, et al (Univ of Aachen, Germany; Leiden Univ Med Ctr, the Netherlands; Massachusetts General Hosp, Boston)
J Bone Joint Surg Am 96:223-230, 2014

Background.—This study addressed risk factors for surgical site infection in patients who had undergone orthopaedic oncology surgical procedures.

Methods.—We retrospectively reviewed data on 1521 orthopaedic oncologic surgical procedures in 1304 patients. We assessed patient demographics, updated Charlson comorbidity index, surgery-specific data, and treatment-related data and attempted to identify predictors of surgical site infection with bivariate and multivariable analysis.

Results.—Eight factors independently predicted surgical site infection: body mass index (odds ratio [OR]:, 1.03, 95% confidence interval [CI]: 1.00 to 1.07), age (OR: 1.18, 95% CI: 1.05 to 1.33), total number of preceding procedures (OR: 1.19, 95% CI: 1.07 to 1.34), preexisting implants (OR: 1.94, 95% CI: 1.17 to 3.21), infection at another site on the date of the surgery (OR: 4.13, 95% CI: 1.57 to 10.85), malignant disease (OR: 1.46, 95% CI: 0.94 to 2.26), hip region affected (OR: 1.96, 95% CI: 1.35 to 2.84), and duration of the procedure (OR: 1.16, 95% CI: 1.07 to 1.25).

Conclusions.—These factors can inform patients and surgeons of the probability of surgical site infection after orthopaedic oncologic surgery. While most risk factors are unmodifiable or related to the complexity of the case, infection at another site on the date of the surgery is one factor amenable to intervention.

Level of Evidence.—Prognostic Level IV. See Instructions for Authors for a complete description of levels of evidence.

▶ This is a large retrospective review of surgical site infection from the Massachusetts General Hospital group analyzing more than 1500 orthopedic oncology procedures in 1300 patients spanning nearly a decade.

The authors found a 10.1% incidence in surgical site infections. Additionally, they found that surgical site infection was correlated with a number of patient and oncologic variables. Oncologic variables that were associated were the use of radiotherapy and chemotherapy, which is not surprising. Several patient-related variables were also noted (body mass index, increase in age, number of preceding procedures, and the use of implants). Interestingly, surgery about the hip had a higher rate than other areas; duration of the procedure, not surprisingly, also influenced infection.

We all recognize the increased risk of infection that tumor patients have in clinical practice. This study is helpful in quantifying infection risk in an era of close (but often uninformed) scrutiny of infection as an outcome and quality measure. The data the authors provide on the use of radiation therapy and its influence on the apparent risk of infection is helpful for surgeons as they try to chart the best course for treatment for their patients, balancing the oncologic needs with the need to not interrupt treatment. There is relatively little literature on this subject, and this article provides a good addition to it. Readers should know that this is a retrospective study. As such, it likely underestimates the instance of infection compared with what would be seen in a prospective study, and these results are probably a low estimate for the instance of infection. The associated factors are likely to remain valid given the large numbers involved despite the retrospective nature.

P. S. Rose, MD

Analysis of Surgical Site Infection after Musculoskeletal Tumor Surgery: Risk Assessment Using a New Scoring System

Nagano S, Yokouchi M, Setoguchi T, et al (Kagoshima Univ, Japan; et al)
Sarcoma 2014:645496, 2014

Surgical site infection (SSI) has not been extensively studied in musculoskeletal tumors (MST) owing to the rarity of the disease. We analyzed incidence and risk factors of SSI in MST. SSI incidence was evaluated in consecutive 457 MST cases (benign, 310 cases and malignant, 147 cases) treated at our institution. A detailed analysis of the clinical background of the patients, pre- and postoperative hematological data, and other factors that might be associated with SSI incidence was performed for malignant MST cases. SSI occurred in 0.32% and 12.2% of benign and malignant MST cases, respectively. The duration of the surgery ($P = 0.0002$) and intraoperative blood loss ($P = 0.0005$) was significantly more in the SSI group than in the non-SSI group. We established the musculoskeletal oncological surgery invasiveness (MOSI) index by combining 4 risk factors (blood loss, operation duration, preoperative chemotherapy, and the use of artificial materials). The MOSI index (0—4 points) score significantly correlated with the risk of SSI, as demonstrated by an SSI incidence of 38.5% in the group with a high score (3-4 points). The MOSI index score and laboratory data at 1 week after surgery could facilitate risk evaluation and prompt diagnosis of SSI.

▶ This is an article that can be read as a companion to the MGH retrospective series reviewed in an adjacent reference. These authors from Japan prospectively evaluated the risk of surgical site infection in a cohort of patients undergoing surgery for benign and malignant musculoskeletal disease. Additionally, they derived a musculoskeletal oncology surgery invasiveness index (MOSI index) that combined blood loss, operative duration, the use of preoperative chemotherapy, and the use of implants to stratify patients for risk. Note that this study comes from an area where the use of radiotherapy is relatively rare, and thus radiation therapy did not play into their risk assessment. Contemporary North American practice would include radiation therapy in the treatment of many of the patients in this cohort and would likely identify radiotherapy as a risk factor for infection.

In this manner, surgical site infection was seen in less than 1% of patients undergoing benign procedures and 12.2% of patients undergoing malignant procedures. There was face validity to the MOSI index in that patients with high scores had surgical site infections approaching 40%. The authors suggest that this is a way to risk stratify patients in this manner.

This article is valuable in that it provides a more rigorous evaluation (admittedly of a smaller cohort) than that seen in the adjacent article. It remains to be seen whether the MOSI index will be incorporated into orthopedic practice. Its exclusion of radiotherapy would make it less directly applicable to contemporary

North American practice. However, it is a reasonable start at identifying patients at elevated risk in this manner.

P. S. Rose, MD

Histopathological Diagnostic Discrepancies in Soft Tissue Tumours Referred to a Specialist Centre: Reassessment in the Era of Ancillary Molecular Diagnosis

Thway K, Wang J, Mubako T, et al (The Royal Marsden NHS Foundation Trust, London, UK)
Sarcoma 2014:686902, 2014

Introduction.—Soft tissue tumour pathology is a highly specialised area of surgical pathology, but soft tissue neoplasms can occur at virtually all sites and are therefore encountered by a wide population of surgical pathologists. Potential sarcomas require referral to specialist centres for review by pathologists who see a large number of soft tissue lesions and where appropriate ancillary investigations can be performed. We have previously assessed the types of diagnostic discrepancies between referring and final diagnosis for soft tissue lesions referred to our tertiary centre. We now reaudit this 6 years later, assessing changes in discrepancy patterns, particularly in relation to the now widespread use of ancillary molecular diagnostic techniques which were not prevalent in our original study.

Materials and Methods.—We compared the sarcoma unit's histopathology reports with referring reports on 348 specimens from 286 patients with suspected or proven soft tissue tumours in a one-year period.

Results.—Diagnostic agreement was seen in 250 cases (71.8%), with 57 (16.4%) major and 41 (11.8%) minor discrepancies. There were 23 cases of benign/malignant discrepancies (23.5% of all discrepancies). 50 ancillary molecular tests were performed, 33 for aiding diagnosis and 17 mutational analyses for gastrointestinal stromal tumour to guide therapy. Findings from ancillary techniques contributed to 3 major and 4 minor discrepancies. While the results were broadly similar to those of the previous study, there was an increase in frequency of major discrepancies.

Conclusion.—Six years following our previous study and notably now in an era of widespread ancillary molecular diagnosis, the overall discrepancy rate between referral and tertiary centre diagnosis remains similar, but there is an increase in frequency of major discrepancies likely to alter patient management. A possible reason for the increase in major discrepancies is the increasing lack of exposure to soft tissue cases in nonspecialist centres in a time of subspecialisation. The findings support the national guidelines in which all suspected soft tissue tumour pathology specimens should be referred to a specialist sarcoma unit.

▶ This article from London reviews the final diagnoses made at a national referral center for evaluation of soft-tissue sarcomas compared with diagnoses made in the community. Although the results are somewhat specific to the United Kingdom National Health System, they are likely to be generalizable to modern First World practice. This is a follow-up article on one that the authors had performed 6 or more years earlier before the widespread adoption of molecular diagnostic methodologies in their health system.

The overall complete agreement was 72% with 16% of cases having major areas of disagreement between the initial diagnosis and that performed at the referring center. The most common major diagnosis was a discrepancy between benign and malignant lesions.

This article highlights the importance of correct diagnostic ascertainment for soft-tissue sarcomas, a relatively rare field that pathologists may have varying experiences in. There are a number of strong referral centers and pathways in contemporary North American practice to allow review at experienced centers either within or outside of the confines of patients on clinical trial. This article highlights the importance of experienced pathology review if there is any question of center experience or final diagnosis.

P. S. Rose, MD

Cancer Risk from Bone Morphogenetic Protein Exposure in Spinal Arthrodesis

Kelly MP, Savage JW, Bentzen SM et al (Univ of Wisconsin School of Medicine and Public Health, Madison; Northwestern Univ Feinberg School of Medicine, Chicago, IL; et al)
J Bone Joint Surg Am 96:1417-1422, 2014

Background.—The U.S. Food and Drug Administration reported a higher incidence of cancer in patients who had spinal arthrodesis and were exposed to a high dose of recombinant human bone morphogenetic protein-2 (rhBMP-2) compared with the control group in a randomized controlled trial. The purpose of this study was to determine the risk of cancer after spinal arthrodesis with BMP.

Methods.—We retrospectively analyzed the incidence of cancer in 467,916 Medicare patients undergoing spinal arthrodesis from 2005 to 2010. Patients with a preexisting diagnosis of cancer were excluded. The average follow-up duration was 2.85 years for the BMP group and 2.94 years for the control group. The main outcome measure was the relative risk of developing new malignant lesions after spinal arthrodesis with or without exposure to BMP.

Results.—The relative risk of developing cancer after BMP exposure was 0.938 (95% confidence interval [95% CI]: 0.913 to 0.964), which was significant. In the BMP group, 5.9% of the patients developed an invasive cancer compared with 6.5% of the patients in the control group. The relative risk of developing cancer after BMP exposure was 0.98 in males (95% CI: 0.94 to 1.02) and 0.93 (95% CI: 0.90 to 0.97) in females.

The control group showed a higher incidence of each type of cancer except pancreatic cancer.

Conclusions.—Recent clinical use of BMP was not associated with a detectable increase in the risk of cancer within a mean 2.9-year time window.

Level of Evidence.—Therapeutic Level III. See Instructions for Authors for a complete description of levels of evidence.

▶ There has been significant controversy in the potential association between exposure to bone morphogenetic protein (BMP) and the development of cancer. Two studies have been contradictory in the overall literature regarding analysis of the results from randomized trials. Additionally, a high-dose BMP formulation recently failed Food and Drug Administration approval because of a higher incidence of cancer seen in the treatment group at 24- and 60-month follow-up. These authors retrospectively reviewed more than 450 000 Medicare patients undergoing spinal arthrodesis between 2005 and 2010 to assess the development of malignancy.

This study benefits from a large treatment population in a real-world setting. However, it clearly suffers from all of the limitations of a large administrative database study performed in a retrospective fashion. The authors did take great pains to try to minimize this risk and even compared their rates of cancer with those from the Surveillance, Epidemiology, and End Results program database.

In summary, the relative risk of developing a new cancer was actually minimally lower in patients exposed to BMP than in those not exposed to BMP. The average follow-up was only 2.9 years, so it is possible that greater follow-up would be necessary to see an effect. Additionally, we do not have information on the doses that were used in this study or the precise method of application.

Where to place this study in clinical context? Unfortunately, this does not solve the issue or whether BMP exposure is associated with an increased risk of malignancy. The information that has come from other studies certainly raises this question. If such an association does exist, it is likely a subtle one that is dependent on dose, host, and (potentially) method of application. Oncologic surgeons should be aware of this continuing controversy and the varying literature associated with it as they advise colleagues and make treatment decisions for their patients. At this time, I think it is fair to say that there is a lack of scientific consensus as to whether BMP exposure in typical doses increases the risk of cancer at short-term follow-up. However, given the available data that suggests that it may, surgeons should take great care before selecting the use of these agents in any patient with a history or strong predisposition to malignancy.

P. S. Rose, MD

What Is the Use of Imaging Before Referral to an Orthopaedic Oncologist? A Prospective, Multicenter Investigation

Miller BJ, on behalf of the Musculoskeletal Oncology Research Initiative (Univ of Iowa; et al)
Clin Orthop Relat Res 2014 [Epub ahead of print]

Background.—Patients often receive advanced imaging before referral to an orthopaedic oncologist. The few studies that have evaluated the value of these tests have been single-center studies, and there were large discrepancies in the estimated frequencies of unnecessary use of diagnostic tests.

Questions/Purposes.—(1) Is there regional variation in the use of advanced imaging before referral to an orthopaedic oncologist? (2) Are these prereferral studies helpful to the treating orthopaedic oncologist in making a diagnosis or treatment plan? (3) Are orthopaedic surgeons less likely to order unhelpful studies than other specialties? (4) Are there any tumor or patient characteristics that are associated with the ordering of an unhelpful study?

Methods.—We performed an eight-center prospective analysis of patients referred for evaluation by a fellowship-trained orthopaedic oncologist. We recorded patient factors, referral details, advanced imaging performed, and presumptive diagnosis. The treating orthopaedic oncologist determined whether each study was helpful in the diagnosis or treatment of the patient based on objective and subjective criteria used in prior investigations. We analyzed the data using bivariate methods and logistic regression to determine regional variation and risk factors predictive of unhelpful advanced imaging. Of the 371 participants available for analysis, 301 (81%) were referred with an MRI, CT scan, bone scan, ultrasound, or positron emission tomography scan.

Results.—There were no regional differences in the use of advanced imaging (range of patients presenting with advanced imaging 66%–88% across centers, $p = 0.164$). One hundred thirteen patients (30%) had at least one unhelpful study; non-MRI advanced imaging was more likely to be unhelpful than MRIs (88 of 129 [68%] non-MRI imaging versus 46 of 263 [17%] MRIs [$p < 0.001$]). Orthopaedic surgeons were no less likely than nonorthopaedic surgeons to order unhelpful studies before referral to an orthopaedic oncologist (56 of 179 [31%] of patients referred by orthopaedic surgeons versus 35 of 119 [29%] referred by primary care providers and 22 of 73 [30%] referred by nonorthopaedic specialists, $p = 0.940$). After controlling for potential confounding variables, benign bone lesions had an increased odds of referral with an unhelpful study (59 of 145 [41%] of benign bone tumors versus 54 of 226 [24%] of soft tissue tumors and malignant bone tumors; odds ratio, 2.80; 95% confidence interval, 1.68–4.69, $p < 0.001$).

Conclusions.—We found no evidence that the proportion of patients referred with advanced imaging varied dramatically by region. Studies other than MRI were likely to be considered unhelpful and should not be routinely ordered by referring physicians. Diligent education of orthopaedic surgeons and primary care physicians in the judicious use of advanced imaging in benign bone tumors may help mitigate unnecessary imaging.

Level of Evidence.—Level III, diagnostic study. See Guidelines for Authors for a complete description of levels of evidence.

▶ These authors prospectively evaluated the use of advanced imaging before referral to orthopedic oncologists for the evaluation of bone lesions to determine the characteristics of imaging and whether the imaging was felt to be useful for diagnosis. Significantly, 81% of patients were referred with an advanced imaging procedure already completed (magnetic resonance imaging [MRI], computed tomography scan, bone scan, ultrasound, and/or positron emission tomography scan).

Thirty percent had at least 1 advanced imaging scan that was not felt to be helpful in clinical management. Advanced imaging other than MRI was not likely to be helpful in patients. Additionally, patients with benign diagnoses were more likely to have unhelpful advanced imaging studies.

Where to place this study in clinical context? Determining whether imaging studies are necessary or unnecessary is somewhat subjective. Furthermore, as health care changes and standardization increases in the North American practice of orthopedic oncology, it is likely that basic protocols will be adopted to guide imaging before referral. As imaging studies and telemedicine improve, many patients may be managed with a "virtual" orthopedic oncology consultation (with a trained orthopedic oncologist reviewing imaging and clinical records and evaluations provided by a local physician).

As such, this article provides a baseline assessment of the current practice in North America. Additionally, it suggests that protocols to evaluate these lesions should start with plain film radiography and potentially MRI before evaluation by orthopedic oncologists but not include other advanced imaging modalities at this time.

Interested readers are referred to the accompanying commentary by Dr Jones.[1]

P. S. Rose, MD

Reference

1. Jones KB. CORR insights: what is the use of imaging before referral to an orthopaedic oncologist? *Clin Orthop Relat Res.* 2014 [Epub ahead of print].

Sarcoma Mid-Therapy [F-18]Fluorodeoxyglucose Positron Emission Tomography (FDG PET) and Patient Outcome
Eary JF, Conrad EU, O'Sullivan J, et al (Univ of Washington, Seattle; Univ College Cork, Ireland; et al)
J Bone Joint Surg Am 96:152-158, 2014

Background.—Our previous research investigated the ability of [F-18] fluorodeoxyglucose (FDG) positron emission tomography (PET) imaging results to predict outcome in patients with sarcoma. Tumor uptake of FDG before and after neoadjuvant chemotherapy was predictive of patient outcome. With this background, a prospective clinical study was designed to assess whether tumor FDG uptake levels in the middle of neoadjuvant chemotherapy added additional prognostic information to pre-therapy imaging data.

Methods.—Sixty-five patients with either bone or soft-tissue sarcoma were treated with neoadjuvant-based chemotherapy according to the standard clinical practice for each tumor group. All patients had FDG PET studies before therapy, mid-therapy (after two cycles of chemotherapy), and before resection. Tumor FDG uptake (SUVmax, the maximum standardized uptake value) at each imaging time point, tumor type (bone or soft-tissue sarcoma), tumor size, and histopathologic grade were recorded for each patient. The time from the pre-therapy FDG PET study to events of local tumor recurrence, metastasis, or death were extracted from the clinical records for comparison with the imaging data. Univariate and multivariate analyses of the imaging and clinical data were performed.

Results.—Univariate and multivariate data analyses showed that the difference (measured as the percentage reduction) between the pre-therapy and mid-therapy maximum tumor uptake values added prognostic value to patient outcome predictions independently of other patient variables.

Conclusions.—The utility of a tumor pre-therapy FDG PET scan as a biomarker for the outcome of patients with sarcoma was strengthened by a mid-therapy scan to evaluate the interim treatment response (Fig 2).

▶ The use of positron emission tomography (PET) is becoming more common in the staging of patients with high-grade sarcomas; in addition, because of the ability to objectively quantify tumor metabolism, this technique holds the potential to objectively assess tumor response and predict outcome in patients undergoing neoadjuvant therapy. The University of Washington group reports the results of 65 patients with bone or soft-tissue sarcomas treated with

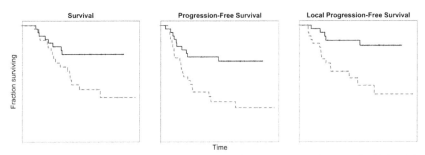

FIGURE 2.—Kaplan-Meier curves of the patient group for three survival end points. The black (solid) lines represent patients with lower risk (below the median) as defined by the survival models. The red (dashed) lines represent patients with higher risk (above the median). For Interpretation of the references to color in this figure legend, the reader is referred to web version of this article. (Reprinted from Eary JF, Conrad EU, O'Sullivan J, et al. Sarcoma mid-therapy [F-18]fluorodeoxyglucose positron emission tomography (FDG PET) and patient outcome. *J Bone Joint Surg Am.* 2014;96:152-158, http://jbjs.org/.)

preoperative chemotherapy and analyzed by PET computed tomography scan at presentation, midtherapy, and before surgical treatment. In reading this article, it is important for surgeons to recognize that it includes both bone and soft-tissue sarcomas in pediatric and adult patients scattered throughout the body. Although the role for and regimens used to treat bone sarcomas are well established, the use of chemotherapy for soft-tissue sarcoma can vary among institutions (both for indications and agents). Some patients with soft-tissue sarcomas also underwent radiotherapy. In generalizing the results of this study to individual practices, these factors need to be kept in mind.

In summary, the authors found that the change in standardized uptake value (SUV) between presentation and mid-chemotherapy was predictive of patient outcome (see Fig 2). The authors stratified patients as being above or below the median value.

Where to place this study in clinical context? When confronting an individual patient, the authors have not provided us with cutoff points to clearly evaluate response (rather, they reported responses for a large group). They do provide a formula in their article, but this is somewhat cumbersome in clinical practice. Additionally, surgeons confronting patients with localized sarcomas will take them to surgery as part of their curative treatment in any event. Although one can imagine a scenario in which a difficult decision is being made between limb salvage and amputation in which an assessment of tumor response might sway treatment one direction or another, the bulk of our decisions regarding the nature and extent of surgery are based on the anatomic extent of an individual lesion. Additionally, no objective data currently suggest a value to shifting chemotherapy regimens based on SUV response in the middle of a preoperative chemotherapy regimen.

As such, this is an interesting article that clinicians should be aware of. As our understanding of PET and its applicability to sarcoma care increases, articles like this will likely lay the groundwork for future evaluation and treatment regimens. At present, these data can help provide prognostic information but will probably not commonly change treatment decisions.

P. S. Rose, MD

Malignant Transformation in Chronic Osteomyelitis: Recognition and Principles of Management
Panteli M, Puttaswamaiah R, Lowenberg DW, et al (Univ of Leeds, West Yorkshire, UK; SPARSH Hosp for Advanced Surgeries, Bangalore, India; Stanford Univ School of Medicine, CA)
J Am Acad Orthop Surg 22:586-594, 2014

Malignant transformation as a result of chronic osteomyelitis represents a relatively rare and late complication with a declining incidence in the modern world. For most patients, the interval between the occurrence of the original bacterial infection and the transformation to malignant degeneration is several years. The diagnosis of malignant transformation in a chronic discharging sinus requires a high index of clinical suspicion. Wound biopsies should be obtained early, especially with the onset of new clinical signs such as increased pain, a foul smell, and changes in wound drainage. Squamous cell carcinoma is the most common presenting malignancy. Definitive treatment is amputation proximal to the tumor or wide local excision, combined with adjuvant chemotherapy and radiation therapy in selected patients. Early diagnosis may sometimes allow for treatment consisting of en bloc excision and limb salvage techniques. However, the most effective treatment is prevention with definitive treatment of the osteomyelitis, including adequate débridement, wide excision of the affected area, and early reconstruction.

▶ Even in an active surgical oncology practice, Marjolin ulcers are infrequently encountered. As well, physicians who pursue missionary or similar work overseas in the developing world may well see patients with malignant transformation secondary to chronic osteomyelitis. I have included this article in the YEAR BOOK because it does a nice job of synthesizing the available literature and clinical understanding that guide treatment of this rare condition. This article may serve as a reference to be consulted when a patient with a suspicion of a Marjolin ulcer is encountered. It also covers basic aspects of orthopedics that are important for students and other learners to be familiar with in our clinical evaluation of chronic wounds.

P. S. Rose, MD

A Translational Study of the Neoplastic Cells of Giant Cell Tumor of Bone Following Neoadjuvant Denosumab

Mak IWY, Evaniew N, Popovic S, et al (McMaster Univ, Hamilton, Ontario, Canada)

J Bone Joint Surg Am 96:e127(1-8), 2014

Background.—Giant cell tumor of bone is a primary bone tumor that is treated surgically and is associated with high morbidity in many cases. This tumor consists of giant cells expressing RANK (receptor activator of nuclear factor-kB) and mesenchymal spindle-like stromal cells expressing RANKL (RANK ligand); the interaction of these cells leads to bone resorption. Denosumab is a monoclonal antibody that binds RANKL and directly inhibits osteoclastogenesis. Clinical studies have suggested clinical and histological improvement when denosumab was administered to patients with a giant cell tumor. However, no studies have yet examined the viability and functional characteristics of tumor cells following denosumab treatment.

Methods.—Specimens were obtained from six patients with a histologically confirmed giant cell tumor. Two of the patients had been treated with denosumab for six months. Primary cultures of stromal cells from fresh tumor tissue were established. Cell proliferation was measured over a two-day time course. The expression of RANKL and osteoprotegerin was analyzed with use of real-time PCR (polymerase chain reaction).

Results.—Histological specimens from both patients who had completed denosumab treatment showed the absence of giant cells but persistence of stromal cells. Cell proliferation studies indicated that proliferation of stromal cells cultured from clinical specimens following denosumab treatment was approximately 50% slower than that of specimens from untreated patients. The expression of RANKL in the specimens from the treated patients was almost completely eliminated.

Conclusions.—Once the giant cell tumor tissue was no longer exposed to denosumab, the stromal cells continued to proliferate in vitro, albeit to a lesser degree. However, they also showed almost complete loss of RANKL expression.

Clinical Relevance.—It is clear that treatment with denosumab only partially addresses the therapeutic need of patients with a giant cell tumor by wiping out the osteoclasts but leaving the neoplastic stromal cells proliferative.

▶ Denosumab treatment has emerged as a therapeutic option in the treatment of patients with giant cell tumor. It may be used as stand-alone treatment for patients with axial tumors that have great functional loss with surgery or may be used as preoperative therapy to "downstage" or "marginate" tumors prior to surgery. The medication is a monoclonal antibody that binds RANK-ligand and inhibits osteoclastogenesis.

No prior studies have looked at the cell culture effects of denosumab on patients with giant cell tumors. Dr Ghert and colleagues from McMaster University analyzed specimens from 6 patients with giant cell tumors (2 who had been treated with denosumab for 6 months).

On the positive side, the expression of RANK-ligand in the patients treated with denosumab was completely normal. Additionally, no real giant cells were seen, although stromal cells persisted. The stromal cells had slower but very much present proliferation in cell culture compared to stromal cells of patients with untreated giant cell tumors.

Where to place this study in clinical context? This is nice basic science confirmation that denosumab does have a clearly identifiable effect histologically that mirrors the clinical effect that can be seen. However, the persistence of stromal cells with slow but present proliferation suggests that denosumab treatment may not be able to eliminate giant cell tumors. This is important because patients currently being treated with denosumab therapy in lieu of surgery do not have a well-defined "stopping point" in treatments. Until additional data accumulate, it is clear that 6 months alone is probably insufficient.

P. S. Rose, MD

Metastatic Disease

Surgical Management of Metastatic Long Bone Fractures: Principles and Techniques
Scolaro JA, Lackman RD (Univ of California, Irvine; Cooper Univ Health Care, Camden, NJ)
J Am Acad Orthop Surg 22:90-100, 2014

Management of metastatic long bone fractures requires identification of the lesion and the use of sound fracture fixation principles to relieve pain and restore function. The treating surgeon must understand the principles of pathologic fracture fixation before initiating treatment. Because these fractures occur in the context of a progressive systemic disease, management typically involves a multidisciplinary approach. When considering surgical stabilization of these fractures, the abnormal (or absent) healing environment associated with diseased bone and the overall condition of the patient must be taken into account. The goal of surgery is to obtain a rigid mechanical construct, which allows for early mobility and weight bearing. This can be achieved using internal fixation with polymethyl methacrylate cement or segmental resection and joint reconstruction. Prosthetic joint arthroplasty is a more reliable means of fracture management when insufficient bone is present for fixation. Prophylactic stabilization of impending pathologic fractures can reduce the morbidity associated with metastatic lesions.

▶ Bony metastatic disease continues to be a significant clinical burden. Although complex cases are often treated by orthopedic oncologists, many patients are appropriately treated by skilled general orthopedic surgeons who are informed on the subject but not necessarily oncologic specialists. Drs Scolaro and Lackman have put together a nice review article that discusses different surgical options and provides management strategies for different anatomic areas of the body. Additionally, the bibliography includes a nice collection of classic articles for interested clinicians to pursue further. Although much of what is discussed is probably already known to active orthopedic oncologists, this is an excellent article to share with trainees or colleagues who will treat these patients.

P. S. Rose, MD

Management of Metastatic Bone Disease of the Acetabulum
Issack PS, Kotwal SY, Lane JM (Weill Med College of Cornell Univ, NY; Univ of Missouri at Kansas City; Hosp for Special Surgery, NY)
J Am Acad Orthop Surg 21:685-695, 2013

Metastatic acetabular disease can be severely painful and may result in loss of mobility. Initial management may consist of diphosphonates, narcotic analgesics, radiation therapy, protected weight bearing, cemento-plasty, and radiofrequency ablation. Patients with disease affecting large weight-bearing regions of the acetabulum and with impending failure of the hip joint are unlikely to gain much relief from nonsurgical treatment and interventional procedures. The profound osteopenia of the acetabu-lum, limited healing potential of the fracture, and projected patient life span and function necessitate surgical techniques that provide immediate stable fixation to reduce pain and restore ambulatory function. Current reconstructive procedures, including cemented total hip arthroplasty, the saddle or periacetabular endoprosthesis, and porous tantalum implants, are based on the quality of remaining acetabular bone as well as the patient's level of function and general health. Well-executed acetabular reconstructions can provide durable hip joints with good pain relief and function.

▶ Similar to metastatic long-bone lesions, metastatic disease of the acetabulum remains a common clinical problem. Additionally, as adjuvant treatments im-prove, patients' life expectancy with periacetabular metastasis is likely improving. Thus, these patients can provide a more difficult clinical problem because of the need to provide a functional reconstruction with at least intermediate-term durability.

Issack and colleagues provide a review of treatment options including more modern percutaneous treatments (cementoplasty) that may be useful for these patients and not familiar to all surgeons. This article is a nice refresher for prac-ticing surgeons as well as a good teaching article to share with students or col-leagues. Additionally, the bibliography includes contemporary references for clinicians who wish to explore the subject further.

P. S. Rose, MD

The Integration of Radiosurgery for the Treatment of Patients With Metastatic Spine Diseases

Sharan AD, Szulc A, Krystal J, et al (Montefiore Med Ctr, Bronx, NY; Albert Einstein College of Medicine, Bronx, NY; et al)
J Am Acad Orthop Surg 22:447-454, 2014

Significant evidence emerging in the spinal oncology literature recom-mends radiosurgery as a primary modality of treatment of spinal metasta-sis. Improvements in the methods of delivering radiation have increased the ability to provide a higher and more exacting dose of radiation to a tumor bed than previously. Using treatment-planning software, radiation is contoured around a specific lesion with the intent of administering a tumoricidal dose. Combined with a minimally invasive, tumor-load reduc-ing surgery, this advanced form of radiation therapy can provide better local control of the tumor compared with conventional external beam radiation.

▶ The spine is the most common site of bony metastases in patients with advanced cancer, and local progression of disease can have devastating consequences for patient outcome. Thus, surgery and radiotherapy are often called on to treat patients.

New, sophisticated methods of radiation delivery can allow relatively high doses to be delivered to the treatment volume (tumor) with sharp dose gradations that can minimize the dose to target organs at risk (most typically the spinal cord, conus medullaris, or cauda equine). This article by Dr Sharan and colleagues reviews the rationale for treatment of this nature as well as the role of advanced radiotherapy (often called radiosurgery) both as a stand-alone treatment or in conjunction with surgical stabilization and decompression. Early results show that this has the potential to lessen the magnitude of the surgical procedure necessary for clinical management and minimalize the likelihood that the patients will experience symptomatic local recurrence during their remaining life span.

The capability to perform advanced radiotherapy techniques is not available at all centers, but its use is rapidly expanding in contemporary North American practice. Additionally, the techniques described here can have implications for the management of patients with lesions in other areas (pelvis and sacrum), and thus the article may be of interest to surgeons who practice outside of the spine as well.

P. S. Rose, MD

Brain Metastasis in Bone and Soft Tissue Cancers: A Review of Incidence, Interventions, and Outcomes
Shweikeh F, Bukavina L, Saeed K, et al (Northeast Ohio Med Univ, Rootstown; Summa Health System, Akron, OH; Rush Univ Med Ctr, Chicago, IL; et al)
Sarcoma 2014:475175, 2014

Bone and soft tissue malignancies account for a small portion of brain metastases. In this review, we characterize their incidence, treatments, and prognosis. Most of the data in the literature is based on case reports and small case series. Less than 5% of brain metastases are from bone and soft tissue sarcomas, occurring most commonly in Ewing's sarcoma, malignant fibrous tumors, and osteosarcoma. Mean interval from initial cancer diagnosis to brain metastasis is in the range of 20—30 months, with most being detected before 24 months (osteosarcoma, Ewing sarcoma, chordoma, angiosarcoma, and rhabdomyosarcoma), some at 24—36 months (malignant fibrous tumors, malignant peripheral nerve sheath tumors, and alveolar soft part sarcoma), and a few after 36 months (chondrosarcoma and liposarcoma). Overall mean survival ranges between 7 and 16 months, with the majority surviving <12 months (Ewing's sarcoma, liposarcoma, malignant fibrous tumors, malignant peripheral nerve sheath tumors, angiosarcoma and chordomas). Management is heterogeneous involving surgery, radiosurgery, radiotherapy, and chemotherapy. While a survival advantage may exist for those given aggressive treatment involving surgical resection, such patients tended to have a favorable preoperative performance status and minimal systemic disease.

▶ Brain metastases are thankfully rare in treating patients with bone and soft tissue sarcoma. However, because of their rarity, there is relatively little in the literature about them. This review article summarizes what is currently understood about the incidence, treatment, and outcomes of patients with brain metastases from primary sarcomas.

The most common histologies observed were Ewing sarcoma, osteosarcoma, and pleomorphic/malignant fibrous histiocytoma. Most patients who presented with brain metastases did so within 2 years of their initial diagnosis of cancer, although there were some late diagnoses in a small number of patients.

The majority of patients died from disease within 12 months, and there is no clearly defined preferred treatment modality (obviously, treatment selections were biased for the presentations of the patients). This article is useful for surgeons and clinicians to be aware of so that they understand the full background of this thankfully rare phenomenon and for the careful and exhaustive literature review that the authors included. As such, it is valuable for a practicing oncologist to be aware of and share with their trainees.

P. S. Rose, MD

Patient Outcomes

Can Orthopedic Oncologists Predict Functional Outcome in Patients with Sarcoma after Limb Salvage Surgery in the Lower Limb? A Nationwide Study
Kolk S, Cox K, Weerdesteyn V, et al (Radboud Univ Med Ctr, Nijmegen, The Netherlands; et al)
Sarcoma 2014:436598, 2014

Accurate predictions of functional outcome after limb salvage surgery (LSS) in the lower limb are important for several reasons, including informing the patient preoperatively and, in some cases, deciding between amputation and LSS. This study aimed to elucidate the correlation between surgeon-predicted and patient-reported functional outcome of LSS in the Netherlands. Twenty-three patients (between six months and ten years after surgery) and five independent orthopedic oncologists completed the Toronto Extremity Salvage Score (TESS) and the RAND-36 physical functioning subscale (RAND-36 PFS). The orthopedic oncologists made their predictions based on case descriptions (including MRI scans) that reflected the preoperative status. The correlation between patient-reported and surgeon-predicted functional outcome was "very poor" to "poor" on both scores (r^2 values ranged from 0.014 to 0.354). Patient-reported functional outcome was generally underestimated, by 8.7% on the TESS and 8.3% on the RAND-36 PFS. The most difficult and least difficult tasks on the RAND-36 PFS were also the most difficult and least difficult to predict, respectively. Most questions had a "poor" intersurgeon agreement. It was difficult to accurately predict the patient-reported functional outcome of LSS. Surgeons' ability to predict functional scores can be improved the most by focusing on accurately predicting more demanding tasks.

▶ This interesting article from the Netherlands reinforces the limitations of predicting patients' outcomes through record review only. The authors sought to investigate whether surgeons could predict the functional outcome of patients undergoing limb salvage surgery for sarcomas in the Netherlands. They gathered 23 patient records and had 5 practicing orthopedic oncologists predict the Toronto extremity salvage score and RAND-36 physical function score based on case descriptions and imaging studies alone. These were then correlated with the patient's ultimate function.

The results were poor; surgeons were not able to accurately predict outcome. This is presented in a manner that suggests surgeons are unable to predict clinical outcome, and there is probably some truth to this. However, we must not forget that the surgeons making the predictions were reviewing records only rather than seeing patients. This probably has greater application in the current era of electronic consults where expert surgeons provide case input based on review of records and imaging only without actually examining patients. It is an open question whether an experienced surgeon actually meeting and examining the patient could then make a better prediction of their outcome. This was not the focus of this study and could not be evaluated by its design.

Thus, I think the conclusions are a little more nuanced than the authors put forth. Additionally, I think the implications of this in the evolving electronic medical environment are perhaps different from what the authors suggest.

P. S. Rose, MD

Assessment of Objective Ambulation in Lower Extremity Sarcoma Patients with a Continuous Activity Monitor: Rationale and Validation
Gundle KR, Punt SE, Conrad EU III (Univ of Washington Med Ctr, Seattle)
Sarcoma 2014:947082, 2014

In addition to patient reported outcome measures, accelerometers may provide useful information on the outcome of sarcoma patients treated with limb salvage. The StepWatch (SW) Activity Monitor (SAM) is a two-dimensional accelerometer worn on the ankle that records an objective measure of walking performance. The purpose of this study was to validate the SW in a cross-sectional population of adult patients with lower extremity sarcoma treated with limb salvage. The main outcome was correlation of total steps with the Toronto Extremity Salvage Score

(TESS). In a sample of 29 patients, a mean of 12 days of SW data was collected per patient (range 6–16), with 2767 average total steps (S.D. 1867; range 406–7437). There was a moderate positive correlation between total steps and TESS ($r = 0.56$, $P = 0.002$). Patients with osseous tumors walked significantly less than those with soft tissue sarcoma (1882 versus 3715, $P < 0.01$). This study supports the validity of the SAM as an activity monitor for the objective assessment of real world physical function in sarcoma patients.

▶ Technological advances have allowed real-time activity monitoring to be incorporated into clinical practice as a supplement (or potential replacement) for classic functional outcomes measures such as the MSTS or Toronto extremity salvage scores. The University of Washington group performed an initial pilot study using an activity monitor in 29 patients who had undergone previous lower extremity sarcoma surgery (a combination of both osseous and soft tissue sarcomas). The authors were able to correlate these results to the type of sarcoma (bone vs soft tissue) and correlate them with the TESS score.

This is a great early article on this topic that defines the potential use of these monitors and provides an initial validation for their role in clinical practice. As such, this is important for surgeons engaged in outcomes research to be familiar with as these technologies and techniques are likely to become more prominent in the near future. Although future studies do not need to duplicate the protocol outlined here, it is a starting point for those who wish to engage in this form of functional outcomes research.

P. S. Rose, MD

What Sports Activity Levels Are Achieved in Patients With Modular Tumor Endoprostheses of Osteosarcoma About the Knee?

Lang NW, Hobusch GM, Funovics PT, et al (Med Univ of Vienna, Austria)
Clin Orthop Relat Res 473:847-854, 2015

Background.—Advances in multimodal treatment have improved survival of patients with nonmetastatic osteosarcoma. At the same time, implant design has improved the outcomes of limb salvage with modular endoprostheses. However, little is known about sports activity in long-term survivors with osteosarcoma.

Questions/Purposes.—We wanted to evaluate (1) sports activity levels in long-term survivors of osteosarcoma about the knee who received a modular tumor endoprosthesis; (2) to determine if activity level changed over time from initial reconstruction or (3) was predicted from sports activity level before diagnosis; and (4) if complications that occurred affected sports or contributed to prosthetic failures.

Methods.—Between 1995 and 2005, we treated 120 patients for osteosarcoma about the knee with resection and modular endoprosthetic reconstruction; of those, 25 (21%) have died, six (5%) had an amputation, 39

(32%) did not speak German and so were ineligible, and 14 (12%) were either lost to followup or refused to participate, leaving 27 patients (14 females, 13 males; median age 19 years [range, 12—60 years]; average followup 11 ± 4 years) (54% of the living, German-speaking cohort) for this analysis. Tumors were located in the distal femur (n = 16) and the proximal tibia (n = 11). Sports participation as well as the UCLA Activity Score and the modified Weighted Activity Score were assessed retrospectively. Moreover, postoperative complications were evaluated.

Results.—Before the diagnosis of osteosarcoma and 1, 3, and 5 years and at the latest followup, respectively, after their reconstructions, 24 (89%), nine (33%), 20 (74%), and 24 patients (89%) were able to perform sports activities. There was a reduction in high-impact activities. Those patients with followup longer than 5 years had no changes in sports activity at their latest followup. Patients who had higher levels of sports activity levels before surgery generally had higher levels of activity at last followup (UCLA Activity Score: r = 0.62, p < 0.0005; modified Weighted Activity Score r = 0.49, p < 0.01). Fourteen patients (51%) underwent revision surgery. With the numbers available, complications had no effect on sports activity. No sports activity-related complications were found.

Conclusions.—Some long-term survivors of osteosarcoma can achieve high levels of sports activity. Preoperative activity levels seem to influence the postoperative activity levels. This information is important to give realistic expectations for long-term survivors of osteosarcoma of the knee.

Level of Evidence.—Level IV, therapeutic study. See Guidelines for Authors for a complete description of levels of evidence.

▶ This is a parallel article to the adjacent one on sports activity after treatment for Ewing sarcoma. The same group applied the same protocol to patients with osteosarcoma. The results were quite similar. Specifically, patients achieved a surprisingly high level of activity in the limited cohort that was studied.

Readers are reminded that only a minority of patients in the database of this tumor center participated in this study. Thus, there is almost certainly a selection bias of which patients chose to participate, and these results may well be biased for higher activity (these results probably represent the best-case scenario). Additionally, the study by design is focused on patients who had limb salvage surgery with modular endoprostheses. It is not at all clear whether the athletic activity of these patients is comparable to those patients who may have been treated with amputation or rotationplasty.

For this reason, this is a valuable study for surgeons to be aware of in counseling their patients as to what may or may not be reasonable activities to expect after limb salvage surgery. The authors did not see any complications that they directly attributed to athletic participation postoperatively. However, there are significant caveats in the interpretation as outlined here.

P. S. Rose, MD

Do Patients With Ewing's Sarcoma Continue With Sports Activities After Limb Salvage Surgery of the Lower Extremity?

Hobusch GM, Lang N, Schuh R, et al (Med Univ of Vienna, Austria)
Clin Orthop Relat Res 2014 [Epub ahead of print]

Background.—Limb salvage surgery has evolved to become the standard method of treating sarcomas of the extremities with acceptable oncologic results. However, little information exists relative to the activity level or ability to participate in sports after tumor reconstructions.

Questions/Purposes.—The aims of the study were to answer the following questions: (1) Which sports activity levels and what types of sports can be expected in the long term after tumor reconstruction? (2) Which frequency durations are patients with Ewing's sarcoma able to perform in longterm followup after local control? (3) Do surgical complications affect sports activity level?

Methods.—Thirty patients (13 females, 17 males; mean age, 18 ± 8 years; range, 2—36 years at diagnosis; mean followup 16 ± 6 years [minimum, 5 years]) were included. Tumors were located in the pelvis, femur, tibia, and fibula. Surgical procedures included surgical resections alone (n =8), surgical resection with biological reconstruction (n = 9), or endoprosthetic reconstruction (n = 13). We assessed UCLA sports activity levels, kinds of sports as well as the frequency per week and the duration of each training unit at long term (minimum followup, 5 years).

Results.—In long-term followup 83% patients (25 of 30) were performing athletic activity regularly. The hours/week of sports depended on type of surgery and were highest after resections in the pelvis and femur (5.8) and were lowest after megaprosthetic reconstruction of the pelvis (1.0). Patients undergoing biologic reconstructions were able to perform high-impact sports. UCLA sports activity levels were high after joint-preserving vascularized fibula for tibia reconstruction (7.4) and after megaprosthetic reconstruction of the lower extremity (6.3—6.4) and were low after tumors located in the fibula (4.2). Complications during followup did not significantly influence sports activity in long-term survivors.

Conclusions.—Long-term survivors can achieve high levels of sports activity in many instances. Tumor sites are associated with the postoperative sports activity levels. This information can help surgeons counsel patients in terms of athletic expectations after limb salvage reconstruction for patients with Ewing's sarcoma.

Level of Evidence.—Level III, therapeutic study. See Guidelines for Authors for a complete description of levels of evidence.

▶ These authors from Vienna with a large experience in limb salvage surgery present the athletic participation of patients treated in adolescence and young adulthood for Ewing sarcoma. They define a surprisingly high level of sports activity in patients who are survivors of this malignancy. Not surprisingly, the level of participation varies with the nature of the limb salvage surgery that was performed. Patients with megaprostheses had relatively low sports participation compared with those who had joint-sparing procedures of the fibula or tibia (who had excellent sports participation). The patients who experienced surgical complications had a temporary lowering of their athletic participation but then regained reasonable athletic function. Of note, no complications arising from participation in sports were identified.

Where to place this study in clinical context? A large number of the authors' cohort declined to participate in the study, so this likely represents a "best-case" assessment of participation after limb salvage surgery. Additionally, these patients were all treated with surgery and limb salvage; we do not know the athletic participation of patients treated with primary radiotherapy or those treated with amputation. With modern prostheses, patients undergoing a rotationplasty or lower extremity amputation at the midfemur or lower can often achieve excellent athletic participation. Additionally, much of the data in this study necessarily are from patient recall to define their predisease activity level.

As such, this article nicely outlines what a young and motivated cohort is capable of and highlights the functional benefits of joint-preserving surgeries. In and of itself, it begins to define, but by no means fully captures, athletic activity because of the limitations of the cohort that was studied. These results may be used to counsel patients but, again, should probably be interpreted as a best-case scenario for activity in setting expectations.

P. S. Rose, MD

What Are the Functional Outcomes of Endoprosthestic Reconstructions After Tumor Resection?

Bernthal NM, Greenberg M, Heberer K, et al (David Geffen School of Medicine at UCLA)
Clin Orthop Relat Res 2014 [Epub ahead of print]

Background.—The majority of published functional outcome data for tumor megaprostheses comes in the form of subjective functional outcome scores. Sparse objective data exist demonstrating functional results, activity levels, and efficiency of gait after endoprosthetic reconstruction in patients treated for orthopaedic tumors. Patients embarking on massive surgical operations, often in the setting of debilitating medical therapies, face mortality and a myriad of unknowns. Objective functional outcomes provide patients with reasonable expectations and a means to envision life after treatment. Objective outcomes also provide a means for surgeons to compare techniques, rehabilitation protocols, and implants.

Questions/Purposes.—We asked the following questions: (1) What is the efficiency of gait (ie, oxygen consumption) at final recovery from endoprosthetic reconstruction for oncologic resections? (2) What is the knee strength after lower extremity endoprosthetic reconstruction as compared with the contralateral limb? (3) How active are patients with tumor megaprostheses at home and in the community?

Methods.—Sixty-nine patients with endoprosthetic reconstructions for primary lower extremity bone sarcoma met inclusion criteria and were invited by mailing to undergo oxygen cost study and strength testing. Twenty-four patients (seven proximal femoral replacements, nine distal femoral replacements, and eight proximal tibia replacements) underwent evaluation in the gait laboratory at a mean of 13.2 years after their reconstruction. All patients were then asked to wear step activity monitors at home and in the community for 7 consecutive days.

Results.—Median O_2 consumption (in mL/kg/m) among the endoprosthesis groups was not different from the control patients with the numbers available (proximal femoral replacement 0.17, distal femoral replacement 0.16, proximal tibia replacement 0.18, control 0.15, $p = 0.21$). With the numbers available, there was no difference in walking speed as compared with the control group (proximal femoral replacement 1.20 m/s, distal femoral replacement 1.27 m/s, proximal tibia replacement 1.12 m/s, control 1.27 m/s, $p = 0.08$). Patients with proximal tibia replacements had reduced knee extension and flexion strength compared with patients in other reconstruction groups (84% reduction in extension versus those with proximal femoral replacements, 35%, and distal femoral replacement, 53%, $p = 0.001$, and 43% reduction in flexion versus proximal femoral replacement, 11%, distal femoral replacement, 2%, $p = 0.006$). With the numbers available, mean strides per day were not different among the reconstruction groups (proximal femoral replacement = 4709 strides/day [3094−6696], distal femoral replacement = 2854 [2461−6015], and proximal tibia replacement = 4411 [3093−6215], $p = 0.53$).

Conclusions.—Although knee strength was reduced in patients with proximal tibia replacements compared with femoral reconstructions, all groups had an efficient gait and were active at home and in the community at a mean of 13.2 years after surgery. Despite the magnitude of these surgeries, these patients are similarly active as patients after standard total hip arthroplasty. These findings provide objective data from which patients undergoing tumor megaprosthesis reconstructions of the lower extremity can reasonably base expectations of efficient gait and active lifestyles outside of the hospital setting. These data may provide hope and long-term goals for patients facing the uncertainty of chemotherapy and surgical treatment.

Level of Evidence.—Level III, therapeutic study. See Instructions for Authors for a complete description of levels of evidence.

▶ The UCLA group provides an excellent analysis of objective gait parameters in long-term survivors with megaprosthetic reconstruction about the knee. This experienced oncology group brought back 24 patients for detailed gait laboratory evaluation, including oxygen consumption monitoring and pedometer assessment in the community for 1 week of activity. The authors carefully evaluated patients only a minimum of 2 years after their surgery to be certain they had achieved maximum functional restoration (patients were a mean of 13.2 years after their reconstruction). This study differs from the limited previous literature on this subject in that it includes an assessment of patients' activities in the community and also includes only patients who have arguably made a complete functional recovery (minimum 2-year follow-up) from their surgery.

Surprisingly, the authors found little difference in oxygen consumption between the endoprosthetic group and a control group. This is different from some other studies that have shown as much as a 44% increase in oxygen consumption with gait. Additionally, walking speed was similar to the control group, and the number of steps taken in the community was also similar. The overall pattern of outcome showed these patients to be similar to a contemporary total hip arthroplasty population. Clearly, this is a younger cohort, but these patients do achieve excellent function.

Where to place this study in clinical context? This study certainly benefits by a detailed evaluation from an expert center in patients who have arguably made a complete functional recovery. As such, it can provide surgeons with information to counsel their patients on the anticipated long-term/final functional outcome that may be achieved. It is important to note that only a subset of the surviving UCLA cohort was able to participate in the study (24 of 69 potential patients responded and participated in at least some of the evaluation). As such, this study may be skewed toward a best-case scenario in that there may be a bias in patients who responded positively to the invitation to participate. Additionally, these patients are clearly the result of an expert and experienced sarcoma center with a reputation for excellent functional outcomes.

This study defines a modern functional outcome objectively for patients and sets the bar that other centers may seek to achieve. It provides results for which to counsel patients undergoing surgery by quantifying an attainable if optimistic assessment of their recovery potential.

P. S. Rose, MD

Outcomes and Prognostic Factors for Ewing-Family Tumors of the Extremities

Biswas B, Rastogi S, Khan SA, et al (Dr. B.R. Ambedkar Inst Rotary Cancer Hosp, New Delhi, India)
J Bone Joint Surg Am 96:841-849, 2014

Background.—There are few published studies describing the clinical results of patients uniformly treated for a Ewing-family tumor of an extremity.

Methods.—We performed a review of patients who had received uniform treatment consisting of neoadjuvant chemotherapy, surgery and/or radiation therapy as local treatment, and then adjuvant chemotherapy from June 2003 to November 2011 at a single institution.

Results.—There were 158 patients included in the study. The median age was fifteen years. Sixty-nine (44%) of the patients had metastatic disease at presentation. Fifty-seven patients underwent surgery, and forty-one received radical radiation therapy following neoadjuvant chemotherapy.

After a median of 24.3 months (range, 1.6 to ninety-seven months) of follow-up, the five-year event-free survival, overall survival, and local control rates (and standard error) were 24.1% ± 4.3%, 43.5% ± 6%, and 55% ± 6.8%, respectively, for the entire cohort and 36.4% ± 6.2%, 57.6% ± 7.4%, and 58.2% ± 7.9%, respectively, for patients without metastases. In the multivariate analysis, metastases predicted inferior event-free survival ($p = 0.02$) and overall survival ($p = 0.03$) rates in the entire cohort, whereas radical radiation therapy predicted an inferior local control rate in the entire cohort ($p = 0.001$) and in patients without metastases ($p = 0.04$). In the group with localized disease, there was no difference between the patients who received radical radiation therapy and those who underwent surgery with regard to tumor diameter ($p = 0.8$) or post-neoadjuvant chemotherapy response ($p = 0.1$). A white blood cell count (WBC) of $>11 \times 10^9$/L predicted inferior event-free survival ($p = 0.005$) and local control ($p = 0.02$) rates for patients without metastases.

Conclusions.—To our knowledge, this is the largest study on extremity Ewing-family tumors treated with uniform chemotherapy and either surgical resection or radical radiation therapy in Asia. All possible efforts should be made to resect a primary tumor after neoadjuvant chemotherapy, as radical radiation therapy alone results in a poor local control rate despite a good post-neoadjuvant chemotherapy response. Patients without metastases but with a high WBC had inferior event-free survival and local control rates and may require more aggressive therapy.

Level of Evidence.—Therapeutic Level IV. See Instructions for Authors for a complete description of levels of evidence (Fig 3).

▶ These authors present the results of a large series of extremity Ewing sarcoma patients comparing the results treated with surgery radiation for local control or radiation alone. They also provide data on the oncologic outcomes of patients and predictive factors that are obtained.

There are several things to note in evaluating this study. The vast majority of the patients included were analyzed retrospectively; although this is stated in the Methods section, it is not brought out elsewhere in the article. Additionally, 20% of patients were lost to follow-up. The presenting characteristics of the patients (44% with clinically detectable metastases at presentation and a large median tumor size) suggest that these patients from New Delhi, India, may have come to medical attention later than is commonly seen in contemporary North American practice.

Given these limitations, why include this article in the YEAR BOOK? The authors have nonetheless done an admirable job of assembling "hard data" on oncologic outcomes in these patients, which partially overcomes the retrospective nature of the series and other limitations. They do present complication data from chemotherapy, and readers should keep in mind that this almost certainly underestimates the complication given the retrospective nature of the analysis.

There was a clear selection bias for the use of radiation in patients who have metastases on presentation, and this is certainly reasonable in clinical practice.

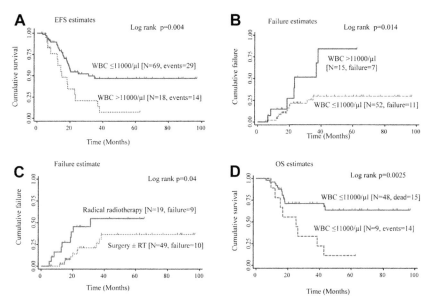

FIGURE 3.—A The five-year event-free survival (EFS) rate in the group with localized disease (n = 87) was 46.8% ± 7.1% for patients with a WBC of ≤11 × 10^9/L compared with 6.9% ± 6.6% for those with a WBC of >11 × 10^9/L. B The five-year local failure rate in the group with localized disease (n = 67) was 29.5% ± 7.9% for patients with a WBC of ≤11 × 10^9/L compared with 83.8% ± 14.4% for those with a WBC of >11 × 10^9/L. C The five-year local failure rate was 36.4% ± 9.9% for the patients who underwent surgery with or without postoperative radiation therapy (RT) compared with 54.6% ± 13% for those who received radical radiation therapy only in the group with localized disease (n = 68). D The five-year overall survival (OS) rate in the group with localized disease (n = 89) was 63.4% ± 8% for patients with a WBC of ≤11 × 10^9/L compared with 11.1% ± 10.5% for those with a WBC of >11 × 10^9/L after exclusion of patients whose survival status could not be assessed (n = 32). (Reprinted from Biswas B, Rastogi S, Khan SA, et al. Outcomes and prognostic factors for ewing-family tumors of the extremities. *J Bone Joint Surg Am.* 2014;96:841-849, http://jbjs.org/.)

However, the authors also analyzed a group of patients who did not have metastases and underwent either surgery radiation or radiation alone for local control. Keeping in mind that these were all extremity tumors (and not subject to the usual selection bias of radiotherapy for axial Ewing sarcoma), the gross presenting characteristics between the surgery and radiation groups were similar. However, the outcomes oncologically favored patients who underwent surgery as a part of their treatment. The aspects of this study are summarized in Fig 3.

Where to place this study in clinical context? The median radiation dose administered was only 45 Gy, less than would typically be used for treatment dose in contemporary North American practice. However, a number of patients were still treated to 60 Gy, more typical of what might be used. The results clearly favored surgery allowing for the caveats of a retrospective study and potential bias in treatment selection that could not be accounted for. Other studies have documented long-term complications in patients who undergo primary radiotherapy for Ewing tumor of the extremities as well.

This study is valuable in that it limits itself to extremity tumors whereas most series of this nature include patients with axial tumors. Although not definitive, these data are similar to what have been seen in other studies, suggesting a beneficial role for surgical treatment of patients with Ewing sarcoma. Given this and the known long-term complications after radiotherapy alone for local control of extremity Ewing's tumors, it is reasonable that the default treatment for patients with extremity Ewing's sarcoma be surgery radiotherapy.

P. S. Rose, MD

Tumor Resection/Reconstruction

Pelvic Resection: Current Concepts

Mayerson JL, Wooldridge AN, Scharschmidt TJ (The Ohio State Univ Wexner Med Ctr, Columbus; Texas Tech Univ Health Sciences Ctr, El Paso)
J Am Acad Orthop Surg 22:214-222, 2014

Pelvic resection is a technique that involves surgical resection of portions of the pelvic girdle. Historically, this procedure was known as internal hemipelvectomy. Hemipelvectomy is a resection that includes the ipsilateral limb. The main indication for these procedures is primary malignant tumors of the pelvis, but in rare cases they are indicated for metastatic lesions, infection, or trauma. Reconstruction is dictated by the extent of the resection and the remaining structures. Surgical technique is dictated by histology of the tumor and location of the lesion. A multidisciplinary team is required. The patient and family should undergo counseling preoperatively to discuss morbidity and mortality, the extensive rehabilitation process, and life expectancy.

▶ I have included this article from the Ohio State group in the YEAR BOOK as a general review of our current understanding of oncologic pelvic resections. Even in busy centers, pelvic resections can present formidable surgical challenges. Additionally, a wide spectrum of reconstructive options are available but not standardized in current oncologic practice. For the experienced surgeon, this article provides a nice review as well as a current reference list to explore areas in further detail. For those residents, fellows, and students, it puts forth in a very readable fashion the background that guides our treatment of pelvic malignancies.

P. S. Rose, MD

What Are the 5-year Survivorship Outcomes of Compressive Endoprosthetic Osseointegration Fixation of the Femur?
Monument MJ, Bernthal NM, Bowles AJ, et al (Univ of Utah, Salt Lake City; UCLA School of Medicine, Santa Monica; Univ of Pittsburgh, PA)
Clin Orthop Relat Res 473:883-890, 2015

Background.—Aseptic complications such as stress shielding leading to bone loss are major problems associated with revision of cemented and uncemented long-stem tumor endoprostheses. Endoprosthetic reconstruction using compressive osseointegration fixation is a relatively new limb salvage technology designed to enhance osseointegration, prevent stress shielding, and provide fixation for short endsegments.

Questions/Purposes.—(1) What is the survivorship of this technique at minimum 5-year followup? (2) Were patient factors (age, sex, body mass index), oncological factors, or anatomic locations associated with implant failure? (3) Were there any prosthesis-related variables associated with failure?

Methods.—A single-center, retrospective review of patients with a minimum 5-year followup (mean, 8 years; range, 5—12 years) treated with an osseointegration compressive device for endoprosthetic fixation of proximal and distal femoral limb salvage reconstructions was performed. We have previously published the implant survivorship of this patient cohort with a minimum 2-year followup and are now reporting on the 5-year survivorship data. From 2002 to 2008, we performed 22 such procedures in 22 patients. Four patients died of their disease within 5 years of surgery and all surviving patients (n = 18) had complete followup data at a minimum of 5 years. General indications for this device during that time were pediatric and adult patients requiring primary endoprosthetic reconstructions of the proximal or distal femur for benign and malignant bone lesions. The primary outcome was reoperations for mechanical (aseptic) failures. Secondary outcomes included implant removal for nonmechanical failures and any patient-, oncological-, or implant-related variables associated with implant removal.

Results.—At a minimum of 5 years followup, overall mechanical (aseptic) implant survivorship was 16 of 18. Survivorship for all modes of failure (oncological failure, infection, arthrofibrosis, and mechanical failure) was 12 of 18. All mechanical failures occurred early, within the first 30 months. We identified no patient-, oncological-, or implant-related features predictive of failure.

Conclusions.—Our intermediate-term experience with compressive osseointegration fixation for endoprosthetic limb reconstructions demonstrates with longer clinical followup, no additional mechanical failures were observed as compared with our early analysis. Our experience with this fixation at a minimum of 5-years followup adds to a very limited but increasing body of literature demonstrating that after a transient period of increased risk for implant failures, survivorship stabilizes. Assessment of this fixation strategy beyond 10 years of clinical followup is needed.

Level of Evidence.—Level IV, therapeutic study. See Guidelines for Authors for a complete description of levels of evidence (Fig 2).

▶ This report from the Huntsman Cancer Institution adds to the small but growing body of literature on the outcomes of compress fixation for limb salvage surgery. This article has a modest number of patients (18) but reports

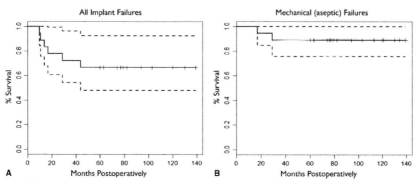

FIGURE 2.—A–B Kaplan-Meier plots demonstrating survivorship of compressive osseointegration fixation at a minimum 5 years clinical followup. When considering all modes of implant failure (infection, oncological failure, arthrofibrosis, and aseptic failures), survivorship was 67% (**A**). Looking only at aseptic (mechanical) failures, survivorship was 89% at a minimum 5 years clinical followup (**B**). All mechanical failures occurred within 30 months and survivorship was stable afterward. (With kind permission from Springer Science+Business Media: Monument MJ, Bernthal NM, Bowles AJ, et al. What are the 5-year survivorship outcomes of compressive endoprosthetic osseointegration fixation of the femur? *Clin Orthop Relat Res.* 2015;473:883-890, with permission from The Association of Bone and Joint Surgeons.)

the minimum 5-year outcome. This group had previously reported the minimum 2-year outcome of a similar cohort.

Failure of the compress mechanism occurred in 2 of 18 patients, both at less than 30 months. Subsequently, there were no instances of mechanical failure of the prosthesis (Fig 2). An additional 4 patients underwent removal of the prosthesis for other reasons for a total prosthetic survival of 12 of 18 patients. Readers should note that most patients in this series were treated with postoperative chemotherapy, and the rehabilitation regimen (6 weeks non-weight bearing and then progressive weight bearing as tolerated) did not vary based on whether patients did or did not receive postoperative chemotherapy. Antirotation pins were used in most but not all patients. Given the small number of failures observed, the authors were not able to identify factors associated with failure.

This study continues to report a pattern that has been observed with this implant in which a modest number of patients will not achieve ingrowth and have early mechanical failure. After this, mechanical failure is rare. This is in contrast to conventional stems in which early fixation is nearly assured but fixation fails over time. The overall mechanical failure profile for this implant appears to be identical to that of other implants. These data support this device as an option for surgeons to consider, particularly in younger patients or those with long resections for which the conventional stem might not work well.

P. S. Rose, MD

Survival of Modern Knee Tumor Megaprostheses: Failures, Functional Results, and a Comparative Statistical Analysis

Pala E, Trovarelli G, Calabrò T, et al (Univ of Bologna, Italy)
Clin Orthop Relat Res 473:891-899, 2015

Background.—Modular megaprostheses are now the most common method of reconstruction after segmental resection of the long bones in the lower extremities. Previous studies reported variable outcome and failure rates after knee megaprosthetic reconstructions.

Questions/Purposes.—The objectives of this study were to analyze the results of a modular tumor prosthesis after resection of bone tumor around the knee with respect to (1) survivorship; (2) failure rate; (3) comparative survivorship against different sites of reconstructions and of primary and revision implants; and (4) functional results on the Musculoskeletal Tumor Society (MSTS) scoring system.

Methods.—Between 2003 and 2010, 247 rotating-hinge Global Modular Reconstruction System (GMRS) knee prostheses were implanted in our institute for malignant and aggressive benign tumors. During this time, that group represented 23% of the patients who had oncologic megaprosthesis reconstruction about the knee after resection of primary or metastatic bone tumors (247 of 1086 patients). In the other 77% of cases we used other types of oncologic prostheses. Before 2003 we used the older Howmedica Modular Resection System and Kotz Modular Femur/Tibia Replacement from 2003 we used mostly the GMRS but we continued to use the HMRS in some cases such as patients with poor prognoses, elderly patients, or metastatic patients. Sites included 187 distal femurs and 60 proximal tibias. Causes of megaprosthesis failure were classified according to Henderson et al. in five types: Type 1 (soft tissue failure), Type 2 (aseptic loosening), Type 3 (structural failure), Type 4 (infection), and Type 5 (tumor progression). Followup was at a minimum oncologic followup of 2 years (mean, 4 years; range, 2—8 years). Kaplan-Meier actuarial curves of implant survival to major failures were done. Functional results were analyzed according to the MSTS II system; 223 of the 247 were available for functional scoring (81%).

Results.—At latest followup, among 175 treated patients for primary reconstruction, 117 are continuously disease-free, 26 have no evidence of disease after treatment of relapse, eight are alive with disease, and 24 died from disease. The overall failure rate of the megaprostheses in our series was 29.1% (72 of 247). Type 1 failure occurred in 8.5% (21 of 247) cases, Type 2 in 5.6% (14 of 247), Type 3 in 0%, Type 4 in 9.3% (23 of 247), and Type 5 in 5.6% (14 of 247). Kaplan-Meier curve showed an overall implant survival rate for all types of failures of 70% at 4 years and 58% at 8 years. Prosthetic survivorship for revisions was 80% at 5 years and for primary reconstructions was 60% at 5 years ($p = 0.013$). Survivorship to infection was 95% at 5 years for revision patients and 84% at 5 years for primary patients ($p = 0.475$). The mean MSTS score was 84 (25.2; range, 8—30) with no difference between sites of localization (24.7 in proximal tibia versus 25.4 in distal femur reconstruction; $p = 0.306$).

Conclusions.—Results at a minimum of 2 years with this modular prosthesis are satisfactory in terms of survivorship (both oncologic and reconstructive) and causes and rates of failure. Although these results seem comparable with other like implants, we will continue to follow this cohort, and we believe that comparative trials among the available megaprosthesis designs are called for.

Level of Evidence.—Level IV, therapeutic study. See Guidelines for Authors for a complete description of levels of evidence (Fig 1).

▶ This report from the Rizzoli Institution was selected for the CORR symposium issue from the 2013 meeting of the Musculoskeletal Tumor Society (MSTS). These authors report a large series of Global Modular Reconstruction System (GMRS) prostheses and their failure mechanisms. These come from a very busy tumor service in which 247 of these were implanted between 2003 and 2010. The authors describe failure using the Henderson classification; they do provide some minimal functional results using the MSTS scoring system as well. Although some oncologic results are presented, they are very difficult to interpret given the heterogeneity of diagnosis for which these were implanted (spanning from aggressive benign tumors to patients with metastatic disease).

Overall implant survival rate was 70% at 4 years and 58% at 8 years (Fig 1). Interestingly, prostheses placed for revision had a higher survival than those

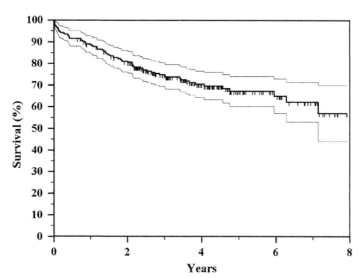

FIGURE 1.—The Kaplan-Meier actuarial curve shows overall implant survival to all types of failure of 70% and 58%, respectively, at 4 and 8 years. (With kind permission from Springer Science+Business Media: Pala E, Trovarelli G, Calabrò T, et al. Survival of modern knee tumor megaprostheses: failures, functional results, and a comparative statistical analysis. *Clin Orthop Relat Res.* 2015;473:891-899, with permission from The Association of Bone and Joint Surgeons.)

placed for primary disease. Most patients in this cohort received uncemented stems.

Where to place this study in clinical context? On the plus side, this is a large series using a uniform implant that is now in common clinical practice. These results seem reasonable and comparable to other large series that have been reported using either previous-generation implants or a variety of implants. Unfortunately, the results mix indications with prosthetic implantation and mix those placed in the primary or revision setting with a relatively limited discussion. Additionally, perhaps one of the most difficult clinical problems is how to deal with prosthetic failure. The authors' discussion of this is relatively limited as well.

I think this report validates the outcome and use of the GMRS prosthesis, which is in common clinical practice. There is no glaring deficiency that has come to light with longer follow-up of an extended series. Readers should recognize that these implants were all placed by an expert group in a high-volume oncology center. These results may represent a best-case scenario given the recognized experience and skill of the surgeons involved.

P. S. Rose, MD

What Was the Survival of Megaprostheses in Lower Limb Reconstructions After Tumor Resections?

Capanna R, Scoccianti G, Frenos F, et al (Azienda Ospedaliera Universitaria Careggi, Firenze, Italy; et al)
Clin Orthop Relat Res 473:820-830, 2015

Background.—Prosthetic replacement is the most commonly used option for reconstruction of osteoarticular bone loss resulting from bone neoplasm resection or prosthetic failure. Starting in late 2001, we began exclusively using a single system for large-segment osteoarticular reconstruction after tumor resection; to our knowledge, there are no published series from one center evaluating the use of this implant.

Questions/Purposes.—We investigated the following issues: (1) What is the overall survival, excluding local tumor recurrence, for these endoprostheses used for tumor reconstructions of the lower extremities (knee and hip)? (2) What types of failure were observed in these reconstructions? (3) Do the survival and complications vary according to site of implant?

Methods.—Between September 2001 and March 2012, we exclusively used this implant for tumor reconstructions. During that time, 278 patients underwent tumor reconstructions of the hip or knee, of whom 200 (72%) were available at a minimum 2 years followup. Seventy-eight patients were excluded from the study for insufficient followup as a result of early death (42) or loss at followup (36). The reconstruction types were the following: proximal femur (69 cases), distal femur (87), proximal tibia (32), and total knee (12). Failures were classified according to the Henderson classification. Nine patients among those with followup shorter than

2 years had presented one or more failures and they were included in our analysis but separately evaluated.

Results.—Overall survival (no further surgical procedures of any type after primary surgery), excluding Type 5 failure (tumor recurrence), was 75.9% at 5 years and 66.2% at 10 years. Seventy-one failures occurred in 58 implants (29%). Mechanical failures accounted for 59.2% and non-mechanical failures for 40.8%. The first causes of failure of the implants were the result of soft tissue failure in 6%, aseptic loosening in 3%, structural failure in 7%, infection in 8.5%, and tumor recurrence in 4.5% of the whole series. Nine implants sustained two or more failures. Overall incidence of infection was 9.5%. No statistically significant differences were observed according to anatomical site.

Conclusions.—Like in the case with many such complex oncologic reconstructions, the failure rate at short- to midterm in this group was over 20%. Comparative trials are called for to ascertain whether one implant is superior to another. Infection and structural failure were the most frequent modes of failure in our experience.

Level of Evidence.—Level IV, therapeutic study. See Instructions for Authors for a complete description of levels of evidence.

▶ As another article from the 2013 Musculoskeletal Tumor Society/International Society of Limb Salvage symposium, these authors report the outcomes of a recently released prostheses from Link (the Megaprosthesis-C). This is a study that can be read in parallel to the adjacent study on the Global Modular Reconstruction System from the Rizzoli Institution.

The results were quite similar. Overall prosthetic survival (excluding those removed for tumor recurrence) was 76% at 5 years and 66% at 10 years. The authors include a nice discussion of modification of the implant over time, noting that there have been 2 modifications to address concerns about mechanical failure at the junction. The initial design had a set screw that served as a stress riser; this was removed in favor of a more standard Morris taper that was later modified further to unify stresses with good apparent results in this setting (obviously there is a shorter follow-up on the more recent modifications).

Where to place this study in clinical context? This demonstrates that a modern prosthesis more commonly distributed in Europe but becoming available in the United States can have a track record that parallels other implants. There are some technical reasons why a surgeon might consider this implant in some or all of his or her patients; specifically, there are features of this system that allow ready adaptation to an allograft prosthetic composite, which may be an option that surgeons wish to have for their cases. As such, this is of interest to North American surgeons despite the current limited market share and availability of this implant outside of Europe.

P. S. Rose, MD

Intercalary Allograft Reconstructions Following Resection of Primary Bone Tumors: A Nationwide Multicenter Study

Bus MPA, Dijkstra PDS, van de Sande MAJ, et al (Academic Med Ctr, Amsterdam, The Netherlands; Leiden Univ Med Ctr, The Netherlands; et al)
J Bone Joint Surg Am 96:e26(1-11), 2014

Background.—Favorable reports on the use of massive allografts to reconstruct intercalary defects underline their place in limb-salvage surgery. However, little is known about optimal indications as reports on failure and complication rates in larger populations remain scarce. We evaluated the incidence of and risk factors for failure and complications, time to full weight-bearing, and optimal fixation methods for intercalary allografts after tumor resection.

Methods.—A retrospective study was performed in all four centers of orthopaedic oncology in the Netherlands. All consecutive patients reconstructed with intercalary (whole-circumference) allografts after tumor resection in the long bones during 1989 to 2009 were evaluated. The minimum follow-up was twenty-four months. Eighty-seven patients with a median age of seventeen years (range, 1.5 to 77.5 years) matched inclusion criteria. The most common diagnoses were osteosarcoma, Ewing sarcoma, adamantinoma, and chondrosarcoma. The median follow-up period was eighty-four months (range, twenty-five to 262 months). Ninety percent of tumors were localized in the femur or the tibia.

Results.—Fifteen percent of our patients experienced a graft-related failure. The major complications were nonunion (40%), fracture (29%), and infection (14%). Complications occurred in 76% of patients and reoperations were necessary in 70% of patients. The median time to the latest complication was thirty-two months (range, zero to 200 months). The median time to full weight-bearing was nine months (range, one to eighty months). Fifteen grafts failed, twelve of which failed in the first four years. None of the thirty-four tibial reconstructions failed. Reconstruction site, patient age, allograft length, nail-only fixation, and non-bridging osteosynthesis were the most important risk factors for complications. Adjuvant chemotherapy and irradiation had no effects on complication rates.

Conclusions.—We report high complication rates and considerable failure rates for the use of intercalary allografts; complications primarily occurred in the first years after surgery, but some occurred much later after surgery. To reduce the number of failures, we recommend reconsidering the use of allografts for reconstructions of defects that are ≥15 cm, especially in older patients, and applying bridging osteosynthesis with use of plate fixation.

▶ These authors respectively reviewed all intercalary allografts used in the Netherlands between 1989 and 2009. They were able to do this because all sarcomas are treated in 1 of 4 centers there. Although this study does suffer from a retrospective nature, the national practice environment does help to overcome some of these limitations.

Complications were seen in more than three-quarters of patients and reoperation was necessary in 70% of patients. Pediatric patients had a much more favorably prognosis for uncomplicated graft incorporation. The authors found that reconstruction site, length of allograft greater than 15 cm, and nail only fixation were associated with a higher risk of complication. Use of radiation and chemotherapy do not clearly affect complication rates, although this is hard to understand given clinical experience.

Where to place this study in clinical context? Intercalary allografts remain a valuable technique for diaphyseal resections. The authors have identified several risk factors for failure, but most of them are not modifiable by surgeons (eg., the age of the presenting patient or the length of resection which needs to be done). However, the finding that plate osteosynthesis is protective compared with nail fixation is useful and can directly influence surgical treatment. As well, in patients at high risk for failure, surgeons may wish to consider other treatment modalities. Intercalary prostheses can be used as a pasteurized or extracorporeally irradiated autograft. Although these also have high complication profiles, this may partially alleviate the inferior results found in some groups in this study.

P. S. Rose, MD

Should Fractures in Massive Intercalary Bone Allografts of the Lower Limb Be Treated With ORIF or With a New Allograft?
Aponte-Tinao LA, Ayerza MA, Muscolo DL, et al (Italian Hosp of Buenos Aires, Argentina)
Clin Orthop Relat Res 2014 [Epub ahead of print]

Background.—Massive bone allografts have been used for limb salvage of bone tumor resections as an alternative to endoprostheses, although they have different outcomes and risks. There is no general consensus about when to use these alternatives, but when it is possible to save the native joints after the resection of a long bone tumor, intercalary allografts offer some advantages despite complications, such as fracture. The management and outcomes of this complication deserve more study.

Questions/Purposes.—The purposes of this study were to (1) analyze the fracture frequency in a group of patients treated with massive intercalary bone allografts of the femur and tibia; (2) compare the results of allografts treated with open reduction and internal fixation (ORIF) with those treated with resection and repeat allograft reconstruction; and (3) determine the likelihood that treatment of a fracture resulted in a healed intercalary reconstruction.

Methods.—We reviewed patients treated with intercalary bone allografts between 1991 and 2011. During this period, patients were generally treated with intercalary allografts when after tumor resection at least 1 cm of residual epiphysis remained to allow fixation of the osteotomy junction. To obtain a homogeneous group of patients, we excluded allograft-prosthesis composites and osteoarticular and hemicylindrical intercalary allografts from this study. We analyzed the fracture rate of 135 patients reconstructed with segmental intercalary bone allografts of the lower extremities (98 femurs and 37 tibias). In patients whose grafts fractured were treated either by internal fixation or a second allograft, ORIF generally was attempted but after early failures in femur fractures, these fractures were treated with a second allograft. Using a chart review, we ascertained the frequency of osseous union, complications, and reoperations after the treatment of fractured intercalary allografts. Followup was at a mean of 101 months (range, 24–260 months); of the original 135 patients, no patient was lost to followup.

Results.—At latest followup, 19 patients (14%) had an allograft fracture (16 femurs [16%] and three tibias [8%]). Six patients were treated with internal fixation and addition of autologous graft (three femurs and three tibias) and 13 patients were treated with a second intercalary allograft (13 femurs). The three patients with femoral allograft fractures treated with internal fixation and autologous grafts failed and were treated with a second allograft, whereas those patients with tibia allograft fractures treated by the same procedure healed without secondary complications. When we analyzed the 16 patients with a second intercalary allograft (13 as primary treatment of the fracture and three as secondary treatment of the fracture), five failed (31%) and were treated with resection of the allograft and reconstructed with an endoprosthesis (four patients) or an osteoarticular allograft (one patient).

Conclusions.—Fractures of intercalary allografts of the tibia could successfully be treated with internal fixation and autologous iliac crest bone graft; however, this treatment failed when used for femur allograft fractures. Femoral fractures could be treated with resection and repeat allograft reconstruction, however, with a higher refracture frequency. The addition of a vascularized fibular graft in the second attempt should be considered.

Level of Evidence.—Level IV, therapeutic study. See the Guidelines for Authors for a complete description of levels of evidence.

▶ This Argentine group provides us with an article on intercalary allografts of the femur and tibia that yields several pertinent facts for orthopedic surgeons. It defines the fracture rate of intercalary allografts in the femur and tibia, time to fracture, the results of treatment with open reduction and internal fixation (ORIF) or repeat segmental allograft, and the overall complication profile of this operation in the hands of an expert group. The authors review 135 patients treated with this method of reconstruction between 1991 and 2011.

The overall complication rate is, of course, formidable (59 of 135 patients). The rate of fracture was 14%, and the mean time to fracture was 53 months after surgery. In patients treated with repeat fixation and iliac crest bone grafting, 3 of 3 tibial patients healed whereas none of 3 femur patients healed. In patients treated with a second intercalary allograft, 31% failed.

This is a good study of a large series of patients to help inform this aspect of clinical practice. The majority of patients received chemotherapy, but the group reported is relatively heterogeneous. Additionally, the authors do not provide us with a clear follow-up timeframe of the patients treated with ORIF and the time to healing or the number of patients treated with repeat intercalary allografts after their revision procedures. The study does suffer from its retrospective nature, although it is drawn from a group with a well-established database.

Where to place this study in clinical context? The authors give us evidence that tibial fractures in allografts may be successfully salvaged with ORIF. Readers must keep in mind that this is based on 3 patients only with unclear final follow-up. Surgeons must carefully consider the role of ORIF with iliac crest bone grafting compared with vascularized bone grafting or other methods and individualize treatment to their patients. The small numbers involved (even from the group with arguably the largest experience in the world) gives us some guidance, but it is necessarily incomplete information on such a rare topic. I appreciated this article for the data it provides on the overall performance of intercalary allografts as much as I did for the focused results it gave toward the questions stated in the title.

P. S. Rose, MD

Does Total Humeral Endoprosthetic Replacement Provide Reliable Reconstruction With Preservation of a Useful Extremity?
Wafa H, Reddy K, Grimer R, et al (The Royal Orthopaedic Hosp NHS Trust, Birmingham, UK)
Clin Orthop Relat Res 2014 [Epub ahead of print]

Background.—Controversy exists regarding the ideal method of reconstruction after proximal humeral resection and several reconstructive techniques have been reported. The reconstructive options are very limited when resection of the entire humerus is required. One option is endoprosthetic reconstruction, but there have been few published studies on the outcome of total humeral endoprosthetic reconstruction.

Questions/Purposes.—The purposes of this study were (1) to assess the longevity of total humerus prostheses in those patients who survived their disease; (2) to review the complications associated with this prosthesis; and (3) to assess the Musculoskeletal Tumor Society functional score in survivors.

Methods.—Thirty-four patients (10 males, 24 females) with a mean age of 26 years (range, 7–86 years) were included in this study. Histological diagnosis was osteosarcoma in 15 patients, chondrosarcoma in seven, Ewing's sarcoma in seven, metastatic carcinoma in three, liposarcoma in one, and giant cell tumor of bone in one remaining patient. Twenty-nine patients had their total humeral endoprosthetic replacement for primary reconstruction, whereas the remaining five patients received their implants for failures with other reconstructive techniques. At a minimum followup of 3 months (mean, 8.2 years; range, 3 months to 29 years), 16 patients were alive with no evidence of disease, whereas 13 of the remaining 18 died with metastatic disease. Local recurrence was seen in five patients and all eventually died of disease progression.

Results.—According to the Kaplan-Meier survival analysis, the cumulative 10-year implant survival rate was 90%. Periprosthetic infection was seen in four patients, postoperative radial nerve palsy in one, and proximal migration of the prosthesis in three, whereas three patients needed a change of the articular elbow bushings at a mean of 16 years after the implant insertion. The mean Musculoskeletal Tumor Society functional score of the 28 patients who survived their disease for more than 12 months after the index procedure and could therefore be functionally assessed was 83% (range, 60%–93%).

Conclusions.—From this small, preliminary report, we suggest that total humeral endoprosthetic replacement may be a reasonable option of reconstruction after tumor resection. We have shown that this prosthesis preserves the function of the hand. The local recurrence rate observed suggests that careful selection of patients is crucial. Infection was our most common surgical complication, but we showed that in those who survived their tumor, this prosthesis offers a method to preserve a functional upper extremity in some patients. Further study with more patients is necessary to confirm the value of this reconstruction method.

Level of Evidence.—Level IV, therapeutic study. See Guidelines for Authors for a complete description of levels of evidence.

▶ It is rare in clinical practice to implant a total humerus prostheses, and there is relatively little literature on the outcome of these patients. The Birmingham group provides a retrospective review of 34 patients treated with a total humerus replacement from 1970 through 2012. The rarity of this procedure is highlighted in that it is performed less than once a year at one of the busiest sarcoma centers in the world.

The overall outcomes were probably better than would have been expected. The 10-year implant survival rate was 90%, and complication profile was modest given such a large operation (4 infections, 1 radial nerve palsy, and proximal humerus migration in 3 patients). The authors report Musculoskeletal Tumor Society functional scores for 28 patients who survived more than 1 year, but it is not clear how these were ascertained; they were likely obtained retrospectively from chart review based on the available manuscript and as such may be overly optimistic. The authors readily acknowledge that patients had limited motion about the shoulder, as would be expected, but did maintain reasonable function of the hand and wrist. Given the nature of this resection and reconstruction, this is probably appropriate to expect and thus to counsel patients in this regard.

Interestingly, a small number of patients had reverse articulations, although the authors anecdotally state that no improved outcome was seen. They did see better outcomes in patients who had mesh capture of the proximal humerus. Surprisingly, 29% of their implants were expandable implants. By and large, these seemed to fare well, although 1 patient did have subluxation of the proximal joint with expansion.

This is a rare procedure that most surgeons will do a handful of times in their career. As such, it is useful to have a report of a relatively large cohort from an experienced center to reference.

P. S. Rose, MD

Is Claviculo Pro Humeri of Value for Limb Salvage of Pediatric Proximal Humerus Sarcomas?
Calvert GT, Wright J, Agarwal J, et al (Univ of Utah, Salt Lake City)
Clin Orthop Relat Res 473:877-882, 2015

Background.—There are several options for proximal humerus reconstruction in young children after resection of a malignant tumor and no one technique has been definitively shown to be superior to others, leaving the decision to surgeon and patient choice. Claviculo pro humeri (CPH) is a biologic reconstruction of the proximal humerus using the patient's ipsilateral clavicle as a rotational osseous flap. CPH represents a potential option for this complicated clinical problem in very young children, but little is known about it because the indications for its use are so uncommon.

Questions/Purposes.—The purposes of this study were to (1) assess the oncologic outcomes of CPH at a minimum of 2 years in a small series of patients; (2) elicit the complications associated with this procedure; and (3) show the Musculoskeletal Tumor Society (MSTS) functional score of these patients.

Methods.—Four patients (average age, 5 years 11 months; range, 4 years 5 months to 8 years 9 months at the time of surgery) were treated with CPH for reconstruction after resection of a proximal humerus sarcoma; this represented all of the patients treated with this approach for this problem between January 2008 and April 2011 at one institution. During this period, the general indications for using CPH were the need to reconstruct a proximal humerus defect in a child younger than 10 years of age. During this time, CPH was used for all patients treated for proximal humerus sarcomas meeting these criteria. Patient demographics, diagnosis, tumor size and extent, operative details, radiographs and MRIs, complications, and functional outcomes were assessed.

Results.—All are alive with no evidence of disease at a minimum followup of 31 months (average, 43 months; range, 31–58 months). Two patients developed nonunion and underwent revision surgery. Osseous union and a stable neoshoulder articulation were ultimately obtained in all patients. Limited shoulder motion was the only functional deficit noted with forward elevation ranging between 30° and 90°. MSTS functional scores were excellent with a range of 87% to 90%.

Conclusions.—This is a rarely used procedure in North America but we achieved functional limb salvage in all four patients. Consistent with prior literature, nonunion was the major complication in this series. The two nonunions were successfully treated without interruption of chemotherapy or significant bone graft donor site morbidity. Based on these results, the authors suggest that this procedure is a reasonable reconstruction option to consider after proximal humerus resection in patients younger than 10 years of age. Further followup will be required to assess long-term results and to determine how this procedure compares with the alternatives.

Level of Evidence.—Level IV, therapeutic study. See Guidelines for Authors for a complete description of levels of evidence.

▶ This report from the Huntsman Cancer Institute outlines the results in 4 children who underwent a claviculo pro humeri reconstruction after resection for proximal humerus sarcomas. The authors performed this procedure in children under 10 years of age who required an oncologic resection in this area.

This is a small case series of a rare procedure. It has value in its discussion of the various options for treatment of tumors of this nature and in the description of the operative technique so that surgeons who consider this option will have a reference. The volume of children who would even be considered candidates for such a procedure is necessarily low, and the world literature on this subject is quite limited. For this reason, this is a valuable publication to remind surgeons of this option and to convey the experience of a team that has carried it out. It is likely a good option when compared with the other techniques that may be used to address this problem even in patients who are slightly older. Although there is a natural hesitation to proceed with this technique in many circumstances, such as rotationplasty, it is probably an underutilized procedure.

P. S. Rose, MD

Prognostic Risk Factors for the Development of Scoliosis After Chest Wall Resection for Malignant Tumors in Children
Scalabre A, Parot R, Hameury F, et al (Hôpital Femme Mère Enfant, Bron, France; Clinique du Val d'Ouest, Ecully, France; et al)
J Bone Joint Surg Am 96:e10(1-7), 2014

Background.—Surgical resection of a malignant tumor of the chest wall in children may result in the development of progressive scoliosis. The aim of this study was to identify the risk factors associated with scoliosis following resection of a tumor of the chest wall and to evaluate the prevalence and characteristics of the scoliosis.

Methods.—Forty children who underwent resection of a malignant tumor of the chest wall from 1984 to 2005 were included in a multicenter, retrospective cohort study. The mean age of the patients at the time of surgery was 9.8 years (range, 0.2 to nineteen years). Resections were classified with the use of the following scheme: the number of resected ribs was noted in Roman numerals, and the level of the resection was identified by dividing the thorax into three sectors (A [anterior], B [lateral], and C [posterior]) in the horizontal plane. One to five ribs (mean, 2.3 ribs) were resected. Patients with scoliosis were compared with patients who did not have scoliosis through the use of univariate and multivariate analyses. The mean duration of follow-up was 8.5 years (range, three to twenty-three years).

Results.—Patients who had a tumor resection during a rapid-growth period (patient age of less than six years or between twelve and fifteen years) had a 5.8 times higher risk of scoliosis. The resection of three or more ribs in the posterior sector (C) was the primary risk factor for scoliosis, with an odds ratio of 18.9. Seventeen (43%) of the children developed scoliosis, which was convex toward the resection side without vertebral rotation in all of them.

Conclusions.—The risk of scoliosis following the resection of a primary malignant tumor of the chest wall in children was shown to be higher when resection was performed during a rapid-growth period and when the resection involved three or more ribs in the posterior sector.

▶ Spine deformity surgeons have experience with the interaction of the chest wall in spinal deformities, but tumor surgeons less frequently do. This multicenter retrospective study reports on the development of spinal deformity after chest wall resection in 40 children. In summary, the resection of 3 or more ribs, particularly in the posterior aspect of the thoracic cage, increases the risk for development of spinal deformity. Additionally, children in rapid growth phases (less than 6 or between 12 and 15 years old) at the time of surgery had a higher risk of deformity. In total, 43% of the children in this series developed scoliosis. Over half who did not have a spinal arthrodesis at the time of their resection required subsequent spine fusion.

How to apply this to clinical practice? When surgeons are presented with a child with a chest wall malignancy, there is no question that it needs to be resected. One option would be to consider spinal arthrodesis at the time of the resection. However, it is not clear that this is necessary in all patients; this could be problematic for young patients (who can develop secondary spinal deformities from unbalanced growth of a fused spinal column) and would also extend the magnitude of an already complex operation. Another option would be bracing and monitoring patients. The average Cobb angle at final follow-up was 34 degrees, and the maximum was 62 degrees. Additionally, the spinal deformity observed was different from that in typical scoliosis in that no rotation was seen. Thus, it is unclear whether the curves that resulted would be progressive and how aggressively they would require treatment.

Thankfully, it is relatively rare to have to perform these resections in children, and treatment must be individualized. Absent a formal spine resection with the chest wall, it is probably reasonable in most cases to observe the child and consider subsequent intervention if significant progressive spinal deformity develops. One caveat would be that in very young children, rib distraction devices could likely counteract and minimize deformity if used early after recognition of scoliosis development.

P. S. Rose, MD

Multilevel En Bloc Spondylectomy for Tumors of the Thoracic and Lumbar Spine Is Challenging But Rewarding

Luzzati AD, Shah S, Gagliano F, et al (IRCCS Istituto Ortopedico Galeazzi, Via Riccardo Galeazzi, Milan, Italy; et al)
Clin Orthop Relat Res 2014 [Epub ahead of print]

Background.—Over the years, en bloc spondylectomy has proven its efficacy in controlling spinal tumors and improving survival rates. However, there are few reports of large series that critically evaluate the results of multilevel en bloc spondylectomies for spinal neoplasms.

Questions/Purposes.—Using data from a large spine tumor center, we answered the following questions: (1) Does multilevel total en bloc spondylectomy result in acceptable function, survival rates, and local control in spinal neoplasms? (2) Is reconstruction after this procedure feasible? (3) What complications are associated with this procedure? (4) is it possible to achieve adequate surgical margins with this procedure?

Methods.—We retrospectively investigated 38 patients undergoing multilevel total en bloc spondylectomy by a single surgeon (AL) from 1994 to 2011. Indications for this procedure were primary spinal sarcomas, solitary metastases, and aggressive primary benign tumors involving multiple segments of the thoracic or lumbar spine. Patients had to be medically fit and have no visceral metastases. Analysis was by chart and radiographic review. Margin quality was classified into intralesional, marginal, and wide. Radiographs, MR images, and CT scans were studied for local recurrence. Graft healing and instrumentation failures at subsequent followup were assessed. Complications were divided into major or minor and further classified as intraoperative and early and late postoperative. We evaluated the oncologic status using cumulative disease-specific and metastases-free survival analysis. Minimum followup was 24 months (mean, 39 months; range, 24–124 months).

Results.—Of the 38 patients, 34 (89%) were alive and walking without support at final followup. Thirty-one (81%) had no evidence of disease. Two patients died postoperatively and another two died of systemic disease (without local recurrence). Only three patients (8%) had a local recurrence. There were 14 major complications and 22 minor complications in 25 patients (65%). Only one patient required revision of implants secondary to mechanical failure. Two cases of cage subsidence were noted but had no clinical significance. Wide margins were achieved in nine patients (23%), marginal in 25 (66%), and intralesional in four (11%).

Conclusions.—In patients with multisegmental spinal tumors, oncologic resections were achieved by multilevel en bloc spondylectomy and led to an acceptable survival rate with reasonable local control. Multilevel en bloc surgery was associated with a high complication rate; however, most patients recovered from their complications. Although the surgical procedure is challenging, our encouraging mid-term results clearly favor and validate this technique.

Level of Evidence.—Level IV, therapeutic study. See Instructions for Authors for a complete description of levels of evidence.

▶ En bloc spondylectomy is a technically challenging procedure that can be applied to select neoplastic conditions in the spine. The literature on this topic is relatively limited. Additionally, several techniques are used with overlapping descriptions; as such, what is commonly reported in the literature as an en bloc resection may in fact have a controlled intralesional transgression and is often applied in patients with metastatic disease. These factors make this body of literature difficult to follow and apply directly to clinical care of sarcoma patients.

In this context, this article by Luzzati and colleagues provides an excellent review of a large series of patients undergoing true en block spondylectomy. The vast majority of patients were treated for sarcomas, typical of what contemporary North American indications would be for a procedure of this nature.

The results are both sobering and refreshing. The complication profile of this operation is significant (2 patients died in the postoperative period, and two-thirds of patients had significant complications). However, 81% of patients remained disease-free at a minimum of 2 years and a mean 39-month follow-up. Additionally, 89% of patients were ambulatory without external support. This is an excellent functional outcome given the magnitude of the procedure that is being undertaken.

As such, I think this is a useful article. It is a description of en bloc spondylectomy from the perspective of a surgical oncologist. For those surgeons who assemble a team and practice in this area, these results are very believable from a complication perspective and demonstrate excellent survival from an oncologic point of view.

P. S. Rose, MD

Benign Tumors

Wait-and-See Policy as a First-Line Management for Extra-Abdominal Desmoid Tumors

Briand S, Barbier O, Biau D, et al (The Univ Hosp of Nantes, France; Begin Military Hosp, Saint Mandé, France; Université Paris Descartes, France)
J Bone Joint Surg Am 96:631-638, 2014

Background.—Extra-abdominal desmoid tumors are rare, locally aggressive neoplasms without metastatic potential. There is no clear consensus regarding their optimal management. The disappointing results of current treatments and the ability of extra-abdominal desmoid tumors to spontaneously stabilize have increasingly drawn interest toward conservative management. The objective of this study was to evaluate a wait-and-see policy as a first-line management for extra-abdominal desmoid tumors.

Methods.—This two-center retrospective study involved fifty-five patients with a histologically proven extra-abdominal desmoid tumor.

The primary outcome was the cumulative probability of dropping out from the wait-and-see policy. The wait-and-see policy included aggressive management of symptoms. We conducted a review of the relevant published series in which a watchful-waiting strategy was used.

Results.—The cumulative probability of dropping out from the wait-and-see policy was 9.6% at the time of the last follow-up. Spontaneous arrest of tumor growth was noted for forty-seven patients (85%) over the course of the study. Half of the tumors were stabilized at one year, and a potential to increase beyond three years was a sporadic event (one case). Regrowth was found in two patients (4%).

Conclusions.—A wait-and-see policy is an effective front-line management for patients with primary or recurrent extra-abdominal desmoid tumor. These tumors tend to stabilize spontaneously, on average after one year of evolution, and the cumulative probability of the failure of a wait-and-see policy is approximately 10%.

▶ Clinicians well recognize the frustrations of dealing with desmoid tumors. As well, trends in clinical management have shifted away from aggressive resection to pharmacologic treatments, potentially limited surgery, and observation. These authors from France report retrospectively 55 patients managed in 2 centers with a "wait-and-see" management strategy and symptomatic treatment only of desmoid tumors.

Almost all tumors (85%) showed growth arrest; approximately half of tumors had no further growth after 1 year, and only 3 total patients showed growth beyond 3 years. Ten percent of patients dropped out of the wait-and-see strategy for other management.

Several points merit discussion. Although the success rate of a wait-and-see policy was high in this study, other studies have seen conservative management fail more frequently. Additionally, essentially half of patients reported functional impairment from their tumor, and more than half reported a painful tumor at the time of their final follow-up. As such, although this treatment regimen may be valid, it too contains significant drawbacks.

This study does demonstrate the safety of a wait-and-see policy in the management of desmoid tumors. Certainly there is no rush for clinicians to settle on any individual treatment, and observation is a reasonable first-line therapy. Treatment decisions based on symptom severity and functional impairment will continue to be individualized toward patients. Additionally, potentially less morbid treatments than open surgery (eg, cryoablation) can also figure into our armamentarium for these tumors.

Readers are also directed to a commentary by Doctors Potter and Fosberg that accompanied this article.[1]

P. S. Rose, MD

Reference

1. Potter BK, Forsberg JA. Is hope a method? Commentary on an article by Sylvain Briand, MD, et al.: "Wait-and-See" Policy as a First-Line Management for Extra-Abdominal Desmoid Tumors". *J Bone Joint Surg Am.* 2014;96:e69.

Unicameral Bone Cysts: General Characteristics and Management Controversies

Pretell-Mazzini J, Murphy RF, Kushare I, et al (Univ of Miami, FL; Univ of Tennessee, Memphis; Children's Natl Med Ctr, Washington, DC; et al)

J Am Acad Orthop Surg 22:295-303, 2014

Unicameral bone cysts are benign bone lesions that are often asymptomatic and commonly develop in the proximal humerus and femur of skeletally immature patients. The etiology of these lesions remains unknown. Most patients present with a pathologic fracture, but these cysts can be discovered incidentally, as well. Radiographically, a unicameral bone cyst appears as a radiolucent lesion with cortical thinning and is centrally located within the metaphysis. Although diagnosis is frequently straightforward, management remains controversial. Because the results of various management methods are heterogeneous, no single method has emerged as the standard of care. New minimally invasive techniques involve cyst decompression with bone grafting and instrumentation. These techniques have yielded promising results, with low rates of complications and recurrence reported; however, prospective clinical trials are needed to compare these techniques with current evidence-based treatments (Tables 1 and 2).

▶ Orthopedic oncologists and pediatric orthopedic surgeons are both called on at times to manage unicameral bone cysts. Although a benign condition with a favorable prognosis, the treatment of these lesions is not standardized, and initial treatment is frequently disappointing. This review article in the *Journal American Academy of Orthopaedic Surgeons* nicely outlines different techniques of injection and surgical management of unicameral bone cysts (see Tables 1 and 2). Although the level of evidence in any individual study is generally level III or IV, this provides a very readable way for surgeons to evaluate the literature and the evidence behind different treatment options. The

TABLE 1.—Summary of Clinical Outcomes of Injections Used to Manage Unicameral Bone Cysts

Study	No. of Patients	Type of Injection	Initial Healing Rate (%)	Recurrence Rate (%)	Level of Evidence
Cho et al[23]	25	DBM	76	8	III
Chang et al[24]	79	ABM: 14, steroid: 65	ABM: 43, steroid: 51	NA	III
Rougraff and Kling[25]	23	ABM and DBM	69	21.7	IV
Di Bella et al[26]	184	ABM and DBM: 41, steroid: 143	ABM and DBM: 58, steroid: 21	NA	III
Thawrani et al[27]	13	α-BSM	38.5	0	IV

ABM = autologous bone marrow, α-BSM = apatitic calcium phosphate bone substitute material, DBM = demineralized bone marrow, NA = not available.

Editor's Note: Please refer to original journal article for full references.

Reprinted from Pretell-Mazzini J, Murphy RF, Kushare I, et al. Unicameral bone cysts: general characteristics and management controversies. *J Am Acad Orthop Surg*. 2014;22:295-303.

TABLE 2.—Summary of Outcomes for Surgical Management of Unicameral Bone Cysts

Study	No. of Patients	Technique	Graft Material	Healing Rate (%)	Recurrence Rate (%)	Level of Evidence
Mik et al[20]	55	Percutaneous curettage, decompression with flexible IM nail	Calcium sulfate pellets	80	0	IV
Brecelj and Suhodolcan[35]	8	Open curettage and bone grafting	50% glucose and bone allograft	25	NA	III
Sung et al[36]	34	Open curettage and bone graft	Corticocancellous allograft bone chips	36	NA	III
Hou et al[37]	12	Open curettage and grafting	Calcium sulfate pellets	66	25	III
	12	Percutaneous curettage; ethanol injections; IM decompression, grafting, and placement of cannulated screw for continuous decompression	Calcium sulfate pellets	91.6	NA	III
Canavese et al[38]	10	Disruption of cyst walls with percutaneous curettage	None	70	NA	III
de Sanctis and Andreacchio[39]	47	Decompression with flexible IM nail	None	65.9	0	IV
Masquijo et al[40]	48	Decompression with flexible IM nail	None	54.2	8.33	IV
Glanzmann and Campos[41]	22	Decompression with flexible IM nail	None	72.7	9	IV
Kanellopoulos et al[42]	9	Decompression with flexible IM nail	DBM/iliac crest bone marrow	77	0	IV
Dormans et al[43]	24	Percutaneous curettage, decompression with flexible IM nail	Calcium sulfate pellets	91.7	9	IV

DBM = demineralized bone marrow, IM = intramedullary, NA = not available.
Editor's Note: Please refer to original journal article for full references.
Reprinted from Pretell-Mazzini J, Murphy RF, Kushare I, et al. Unicameral bone cysts: general characteristics and management controversies. *J Am Acad Orthop Surg.* 2014;22:295-303.

bibliography is thorough and allows the interested reader to pursue the matter in greater detail.

P. S. Rose, MD

Liquid Nitrogen or Phenolization for Giant Cell Tumor of Bone?: A Comparative Cohort Study of Various Standard Treatments at Two Tertiary Referral Centers

van der Heijden L, van der Geest ICM, Schreuder HWB, et al (Leiden Univ Med Ctr, The Netherlands; et al)
J Bone Joint Surg Am 96:e35(1-9), 2014

Background.—The rate of recurrence of giant cell tumor of bone is decreased by use of adjuvant treatments such as phenol, liquid nitrogen, or polymethylmethacrylate (PMMA) during curettage. We assessed recurrence and complication rates and functional outcome after curettage with use of phenol and PMMA, liquid nitrogen and PMMA, and liquid nitrogen and bone grafts.

Methods.—We retrospectively compared the relative effectiveness of treatment of giant cell tumors of bone at two tertiary centers with a regional function from 1990 to 2010. The 132 (of 201) patients who met the inclusion criteria had a mean age of thirty-three years (range, eleven to sixty-nine years). Treatment assignment depended purely on the center, with primary treatment consisting of curettage with use of phenol and PMMA (n = 82) at one center and with use of either liquid nitrogen and PMMA (n = 26) or liquid nitrogen and bone grafts (n = 24) at the other center. Recurrence and complication rates were determined, and functional outcome was assessed on the basis of the Musculoskeletal Tumor Society (MSTS) score.

Results.—The mean duration of follow-up was eight years (range, two to twenty-two years). Recurrence rates were comparable among the groups (28% for phenol and PMMA, 31% for liquid nitrogen and PMMA, and 38% for liquid nitrogen and bone grafts; $p = 0.52$). Soft-tissue extension increased the recurrence risk (hazard ratio [HR] = 2.1, 95% confidence interval [CI] = 1.1 to 4.0, $p = 0.024$). The complication rate was 33% after use of liquid nitrogen and bone grafts, 27% after liquid nitrogen and PMMA, and 11% after phenol and PMMA ($p = 0.019$); complications included osteoarthritis, infection, postoperative fracture, nonunion, transient nerve palsy, and PMMA leakage. The complication risk was increased by the presence of a pathologic fracture (HR = 4.1, 95% CI = 1.7 to 9.5, $p = 0.001$) and use of liquid nitrogen (HR = 3.9, 95% CI = 1.5 to 10, $p = 0.006$ for liquid nitrogen and bone grafts; HR = 3.1, 95% CI = 1.1 to 8.6, $p = 0.028$ for liquid nitrogen and PMMA). The mean MSTS score was 26 (range, 8 to 30) and was comparable among all three groups ($p = 0.52$).

Conclusions.—Recurrence rates were comparable for treatment with phenol and PMMA, liquid nitrogen and PMMA, and liquid nitrogen and bone grafts. Complication rates were higher after use of liquid nitrogen. The functional outcome was excellent in all three cohorts.

▶ Many methods can be used to minimize local recurrence after intralesional curettage of giant cell tumor of bone in function-sparing treatment. Phenol is commonly used as a chemical adjuvant, and liquid nitrogen is commonly used as a thermal adjuvant. Additionally, both polymethylmethacrylate (PMMA) or bone graft may be used to fill the resulting defect.

These authors from Leiden University and Radboud University in the Netherlands compare the results. At 1 center phenol and PMMA were used routinely. At the other, liquid nitrogen and a mixture of PMMA or bone graft were selected. Surgical treatment was otherwise similar, as was patient selection. Note that both groups would indicate patients for intralesional curettage in the presence of pathologic fracture or soft tissue extension; at some centers, such patients are indicated for formal resection.

In summary, the oncologic outcomes were identical in all groups (see Fig 2 in the original article). However, the complication rate was significantly higher in patients treated with liquid nitrogen. The functional outcome (as assessed by Musculoskeletal Tumor Society score) was comparable in all groups and was overall favorable.

Note that this is a retrospective study and the functional outcomes reported were extracted from the chart. As such, it is difficult to know how faithfully this reproduces the current clinical state of the patients. Additionally, the authors do not give us detail as to what strength phenol they used (different concentrations are available).

In the management of giant cell tumor, mechanical, thermal, and chemical adjuvants can be used to minimize the risk of local recurrence. None of these adjuvants are exclusive, and it is reasonable to employ some form of mechanical, chemical, and thermal adjuvants to the treatment of all patients who undergo intralesional curettage. For example, there is no direct contraindication to patients undergoing both liquid nitrogen treatment and phenol treatment. Additionally, the use of the argon beam coagulator as an alternative thermal treatment should be recognized. It is readily available in most institutions, whereas the special equipment needed for liquid nitrogen treatment may not be.

Where to place this study in clinical context? Aggressive treatment of giant cell tumors with intralesional therapy continues to have a high recurrence rate despite the use of phenol or liquid nitrogen. The higher rate of complications in the patients undergoing liquid nitrogen treatment is concerning. However, different centers have developed different treatment protocols for these tumors, and I am personally unaware of any protocol that is convincingly better than others. Surgeons reading this article should recognize the higher reported complication rate in patients treated with liquid nitrogen; if they employ liquid nitrogen in their own practice, they should probably critically evaluate their results to be certain that they are not exposing their patients to any excess morbidity. That said, liquid nitrogen treatment remains a valid thermal adjuvant in the management of these tumors with good reported results in this and other studies.

P. S. Rose, MD

Article Index

Chapter 1: Basic Science

Chapter 2: General Orthopedics

Chapter 3: Forearm, Wrist, and Hand

Chapter 4: Elbow

Chapter 5: Shoulder

Chapter 6: Spine

Chapter 7: Total Hip Arthroplasty

Chapter 8: Total Knee Arthroplasty

Chapter 9: Foot and Ankle

Chapter 10: Sports Medicine

Chapter 11: Trauma and Amputation

Chapter 12: Orthopedic Oncology

Author Index

Printed and bound by CPI Group (UK) Ltd, Croydon, CR0 4YY

08/05/2025

01864679-0003